# Trophoblast Research
## VOLUME 3

# PLACENTAL VASCULARIZATION AND BLOOD FLOW
## Basic Research and Clinical Applications

# Trophoblast Research

Series Editors

## Richard K. Miller and Henry A. Thiede

*University of Rochester Medical Center*
*Rochester, New York*

---

---

A Continuation Order Plan is available for this series. A continuation order will bring delivery of each new volume immediately upon publication. Volumes are billed only upon actual shipment. For further information please contact the publisher.

# Trophoblast Research
## VOLUME 3

---

# PLACENTAL VASCULARIZATION AND BLOOD FLOW
## Basic Research and Clinical Applications

Edited by

## Peter Kaufmann

*RWTH Aachen*
*Aachen, Federal Republic of Germany*

## and

## Richard K. Miller

*University of Rochester Medical Center*
*Rochester, New York*

SPRINGER SCIENCE+BUSINESS MEDIA, LLC

Library of Congress Cataloging in Publication Data

European Placenta Group. Conference (2nd: 1986: Rolduc Monastery, Netherlands)
  Placental vascularization and blood flow.

  (Trophoblast research; v. 3)
  "Derived from the joint session of the Second European Placenta Group Conference with the
Eleventh Rochester Trophoblast Conference, held September 24–26, 1986, at the Rolduc
Monastery, the Netherlands"–T.p. verso.
  Includes bibliographies and index.
  1. Placenta–Blood-vessels–Congresses. 2. Maternal-fetal exchange–Congresses. I. Kauf-
mann, Peter, 1942-    . II. Miller, Richard K. (Richard Kermit), date. III. Rochester Trophoblast
Conference (11th: 1986: Rolduc Monastery, Netherlands) IV. Title. V. Series. [DNLM: 1.
Placenta–blood supply–congresses. W1 TR877 v. 3 / WQ 212 E89 1986p]
QP281.E97  1986                          612'.63                                  88-9846
ISBN 978-1-4615-8111-6        ISBN 978-1-4615-8109-3 (eBook)
DOI 10.1007/978-1-4615-8109-3

Derived from the joint session of the Second European Placenta Group
with the Rochester Trophoblast Conference, held September 24–26, 1986,
at the Rolduc Monastery, The Netherlands


© 1988 Springer Science+Business Media New York
Originally published by Plenum Press, New York in 1988
Softcover reprint of the hardcover 1st edition 1988

# TROPHOBLAST RESEARCH

*Trophoblast Research* publishes contributions concerning the placenta and the extraembryonic membranes as they relate to embryonic and fetal development and to trophoblastic neoplasia. Original articles, reviews, and reports are published in single bound volumes. All articles are peer-reviewed.

## EDITORS

Richard K. Miller
Rochester, New York

Henry A. Thiede
Rochester, New York

## EDITORIAL ADVISORY BOARD

The Editorial Office for *Trophoblast Research*:
Department of Obstetrics and Gynecology
University of Rochester School of Medicine and Dentistry
601 Elmwood Avenue, Rochester, New York USA 14642
(716) 275-3638

# PREFACE

The optimal function of the placenta and thus fetal well being largely depends upon the integrity of both the fetal and maternal circulations of the placenta. Intense basic research concerned with placental vascularization and blood flow has been performed for the past 30 years, beginning with the classical morphological descriptions of the placental vessels by Boe (1953) and Arts (1961), as well as with the radioangiographic studies of maternal placental circulation in the human by Borell (1958) and in the rhesus monkey by Ramsey (1962). The scientific framework presented by these investigators has been filled and completed by numerous investigators, leading to more morphological details, functional considerations, and pathological understanding. For an extended period of time, this research has been of primarily academic interest by increasing our insights into one important system of the placenta, yet having nearly no practical importance.

Recently, this situation has changed dramatically: in vitro studies of the isolated, dually perfused human placenta and in vivo studies of placental circulation for diagnostic purposes have raised an enormous interest in basic research data. New methods like Doppler Ultrasound and NMR became available. These technics have enabled the obstetrician to study fetal and placental hemodynamics in vivo. Meanwhile, such methods are becoming incorporated into the daily obstetrical routine, to some degree without an adequate background knowledge of placental vascularization and blood flow, since such experience is currently available to only a small group of experts.

As it has been stated by Nico Arts, "...the danger exits therefore, that the clinical research is going to lead a life of its own, independent from developments in anatomy, physiology, and animal research. This will lead to incorrect interpretation of the data and incorrect medical actions taken in clinical practice. Therefore, we not only dearly need to correlate the rapid development in clinical technology with the current knowledge and concepts of feto-maternal placental morphology and physiology, but we also very much need an intensive collaboration between the basic sciences themselves such as anatomy, physiology, biochemistry, etc....".

As a consequence of such insights, in Fall of 1986, the European Placenta Group held its IInd meeting as a joint meeting with the Rochester Trophoblast Conference in the Rolduc Monastery, in The Netherlands. Approximately one half of the scientific program was devoted to a major symposium entitled, "Placental Vascularization and Blood Flow". This symposium was intended to be an international and interdisciplinary approach to summarize the state of the art in this critical area of research. About 60 experts in the fields of anatomy, pathology, physiology, immunology, pharmacology, radiology, and obstetrics were invited to present state of the art interpretations of the field.

From 22 lectures and 17 posters, a total of 26 presentations have been selected for publication in this volume. This volume is not entirely comprehensive, but it draws special attention to amplify not only basic research but also its clinical implications and counterparts. It is hoped that this volume reviews not only our present knowledge of placental vessels and hemodynamics, but offers hints for promising and exciting future research investigations.

In reviewing the list of contributors, one will realize that several chapters are already the result of interdisciplinary and/or international cooperation. Such efforts demonstrate that collaborative efforts as one goal of this joint meeting was a success. This initiative will be continued. The above mentioned meeting in Rolduc was the first opportunity to coordinate the meetings of the major conference series dealing with trophoblast and placenta. This has resulted in the establishment of joint meetings at regular intervals. Following an extended series of 10 Rochester Trophoblast Conferences dating from 1961 through 1985 and a very young series of meetings of the European Placenta Group (pilot meeting in 1981 in Hamburg, Ist official meeting 1984 in Cambridge), the IInd meeting of the EPG, first joint meeting with the Rochester group, was the first essential step in this direction. Both groups, the Rochester Trophoblast Conference and the European Placenta Group, have agreed to hold their future meetings in two year intervals, i.e., the Rochester Trophoblast Conference in 1988, 1990, and 1992 in the United States, and the European Placenta Group in 1989 (France), 1991 (Switzerland), and 1993 etc., with joint meetings every three years.

As it was true for the foregoing meetings of both programs, the future meetings too shall focus on a main subject. It is intended to publish monographs in the series, *Trophoblast Research* under the heading of those subjects, emerging from the single Rochester and European meetings. The 11th Rochester Trophoblast Conference joint meeting with the European Placenta Group will focus on the molecular biology and cell regulation of the placenta on 9-12 October 1988. The IIIrd meeting of the European Placenta Group which is scheduled for 27-29 September 1989 in Dourdan, France (near Paris), will be devoted to placental signals. *Trophoblast Research* in due time hopefully will represent a continuously actualized state of the art in placental research.

Finally, the editors wish to express their gratitude to those numerous people and institutions who provided the scientific, technical, and financial basis for this volume. Since it is a result of the joint meeting of the European Placenta Group and the Rochester Trophoblast Conference, we are indebted to Ralph Wynn who helped us catalyzing the cooperation of both groups; to Ulysse Gaspard, Ruldolf Leiser, and Henry Thiede as our co-organizers of the joint meeting; to Anthony Firth, Harold Fox, Jean Hustin, Heinz-Peter Leichtweiss, Andre Malassine, Hobe Schröder, Colin Sibley, and Maureen Young who provided ample and expert advice. Both the meeting as well as the volume would not have been possible without the dedication and care of our secretaries and coworkers Jutta Jacobs, Linda Philippens, Jacqulyn White, Barbara Witte, and Sean Logghe for his computer expertise. We also gratefully acknowledge the considerable financial support provided by Bayer AG, Leverkusen, Beecham-Wülfing GmbH, Neuss, Behringwerke AG, Marburg, Duphar Co., Belgium, Kontron AG, Düsseldorf, Nourypharma GmbH, Oberschleissheim, Organon BV, Oss, Plano GmbH, Marburg, R. Jung GmbH, Nussloch, and Schering AG, Berlin. All of the above efforts could not provide this volume without the authors of the following 26 contributions. The reader is invited to explore these contributions for the status of research in the placenta and to gather support for the next generation of studies.

Peter Kaufmann, Aachen and Richard K. Miller, Rochester

# CONTENTS

## MATERNAL CIRCULATION

## FETAL CIRCULATION

# Contents

# MATERNAL CIRCULATION

Trophoblast Research 3:3-16, 1988

# HISTOMETRIC INVESTIGATIONS IN PLACENTONES (MATERNO-FETAL CIRCULATION UNITS) OF HUMAN PLACENTAE

R. Schuhmann[1], F. Stoz, and M. Maier

Section of Gynecology Morphology
Department of Obstetrics and Gynecology
University of Ulm, F.R.Germany

## INTRODUCTION

The placenta comprises a variable number of about 50 (40-60) functional and circulatory units called "placentones" according to the investigations of Crawford (1956), Smart (1962), Wilkin (1965), Panigel et al. (1967), Freese, (1968a, 1968b), Freese and Maciolek (1969), Wigglesworth (1969), Reynolds (1966, 1967, 1971), Ramsey (1962, 1966, 1971), Ramsey et al. (1963) and earlier investigations in our own laboratory (Schuhmann, 1976). Concerning the histologic structure of these units especially their fetal part (lobuli) it was shown by Wigglesworth (1969) and by Crawford (1956a, 1956b) and by own investigations (Maier, 1985; Schuhmann and Wehler, 1971; Schuhmann, 1976; Schuhmann et al., 1979) that the villi in the centers are more loosely arranged than in the periphery. Referring to the histology of the villi in the different areas of the lobuli, Grunwald (1966, 1973) and Wigglesworth (1969) pointed out that there is a marked difference in the degree of differentiation between the central and the peripheral area. These findings were confirmed by Alvarez (1970), Crawford (1956b) and by own earlier investigations (Schuhmann et al., 1971, 1972, 1976, 1977; Schuhmann, 1976). With the development of new technical equipment it is now possible to measure and calculate what were only "impressions" by means of the classical histology. Therefore, this laboratories former histologic results were confirmed by means of histometry.

## MATERIALS AND METHODS

The histometric measurements were performed in three placentones of placentae from week 38 (No. 1), week 35 (No. 2), and week 33 (No. 3) of pregnancy. The reason for the premature deliveries in No 2 and 3 was cervical insufficiency. The histologic slides were prepared in the usual way. They were stained with Haematoxylin and Eosin. The histometric investigations were done with a Videoplan (Kontron, München). The unit was described in detail in former publications (Stoz et al., 1982, 1983).

The present study was arranged to cover whole sections rather than to measure single villi in different regions and compare the data. Therefore, the

[1] To Whom Correspondence Should Be Addressed: Prof. Dr. R. Schuhmann, Frauenklinik am Stadtkrankenhaus Worms, Gabriel-von-Seidl-Str. 31, D-6520 Worms, F.R.Germany

fields of measurement had to be arranged in such a way that all regions of the section were equally investigated. Using a moveable stage, the positioning of the slides under the microscope was done so that the basal plate (B1-B2, see Figure 1) were parallel to the abscissa. The center of the circulation unit was marked by a central point (PZ). To cover the whole slide, the placentone was divided in 10 strips of measurement (Figure 2). Since the histologic slides were not symmetric, the strips were not of equal length. Therefore, 50 villi per strip were examined. Using a transfer program, all data stored in the computer of the Videoplan were transferred to the "TR 440" computer (Siemens) of the Computer Center, University of Ulm. After the data transfer, the following procedures were performed:

1. By using a cross of co-ordinates positioned over the point "PZ", all stored data received new co-ordinates.

2. The cross of co-ordinates was positioned on the point "PZ" in such a way that the line B1-B2 ran parallel to the abscissa.

3. The parameters could now be compared to the point "PZ" which was situated in the middle of the loose center of the placentone.

The following parameters, which were described in detail in earlier publications (Stoz et al., 1982, 1983), were evaluated:

1. Cross sectional surface of the villus
2. Degree of vascularization GF:ZF (Gefaessflaeche:Zottenflaeche)
3. Percentage of villous circumference represented by epithelial plates (EL:ZU) = (Epithelplattenlaenge:Zottenumfang)
4. Percentage of vessels in contact with epithelial plates (EL:GU) = (Epithelplattenlaenge:Gefaessumfang)

In former investigations, it has proved useful to classify the villi in three groups for demonstration of the results as follows:

1. Villi with a cross sectional surface < 4000 µm
2. Villi with a cross sectional surface < 2000 to 4000 µm
3. Villi with a cross sectional surface from 0 to 2000 µm

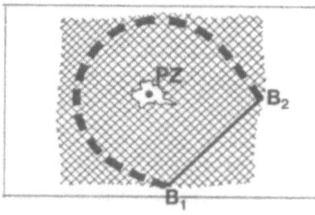

Figure 1. Schematic demonstration of the placentone and indication of the localization of the points B1, B2, and PZ.

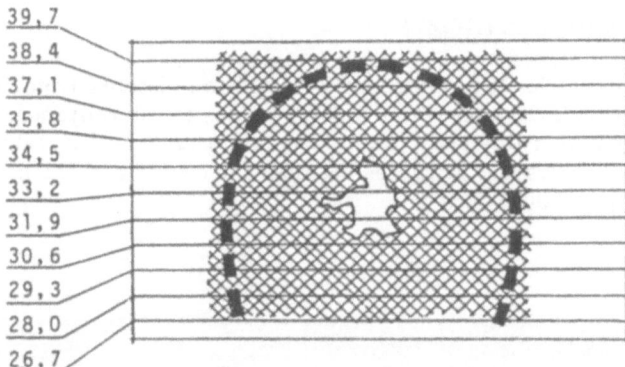

39,7
38,4
37,1
35,8
34,5
33,2
31,9
30,6
29,3
28,0
26,7

Figure 2. Schematic demonstration of the strips in which the section of the placentone was divided.

As there were no symmetric normal distributions the logarithms to the base E were chosen for demonstration of the results. The correlation between the villous parameters (cross-sectional surface, GF:ZF, EL:ZU, EL:GU) and the distance of the villi from the center of the placentone was tested by a regression analysis.

## RESULTS

The three placentones are presented in photomicrographs (Figures 3 - 5). To demonstrate the distances to the central point (PZ), a scattering of points with a regression line was chosen. For the parameter - "cross sectional surface", an additional representation was chosen in which the villi of the different classes were marked by different symbols in the system of co-ordinates. These symbols were plotted according to the stored co-ordinates.

### Cross Sectional Surface

As can be seen in Figures 6, 7, and 8, in comparison to the optic impression when looking at the photomicrograph, the bigger villi (> 4000 μm²) were in the center of the circulation units, whereas the villi with cross sectional surfaces of more than 2000 to 4000 and under 2000 μm were mainly located in the periphery of the placentone. This comparison was most impressive when the photomicrograph and the graphic demonstration in Figures 5 and 8 were compared. The center had the typical feature of a "chimney" reaching from the basal plate to the chorionic plate. In Figures 9A-C, the logarithm of the villous cross sectional area was plotted against the distance to the central point of the circulation unit. The cross sectional villous area decreased with the distance from the center of the circulation unit. The results were statistically significant for all of the three sections (p < 0.001).

### Degree of Vascularization (GF:ZF)

In placentone No. 1, a connection between the distance from the center and the degree of vascularization could not be seen. In placentones No. 2 and 3, however, the regression line showed an ascending course. This value means that the degree of vascularization increases between the center and the periphery of the circulation unit (p < 0.001).

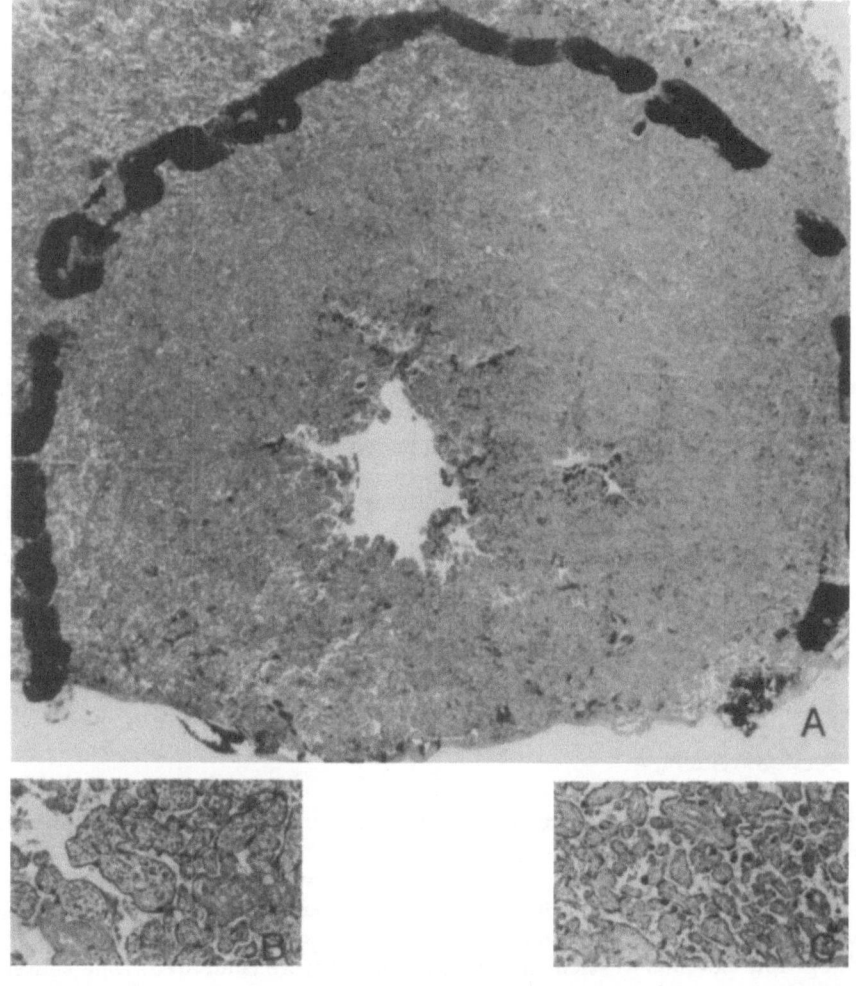

Figure 3. A) (Placentone 1) Placentone from a placenta of week 38 of gestation. Photomicrograph, original magnification 1:5. B) Detail of the center of the placentone. Photomicrograph, original magnification 1:40. C) Detail from the periphery. Photomicrograph, original magnification 1:40.

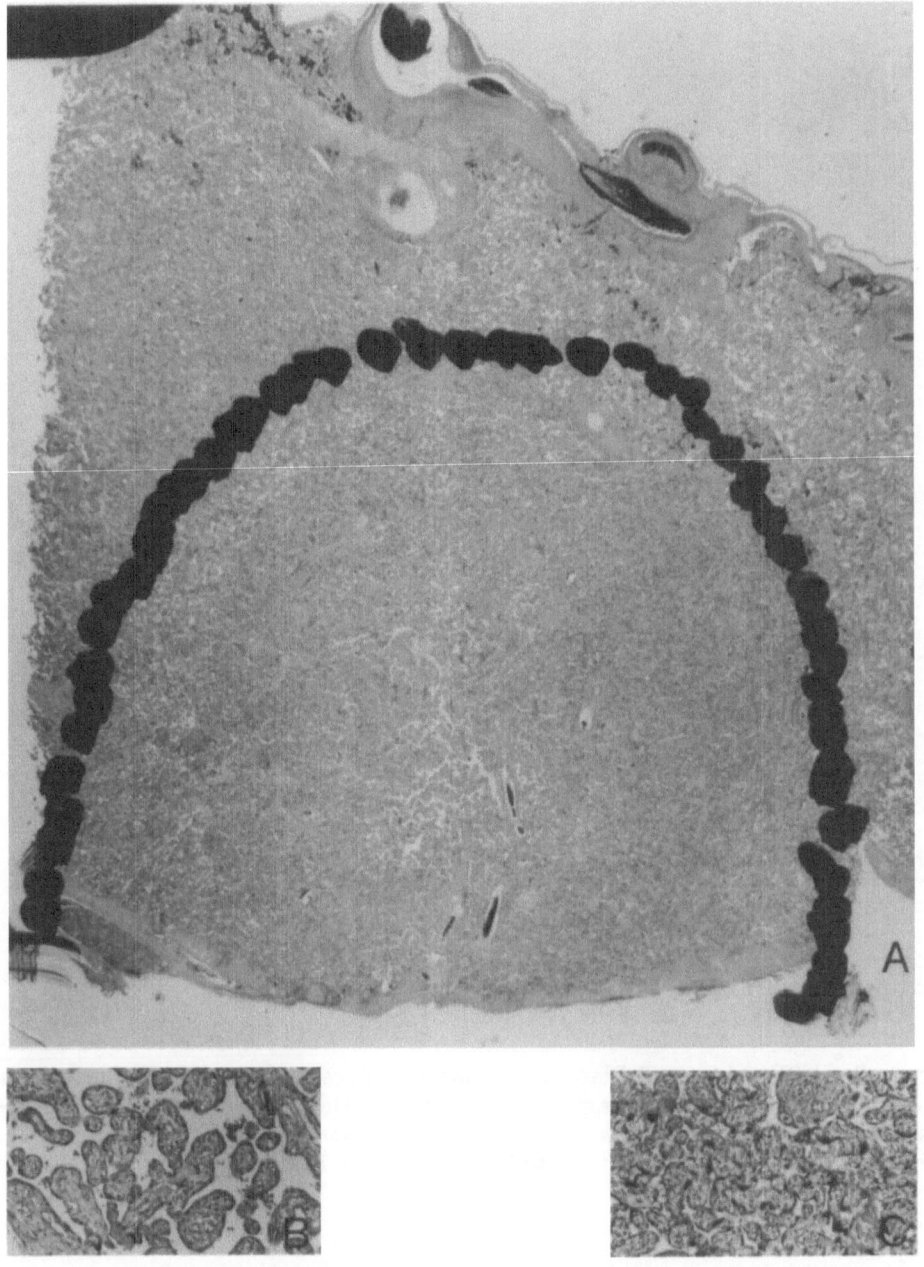

Figure 4. A) (Placentone 2) Placentone from a placenta of week 35 of gestation. Photomicrograph, original magnification 1:5.   B) Detail from the center of the placentone.   Photomicrograph, original magnification 1:40.   C) Detail from the periphery.   Photomicrograph, original magnification 1:40.

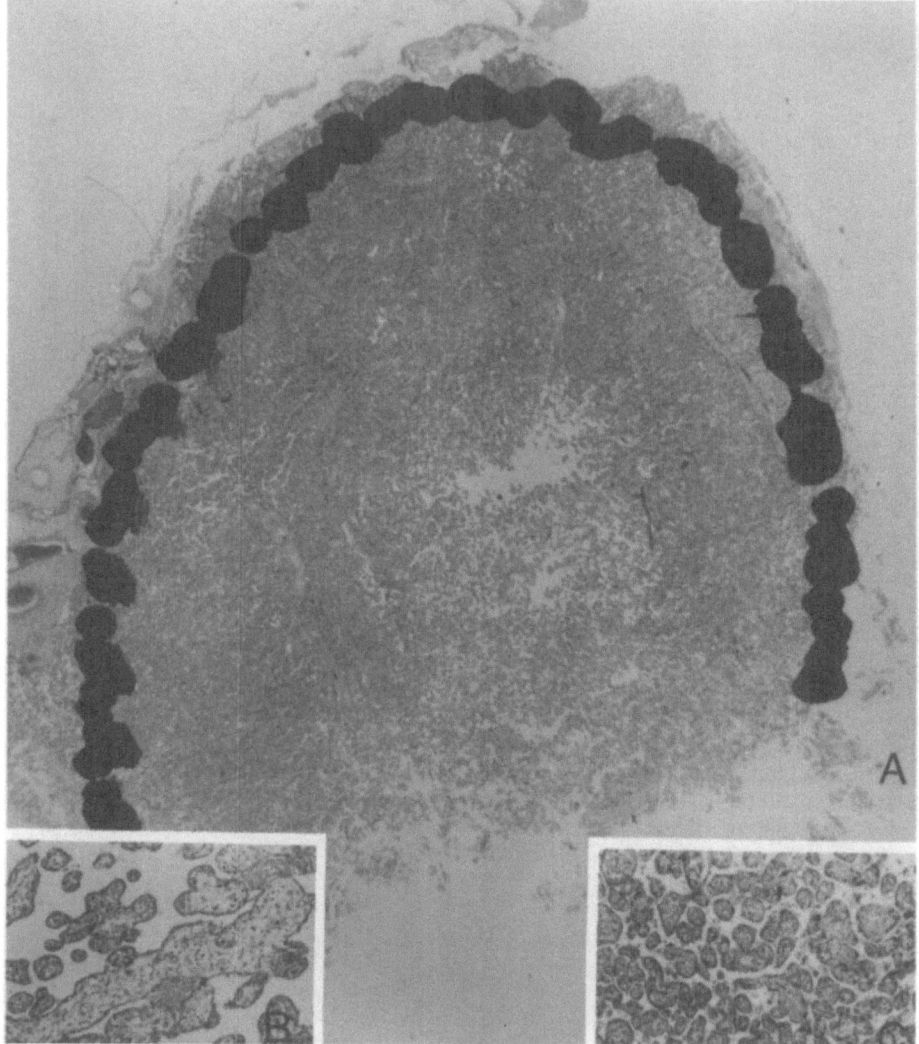

Figure 5. A) (Placentone 3) Placentone from the placenta of week 33 of gestation. Photomicrograph, original magnification 1:5.  B) Detail from the center of the placentone.  Photomicrograph, original magnification 1:40.  C) Detail from the periphery.  Photomicrograph, original magnification 1:40.

## Percentage of Villous Circumference Represented by Epithelial Plates

In all placentones measured, an increase in the regression line was seen. This rise demonstrated that with increasing distance from the center, the percentage of epithelial plates increased (p < 0.001).

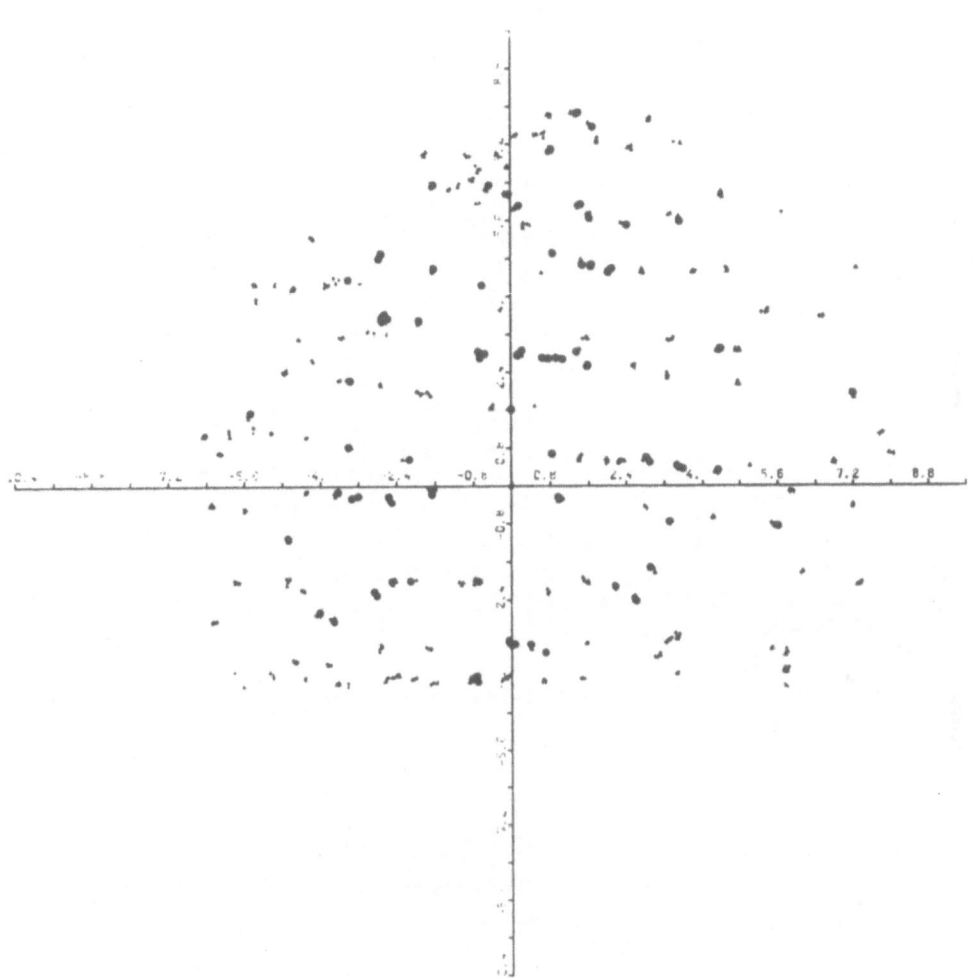

Figure 6. Computer print of the localization of the villi of different size in placentone No. 1. • villi with cross sectional surface of < 4000 µm; X calibration marks referring to B1, B2. PZ in the crossing of the co-ordinates.

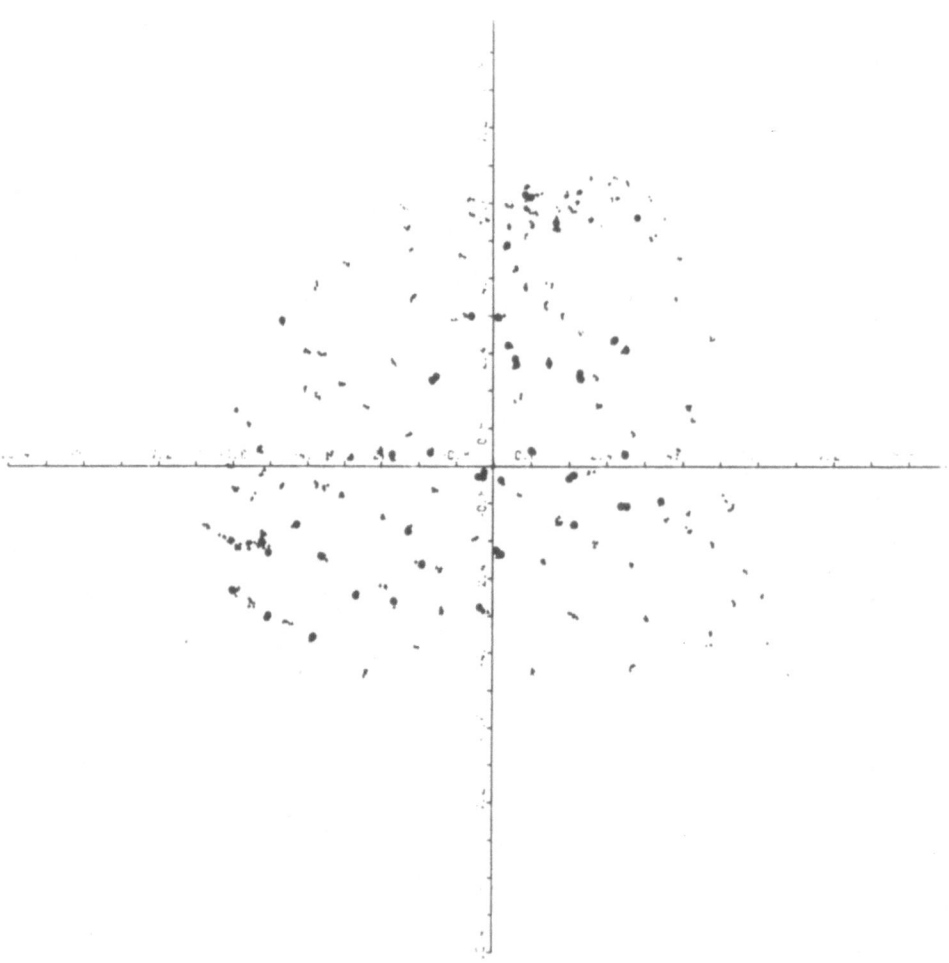

Figure 7. Computer print of the localization of the villi of different size in placentone No. 2.    • villi with cross sectional surface of < 4000 μm; X calibration marks referring to B1, B2. PZ in the crossing of the co-ordinates.

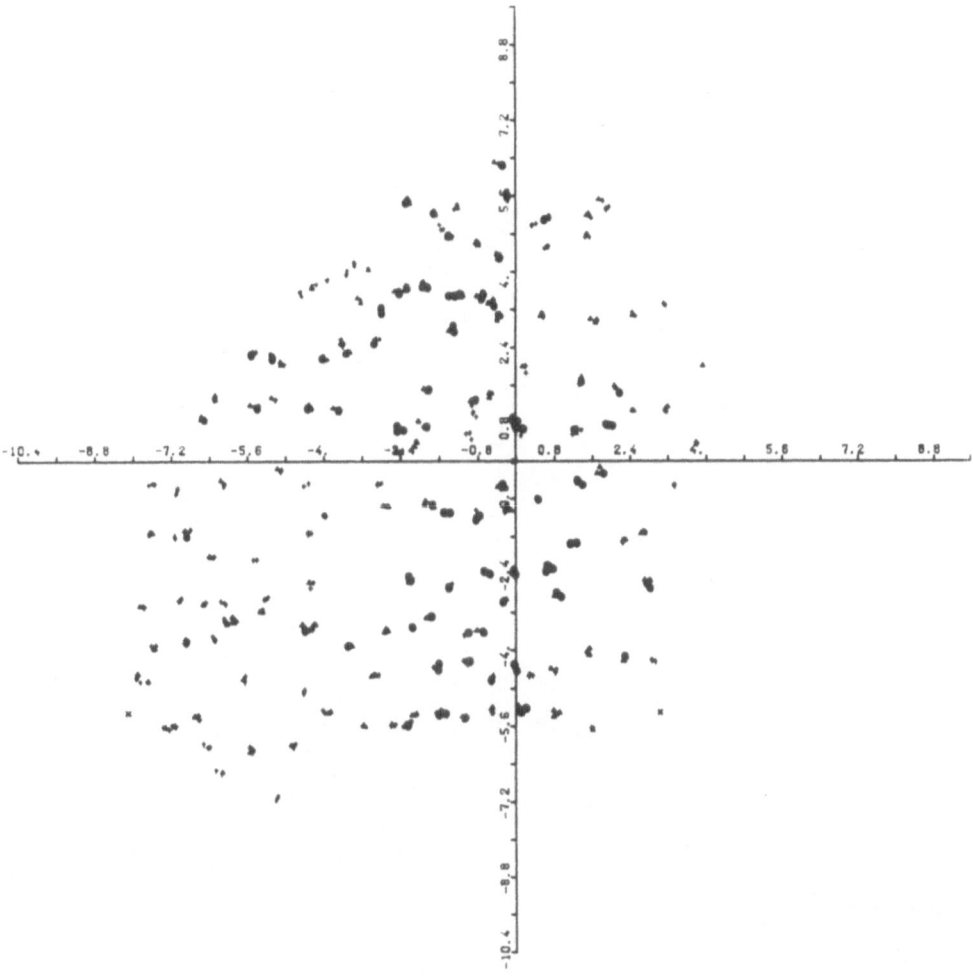

Figure 8. Computer print of the localization of the villi of different size in placentone No. 3. • villi with cross sectional surface of < 4000 μm X calibration marks referring to B1, B2. PZ in the crossing of the co-ordinates.

## Percentage of Vessels in Contact With Epithelial Plates (EL/GU)

For this parameter, a slight rise in the regression line was measured in all placentones. This rise indicates that with increasing distance from the center, the percentage of epithelial plates, in direct contact to the fetal sinusoids increased. The results were only statistically significant in placentones No. 1 and 3 ($p <$ 0.001).

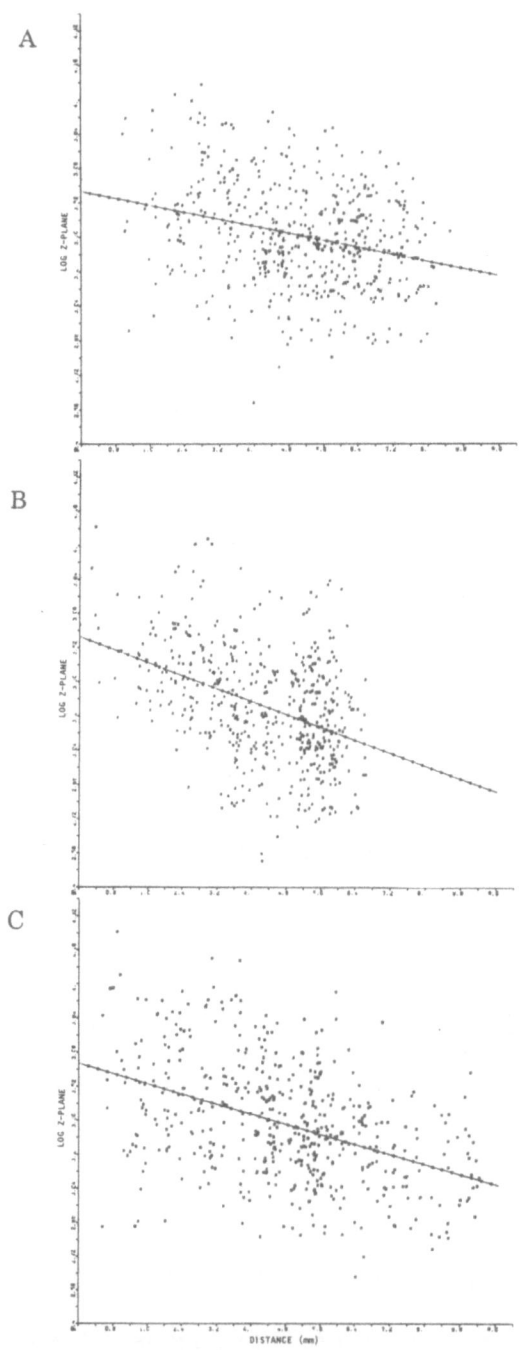

**Figures 9A-C.** Dependence of villous size versus the distance to the central point (PZ). All three placentones show, by the incline of the regression line, that the cross sectional surface of the villi becomes smaller with increasing distance from the center (PZ).

## DISCUSSION

There is a linear relationship between the logarithms of the cross sectional villous area and the distance from the center of the circulation unit in all placentones. Also the logarithms of the degree of vascularization was linearly related to the distance from the center in placentones No. 2 and 3. In placentone No. 1, this relationship could not be demonstrated. Also for the parameter "percentage of villous circumference represented by epithelial plates", there was a linear relationship, and the logarithms of the parameter "percentage of vessels in contact with the epithelial plates" a similar linear relationship in all placentones. In placentone No. 2, a quadric component was observed. All parameters, villous cross sectional surface as well as degree of vascularization and percentage of villous circumference represented by epithelial plates and percentage of vessels in contact with the epithelial plates, indicated the degree of differentiation, i.e., of maturation of the placental villi. This relationship was demonstrated in earlier investigations (Schuhmann et al., 1976; Stoz et al., 1982, 1983). Such a relationship makes it probable that the villi which were described previously as immature or less differentiated villi are rami, ramuli, and especially immature intermediate villi in their nomenclature (Kaufmann et al., 1979; Schweikhart and Kaufmann, 1977, Schweikhart, 1985, Schweikhart et al., 1986, and Sen et al., 1979). Sen and associates (1979) published an average diameter of the immature intermediate villi of 76.6 µm. This diameter corresponded to a cross sectional surface of 2574.47 µm. The middle group of villi in the present study represented an area of overlapping in which terminal villi are located as well asimmature intermediate villi.

The histometric measurements confirm the former histologic investigations in so far as the centers of the circulation units were more "immature" or "juvenile" villi, whereas in the periphery the terminal villi are more numerous. When seeking explanations for this different distribution, it is necessary to consider the circulation of the maternal blood in the placentone. In the previous investigations of Ramsey (1962, 1966, 1971), Ramsey et al. (1963), Freese (1968a, 1968b, 1969), Borell et al. (1958), and Beck (1982a, 1982b), there was agreement that the maternal blood reached the center of the circulation unit from the basal plate as a so-called "jet" or "spurt" and from there the blood was distributed radially to the periphery of the placentone. Oxygen measurements by Reynolds (1971) demonstrated that the oxygen tension in the center of the circulation units was higher than in the periphery. Radiocinematographic investigations (Ramsey et al., 1963) showed a decreasing flow velocity from the center to the periphery. It can be assumed, that terminal villi are formed mainly in an area where a low flow velocity provided for optimal function, e.g., fetomaternal exchange. This phenomenon was analogous to the observation that new capillaries were built in areas of low oxygen tension. In the centers of the circulation units with their higher oxygen tension the stimulus for the formation of terminal villi was missing.

One could compare this situation to that of a tree. A tree produces the majority of leaves in the periphery where the light allows photosynthesis. In the inner part of a tree top, bigger and smaller branches are found, and the leaves are missing. In older forests of pine, only the trees on the edge of the forest show branches to the bottom. On their inner side the branches in the lower parts are missing.

The hypothesis that the relative oxygen deficiency in the periphery of the placentone was the stimulus for the formation of terminal villi was substantiated by the following observation: in placentae of pathologic pregnancies where the maternal placental perfusion was decreased, a premature maturation of the villi was observed. This maturation meant that in these placentae the formation of terminal villi was increased and, as far as premature deliveries are concerned, all too soon induced. Additionally, in these placentae an increased formation of terminal villi is observed also in the centers of the circulation units. Thus, the regional differences between center and periphery were widely neutralized. It will be the task of further studies to analyze the different types of villi in the different areas of the placentone using the classification of Schweikhart (1985) and Schweikhart et al. (1977, 1986). Probably it will be found that also in the periphery an equal or comparable number of intermediate villi per unit area will be found. The difference between center and periphery will probably persist in the finding that intermediate spaces between these "intermediate villi" were empty in the center whereas these spaces were filled with terminal villi in the periphery.

## SUMMARY

Previous investigations have proposed structural differences in terminal villi located in different regions of the human placenta. This study demonstrates via histometry that the villi in the centers of the circulation units are less differentiated than those in the periphery. The results are statistically significant.

## REFERENCES

Alvarez, H. (1970) Trophoblast development gradient and its relationship to placental hemodynamics. *Am. J. Obstet. Gynecol.* 106, 416.

Beck, T. (1982a) Der materne Blutfluss durch die menschliche Plazenta. *Z. Geburtshilfe Perinatol* 186, 65-71.

Beck, T. (1982b) Der venoese Abfluss der intervilloesen Mikrozirkulation in der menschlichen Plazenta. *Z. Geburtshilfe Perinatol.* 186, 114-118.

Borell, U., Fernstrom, I., and Westman, A. (1958) Eine arteriographische Studie des Plazentarkreislaufes. *Geburtshilfe Frauenheilkd.* 18, 1-9.

Crawford, J.M. (1956a) The foetal placental circulation. III. The anatomy of the cotyledons. *J. Obstet. Gynaecol. Br. Emp.* 63, 542-547.

Crawford, J.M. (1956b) The foetal placental circulation. IV. The anatomy of the villus andits capillary structure. *J. Obstet. Gynaecol. Br. Emp.* 63, 548-552.

Freese, U.E. (1968a) The uteroplacental vascular relationship in the human. *Am. J. Obstet. Gynecol.* 101, 8-16.

Freese, U.E. (1968b) The fetal-maternal placental circulation. *J. Reprod. Med.* 1, 161-172.

Freese, U.E. and Maciolek, B.J. (1969) Plastoid injection studies of the uteroplacental vascular relationship in the human. *Obstet. Gynecol.* 33, 160-169.

Gruenwald, P. (1966) The lobular architecture of the human placenta. *Bull. Johns Hopkins Hosp.* 119, 172-190.

Gruenwald, P. (1973) Lobular structure of hemochorial placentas and its relation to maternal vessels. *Am. J. Anat.* 136, 133-151.

Kaufmann, P., Sen, D.K., and Schweikhart, G. (1979) Classification of human placental villi. I. Histology and scanning electron microscopy. *Cell Tissue Res.* 200, 409-423.

Maier, M. (1985) Histometrische Untersuchungen an Plazentonen menschlicher Plazenten. *Dissertation*, Ulm.

Panigel, M., Pascaud, M., and Brun, J.L. (1967) Etude radioangiographique de la circulation dans les villositées et l'espace intervilleux du cotyledon placentaire humain isole maintenu en survie par perfusion. *J. Physiol.* (Paris), 59, 277.

Ramsey, E.M. (1962) Circulation in the intervillous space of primate placenta. *Am. J. Obstet. Gynecol.* 84, 1649-1663.

Ramsey, E.M. (1966) Venous drainage of the placenta in rhesus monkeys; radiographic studies. *Am. J. Obstet. Gynecol.* 95, 948.

Ramsey, E.M. (1971) Maternal and foetal circulation of the placenta. *Ir. J. Med. Sci.* 140, 151-168.

Ramsey, E.M., Corner, G.W., Jr., and Donner, M.W. (1963) Serial and cineradioangiographic visualisation of maternal circulation in the primate (hemochorial) placenta. *Am. J. Obstet. Gynecol.* 86, 213-225.

Reynolds, S.R.M. (1966) Formation of foetal cotyledons in the hemochorial placenta. *Am. J. Obstet. Gynecol.* 94, 425-439.

Reynolds, S.R.M. (1967) Derivation of the vascular elements in the cotyledons of the hemochorial placenta. *Anat. Rec.* 157, 43-46.

Reynolds, S.R.M. (1971) Multiple simultaneous intervillous space pressure recorded in several regions of the hemochorial placenta in relation to functional anatomy of the fetal cotyledon. *Am. J. Obstet. Gynecol.* 109, 63.

Reynolds, S.R.M. (1972) On growth and form in the hemochorial placenta: An essay on the physical forces that shape the chorionic trophoblast. *Am. J. Obstet. Gynecol.* 114, 115-132.

Sen, D.K., Kaufmann, P., and Schweikhart, G. (1979) Classification of human placental villi. II. Morphometry. *Cell Tissue Res.* 200, 425-434.

Smart, P.J.G. (1962) Some observations on the vascular morphology of the foetal side of the human placenta. *J. Obstet. Gynaecol. Br. Cwlth.* 69, 929-933.

Schuhmann, R. and Wehler, V. (1971) Histologische Unterschiede an Plazentazotten innerhalb der materno-fetalen Stroemungseinheit. Ein Beitrag zur funktionellen Morphologie der Plazenta. *Arch. Gynecol.* 210, 425-439.

Schuhmann, R., Borst, H., and Lehmann, W.D. (1972) Regionale Unterschiede der alkalischen Phosphataseaktivitaet innerhalb der materno-fetalen Stroemungseinheiten (Plazentone) der reifen menschlichen Plazenta (histochemische und biochemische Untersuchungen). *Arch. Gynecol.* 213, 93-102.

Schuhmann, R. (1976) Die funktionelle Morphologie der Plazentone reifer menschlicher Plazenten (histologische, histochemische, biochemische und autoradiographische Untersuchungen). *Gestosis Press,* Basel, 3-53.

Schuhmann, R., Kraus, H., Borst, R., and Geier, G. (1976) Regional unterschiedliche Enzymaktivitaet innerhalb der Plazentone reifer menschlicher Plazenten (histochemische und biochemische Untersuchungen). *Arch. Gynecol.* 220, 209-226.

Schuhmann, R., Borst, H., Geier, G., and Kraus, H. (1977) Uber die Plazentone der reifen menschlichen Plazenta. *Z. Geburtshilfe Perinatol.* 8, 13-25.

Schweikhart, G. and Kaufmann, P. (1977) Zur Abgrenzung normaler, artefizieller und pathologischer Strukturen in reifen menschlichen Plazentazotten. I. Ultrastruktur des Syncytiotrophoblasten. *Arch. Gynecol.* 222, 213-230.

Schweikhart, G. (1985) Morphologie des Zottenbaumes der menschlichen Plazenta. Orthologische und pathologische Entwicklung und klinische Relevanz. *Habilitationsschrift,* Mainz.

Schweikhart, G., Kaufmann, P., and Beck, T. (1986) Morphology of placental villi after premature delivery and its clinical relevance. *Arch. Gynecol.* 239, 101-114.

Stoz, F., Schuhmann, R.A., and Noack, E.J. (1982) Morphometrische Plazentabefunde bei EPH-Gestose. *Z Geburtshilfe Perinatol.* 186, 72-75.

Stoz, F., Schuhmann, R.A., and Noack, E.J. (1983) Morphometrische Untersuchungen an Plazenten reifer Mangelgeborener. *Z Geburtshilfe Perinatol.* 187, 142-145.

Wigglesworth, J.S. (1969) Vascular anatomy of the human placenta and its significance for placental pathology. *J. Obstet. Gynaecol. Br. Cmwlth.* 76, 979-989.

Wilkin, P. (1965) Pathologie du placenta. *Masson et Cie,* Paris.

# CONCEPTIONAL PROPOSITION FOR A SPECIFIC MICROCIRCULATORY PROBLEM : MATERNAL BLOOD FLOW IN HEMOCHORIAL MULTIVILLOUS PLACENTAE AS PERCOLATION OF A "POROUS MEDIUM"

Holger Schmid-Schönbein

Department of Physiology
Klinikum der RWTH Aachen
D-5100 Aachen, FR Germany

## INTRODUCTION

### Normal and Abnormal Percolation of the Intervillous Spaces: The Cotyledon as a "Chromatographic Trough"

Recently, it has been convincingly shown by Murphy et al. (1986) that hemoconcentration is a risk factor in severe pre-eclampsia. More specifically, the work of Heilmann et al. (1977, 1984) has shown that the non-Newtonian behavior of blood is distinctly more pronounced in patients suffering from pre-eclampsia and other forms of placental dysfunction. In these pathologic pregnancies, many of which are known to have a high uterine artery impedence to flow (Campbell et al., 1983; Fendel, 1985), there is evidence that curtailed fluidity of maternal blood might critically limit the perfusion of the intervillous spaces (a topic recently covered in an international symposium, cf. Heilman, 1984).

This pathophysiologic hypothesis, which would have considerable therapeutic implications, requires an elaborate presentation of the unique blood flow behavior and microchemodynamics in the intervillous spaces. Even though totally concealed from "flow visualization" as the only objective method to establish unequivocally the micro-fluid-dynamics within an organ, the vascular spaces in the maternal part of the hemochorial, multivillous placentae can be safely classifed as an exception to the fundamental architecture of the vascular tree, in which blood perfuses cylindrical or nearly cylindrical conduits. Instead, the villi are immersed into an open conduit and are "percolated" by the blood. This mode of blood flow can be compared to the motion of water around the rootlets of water plants; its fluid dynamics is closely related to that of the motion of the solvent through the voids of a chromatographic column prepared by sedimenting discreet particles.

It is the aim of this communication to submit for the "placentologic sciences", basic information about pragmatic solutions and their theoretical foundation as applied to "flow in porous media", an important process dealt with in the engineering profession (Muskat, 1949; Greeley and Stanley, 1952).

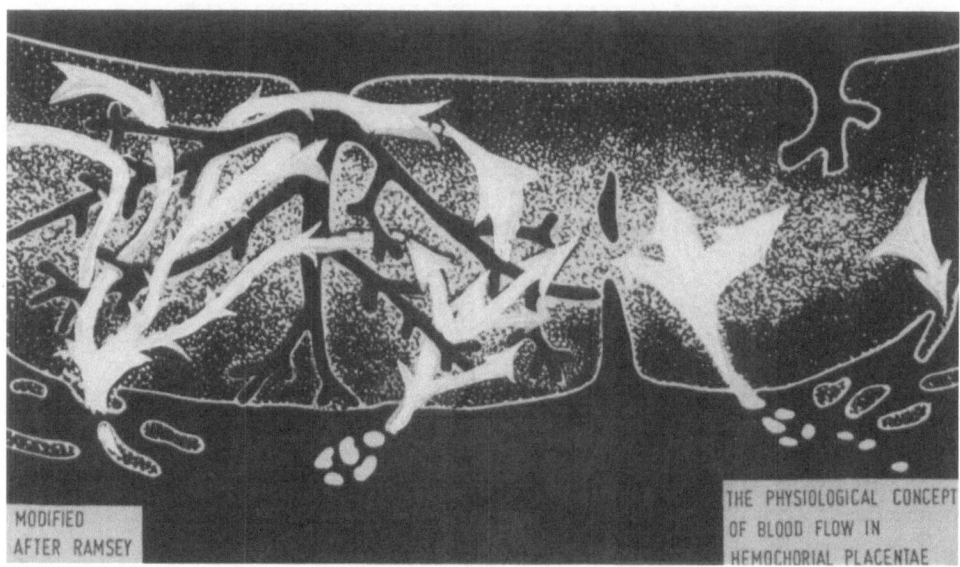

Figure 1. The physiological concept of placental flow illustrated as villus percolation. The maternal blood (depicted in white) shown to be streaming from the spiral artery (well) to the uterine veins (sinks), washing the surfaces of the trophoblastic villus tree much like a river washes the surfaces of the roots of water plants. (Modified after Ramsey et al., 1965)

Owing to the complexity of the fluid dynamic problem under consideration and in light of the fact that many particular aspects of this deviate in principle from conventional hemodynamics, it is necessary to extend conventional terminology. As can be seen in Figure 1 (modified from the classical scheme of Ramsey), the flow of maternal blood in each cotyledon proceeds from the mouth of each spiral artery to the exit ports of the uterine veins in a broad stream that, on a macroscopic scale, is not really "directed" by the trophoblast but proceeds as if it were not there. Microscopically speaking, of course, the villi "stand in the way" of maternal blood. This situation is similar to that observed in many "porous media", e.g., granular, of fibrous filter beds. The hemochorial multivillous placentae, however, are "washed" in a large trough through which maternal blood drains (Figures 1 and 2).

Since the fetal capillaries deliver $CO_2$ and remove $O_2$, steady state concentration gradients for these blood gases (and all other metabolites) can only be maintained if there is blood flow. Flow, in turn, is a process by which a fluid is undergoing a continuous shear deformation at the expense of frictional energy dissipation. The higher the velocity of shear deformation, and the lower the fluidity of the moving liquid, the higher the energy dissipation associated with a deformation process that "spreads out", as if it was a large volume of fluid in a thin layer with a large surface area.

Since frictional work is done in this "spreading" or "dissipation" process, there are important fluid-dynamic differences between the "spreading mode" associated with the washing of villous surfaces and that associated with being funneled through the narrow lumina of narrow cylindrical conduits. Even if the minimum diameter of space and the diameter of the tubes and the fluidity of the liquid are identical, the fluid particles moving past villi are conducted with much less shear than those moving through the narrow cylindrical conduits of identical diameter.

Such differences in shear regime become effective as different "resistances" against fluid motion: a parameter that can be calculated from the ratio of pressure and flow rate. This reciprocal is called conductance. Conductance depends on the geometry of the conduit and the fluidity of the liquid moved; obviously, a more "porous" bed will "conduct" the fluid more readily.

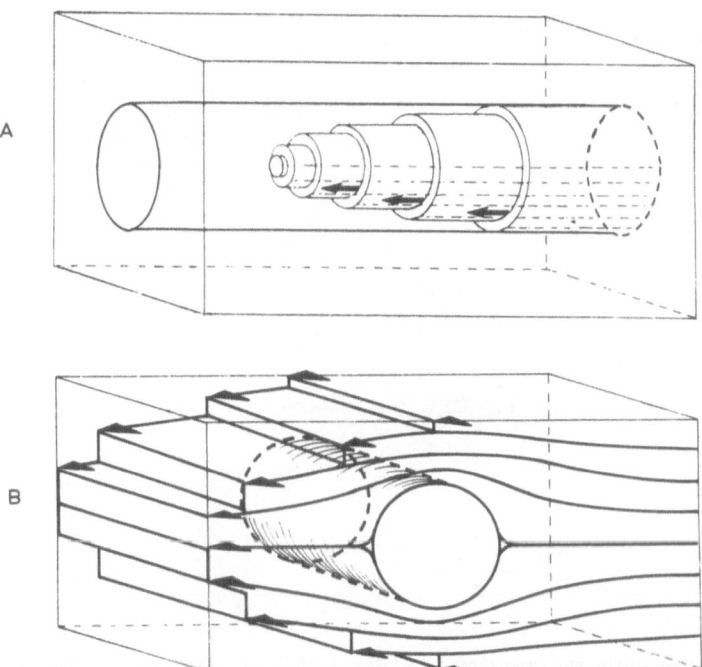

Figure 2. Schematic representation of the flow through the opening of cylindrical hole obstructing a rectangular channel and of flow around a single cylindrical pillar. In tube flow, the stream lines must be condensed. This effect, however, is far more pronounced than in the flow situation created by a pillar as an obstacle. The resistance caused by the additional shearing between fluid lamellae is proportional to the channel length. In flow around a pillar, the stream lines become condensed on both sides of the pillar. The frictional work (for any given flow rate) is increased approximately proportional to the cross sectional area of the pillar and thus proportional to the free space left between cylinder surface and channel wall.

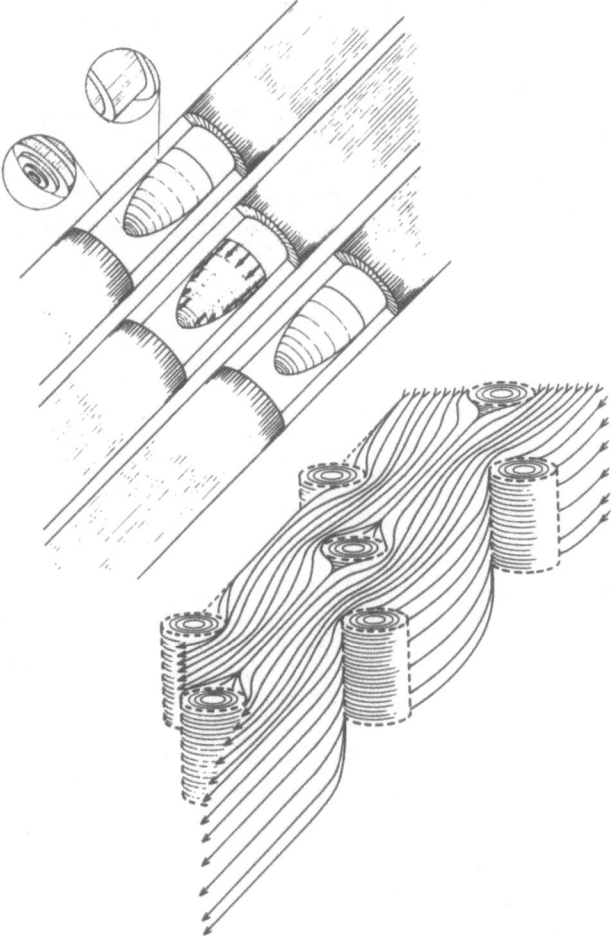

Figure 3. Schematic representation of the fluid dynamics of flow between systems of staggered obstacle rows. Note the wavy path of fluid particles, the periodic increases and decreases in effective cross sectional area. The mean cross sectional area is considerably larger than that predictable from the minimum distance between any two pillars. Poiseuille flow with pronounced shearing of fluid in a set of parallel tubes is shown for comparison.

Thus, there is a direct relationship between "porosity" and conductance. Work in unit time (or power) is the product of pressure and flow rate: less power is required to deform a unit volume of fluid in unit time as it "percolates" through the intervillous spaces than is required to perfuse any other organ. Any design of an exchange system with high conductance thus means to provide favorable conditions for diffusive transport blood gases with less power requirement. It is known from chromatographic columns of granular matrices how little power may be needed to maximize an exchange area if a fluid passes through the voids between small spheres, a typical example of a porous material (Novak, 1984). Many biologists might be more familiar with the macroscopic physics of chromatography columns; it is hoped that despite the marked differences in microscopic detail, familiar terms from every day chemical procedure (like void volume, wet surface, effective cross-sectional area, and geometric conductivity) will, therefore, help the reader to grasp the unique nature of blood flow in the intervillous spaces. It will also be intuitively clear that pores might be clogged by "aggregated matter" under all conditions where cohesive energy between cellular blood components exceeds the dispersive energy of the fluid in shear. This topic is covered in the next sections and the Appendix.

### Fluid Dynamics of Flow Around Obstacles

The gaps between the villi in hemochorial placentae can be looked at as a randomly oriented and shaped labyrinth of narrow, connected slits. The flow of maternal blood in this unique "open" conduit is called a "percolation" (from latin percolare = to sieve) to differentiate it from "perfusion" (from Latin perfundere = to pour through) as it occurs in the capillary networks of all other vascular beds, including those of the maternal side of the epithelio-chorial, endothelio-chorial and labyrinthine placentae. In order to justify this arbitrary distinction, a simple hydrodynamic description of the motion of blood around the villi is necessary.

Flow of a liquid through any container is the consequence of a continuous deformation or "shearing" of fluid elements. Provided the liquid molecules adhere to the wall of the conduit, any driving force (e.g., a pressure difference $P1 - P2 = \Delta P$) will cause the fluid elements to glide past each other in such a fashion that a velocity difference builds up between those elements stationary at the wall and those most distant from it, e.g., those traveling along the axis of the conduit. As detailed in any introductory textbook of fluid dynamics, (e.g., Davis, 1952; Franke, 1971) this process is called laminar shearing (because all elements traveling with equal velocity along a trajectory form a kind of "lamina"), causes the buildup of velocity gradients, also called shear rates (m/s m = $s^{-1}$). These shear rates are, for any given geometry, directly proportional to the incident driving pressure or pressure gradient ($\Delta P/L$, $N/m^2$) acting along the length of the conduit and also the fluidity ($m^2/s \cdot N$ of the fluid medium), i.e., the reciprocal value of its coefficient of viscosity. The shear stress, i.e., a force acting tangentially on the interface between individual laminae, is 1) proportional to the pressure gradient, and 2) proportional to the ratio of shear rate and fluidity of the fluid. At steady state flow (i.e., without net deceleration or acceleration) frictional energy dissipation (work/time, $N \cdot m/s$) is proportional to the product of shear stress ($N/m^2$), shear rate ($s^{-1}$) and volume ($m^3$), or the product of flow rate ($m^3/s$) and driving pressure ($N/m^2$).

$$\Delta E = V \cdot \tau \cdot \gamma = \left[ \frac{Nm}{s} \right]$$

$$\Delta E = \dot{V} \cdot \Delta P \quad \left[ \frac{Nm}{s} \right]$$

When applying these fundamental considerations to perfusion of cylindrical conduits and percolation of spaces between cylindrically shaped obstacles of similar dimension, some fundamental kinematic differences come to light.

For discussion purposes, a villus is reduced to a cylinder (Figures 1 and 2). The above consideration intuitively makes it clear that its effect on the net frictional energy dissipation is restricted to its local effect on the shearing motion. As shown in Figure 2, the laminae (in squeezing past the cylinder as an obstacle) have to be locally condensed, resulting either in a fall of the mean shear rates for any given pressure (slowing down flow) or in a rise of shear stresses (and thus the pressure gradient) for a given flow rate (V). Obviously, there is less fluid displacement for a given energy dissipation, or figuratively speaking, the hydraulic conductance of the conduit is locally lowered by the presence of the obstacle. If one calculates the decrease in conductance, it is immediately clear that it shall be proportional to the aspect area of the cylinder, more precisely the fractional aspect area ($A_D/A_{tot}$)

$$\frac{A_D}{A_{tot}} = \frac{D_{cyl} \cdot H_{cyl}}{W_V \cdot H_V}$$

where $D_{cyl}$ and $H_{cyl}$ are the cylinder diameter and height, $W_V$ and $H_V$ are the width and height of the free space (void).

When many cylinders are arranged in staggered rows, the fluid percolating the interspace (void) has to follow tortuous paths, the moving laminae loosing their parallelism and becoming periodically condensed and expanded. The fractional cross sectional area of the void ($A_{eff}$) within the arrangement of pillars (dead volume) oscillates between a maximum of 1.0 ($A_D$, $D_{cyl} = 0$) and a minimum ($1 - D_{cyl} \cdot H_{cyl}/W_V \cdot H_V$). As the fluid adheres to the walls of each cylinder (the latter being washed, from all sides), its adherence causes a local drop in velocity to zero but nevertheless only a small increase in overall shearing in the neighboring void (Figure 3).

In comparison, fluid elements coming from large reservoirs and being channeled into a single cylindrical conduit of dimensions identical to the pillar just discussed, will all be subjected to rapid shearing during their entire passage through the conduit. The energy dissipation will be increased to a much higher degree (Figure 1). The situation is called Poiseuillian flow. It is based on a telescope-like deformation of fluid laminae and is associated with much higher mean shear rates for any given mean fluid velocity or flow rate: the surface is "washed" at great energy expenditure.

The same arguments apply to a situation where many cylindrical conduits are positioned in parallel. The change in conductance of such an arrangement is no longer simply related to fractional cross sectional area of the conduits. Instead, it is highly dependent upon the individual conduit diameter (since its geometric conductivity is proportional to the 4th power of the diameter, whereas the cross sectional area is only proportional to the square of the diameter. Perfusion of microtube networks obtained increase in washed surface of the expense of very high frictional energy dissipation. This can only be compensated for in part by placing many microtubes in parallel.

Modern microcirculatory research, attempting to cope with a multitude of factors that determine the hydraulics of microvascular beds perfused with a fluid that has a high non-Newtonian viscosity, was forced to extend the traditional vocabulary used in macrocirculatory physiology, which simply calculated the ratio of pressure and flow as a resistance in analogy to OHM's law. As detailed elsewhere (Schmid-Schönbein, 1988), when dealing with networks, it is helpful to refer to conductance rather than resistance. Moreover, since the flow behavior of blood is highly variable and cannot be described by a constant parameter, it is necessary to divide resistance into its geometric part (called vascular hindrance, $\pi D^4/128\ L$) related to diameter (D) and length (L), and viscosity ($Ns/m^2$), or their respective reciprocal values, geometric conductivity ($128\ L/\pi D^4$) and fluidity ($Ns/m^2$). It is immediately obvious that the conductance of an individual conduit (or a network of conduits) can drop to zero when either its diameter or the fluidity of a viscoelastic suspension perfusing it approaches zero. Blood as a perfusate has this very potential, as detailed in the Appendix).

Coming back to the hydrodynamic modeling of the maternal space of multivillous hemochorial placentae, one can conceive of flow as a process of washing thousands of cylinders. In such "void percolation" the conductance of the intervillous spaces will be proportional to the volume of intervillous space and inversely proportional to the volume of the villous tree, expressed as fractional void volume ($V_V/V_V + V_D$) and fractional "dead space" ($V_D/V_V + V_D$).

The intervillous space is a system of randomly shaped and oriented, interconnected clefts (connected voids). With respect to their topology, these clefts lack the regular connectivity seen in dichotomously branching vascular trees, where certain classes of vessels are grown to be positioned in series, others in parallel. Such fixed relationships, which, among other things, orient pressure gradients, are not found in randomly connected voids; here, the local hydraulic forces and the variable conductances determine both direction of flow and energy dissipation associated with it. It is this feature that creates the potential hazards of connected voids when percolated with liquids (and especially with suspensions) of variable fluidity. Whenever the driving force drops, so does energy dissipation and the fluidity of an aggregated suspension. Thus, the conductance can drop locally to zero either because of geometric or because of rheological factors (see Appendix).

These considerations can offer a comprehensive explanation for a number of well established, unique features of the normal human placenta. Its high fractional voidage (porosity) during most of the early pregnancy, in combination with the high fluidity of the perfusate (due to physiological hemodilution, Heilman, 1982) explains its high conductance (Figure 3). As will be discussed in the Appendix, one can anticipate a percolation with high volumetric flow rate, but low local velocities. Such motion, in turn, requires low shear stresses (and energy dissipation). Under most conditions, this is advantageous; most of all, such a system favors diffusive exchange (v.i.) at low viscous energy expenditure. There are, however, serious potential disadvantages of random connectivity. These can be related to its proneness to become clogged by soft materials such as sludges or thixotropic blood elements (see Appendix and Schmid-Schönbein, 1988 for a detailed definition of this term).

## The Placenta as a Non-Uniform Porous Continuum: "Dead Space" Separated by "Void Space"

As one looks at the entire cotyledon (trophoblast and its bed), it can be likened to a porous continuum, a pervious material percolated by maternal blood. There is nothing new in such a description. It does, however, open a new perspective for its fluid dynamic analysis in semantic and conceptual terms that are well established (e.g., in Darcy's law, v.i.) and that should be tried and tested with presently available techniques in human placentology. Instead of microscopic details, macroscopic "porosity" is placed in the center of consideration, leading to a novel, coherent concept for the unique motion of maternal blood in hemochorial placentae. In its initial application, this concept deliberately disregards geometrical details of the villus structure and accepts the whole of the intervillous spaces as a system of connected pores of unknown, but highly variable diameters. It can be predicted from known morphological data (e.g., Kaufmann et al., 1988) that porosity differs in the different stages of placental maturation, in different locations within each individual cotyledon and in different parts of the individual villous tree. In the future development of strategies to comprehend the overall trophoblast influence on cotyledonal flow, emphasis must be extended from individual variabilities in villus configuration assessment to that of the distribution of intervillous distances. In analogy to conventions in the engineering sciences (Dullian, 1979 and Scheidegger, 1960), the trophoblast proper can be taken as a variable "dead volume", which locally determines the hydraulic conductivity (permeability, v.i.) of the intervillous or "void space" (for any given fluidity of the perfusing medium). For discussion purposes, it can be said that porosity or voidage is highest near the mouth of the spiral artery and lowest near the uterine veins (Ramsey et al., 1965). This distribution of voidage is bound to create a gradient of conductancies which, even in randomly connected voids, necessarily determines overall cotyledonal flow rate as well as flow rate distribution in different parts of the cotyledon.

In other words, in applying abstractions developed in Darcian systems, the growth process of trophoblast maturation (as well as its pathological deviations, see Kaufmann et al., 1988) can in principle be described in terms of fractional volume of void space ($\kappa$) and fractional volume of "dead space" ($1-\kappa$). Obviously, the effect of any type of additional material deposited in the intervillous space (e.g., fibrin and fibrinoid), cell aggregates and infarcts can be interpreted as a shift of original void space to functional "dead space".

At present, one is faced with a lack of reliable in situ data on: 1) the geometry, 2) the topology of the trophoblast tree, and 3) most of the voidage, due to the collapse of the intervillous spaces during detachment and delivery of the placenta. No useful direct knowledge about intervillous distances in situ is available. Despite such ignorance about the real hydraulics, the formalities developed for analyzing the percolation of other types of non-biological gross porous media (Muskat, 1949; Dullian, 1979) are of theoretical interest to comprehend intervillous flow. This work attempts to extrapolate formalities successfully applied by engineers for analyzing flow processes (such as the washout of fluids from concealed granular or fibrous beds), interaction of convective transport (flow), and diffusive transport (exchange). Such problems have to be solved in sewage technology (e.g., Greely and Stanley, 1952), in the geophysics of crude oil sedimentation (Muskat, 1949), and last but not least, in the chromatographic flow, through analytic or preparative gel filter columns.

### Darcy's Law Applied to the Entire Placenta

Many naturally occurring porous media are extremely difficult to quantify morphologically, but can still be described fluid-dynamically. The fundamental equations describing perfusion of porous media are formulated by Darcy's law, which describes the ratio of flow rate and driving forces in containers of known geometry, filled with a porous medium of unknown properties. Darcy's law can be stated as follows:

$$\dot{V}_D = \frac{\Delta P}{L} \cdot C_D$$

or

$$\dot{V}_D = \frac{\Delta P}{L} \cdot \varphi \cdot k_D$$

$$\text{where } k_D \stackrel{\wedge}{=} f(A_{eff}, D^2, \alpha, T)$$

$C_D$ is defined as the ratio of flow rate and pressure gradient ($\Delta P/L$) and depends on the total cross sectional area ($A_{eff}$), the porosity ($\kappa$) and the fluidity of the perfusate. In hydrology, the term "fluid permeability" (Dullian, 1979) of a porous rock, a sand filter, or a fibrous bed is customary, which depends on the shape factor $\alpha$ of the pores, determinable if all other factors in Darcy's law can be measured. Strictly speaking, Darcy's law applies only to Newtonian fluids of constant viscosity, for porous media perfused with a non-Newtonian fluid it is useful to separate this entity in its determining factor kd (geometric conductivity, which is a function of porosity) and apparent fluidity. Flow rate obviously depends on the pressure gradient ($\Delta P/L_{eff}$), that is to say the pressure between the upper and the lower end of the container, divided by the effective length of the pores. If these paths are tortuous, $L_{eff}$ can be considerably greater than the nomimal length (L). An essential feature of Darcian systems is the empirical observation that in porous media conductivity is proportional to the square of either pore diameter $D^2$ or equivalent hydraulic diameter (v.i.).

Strictly speaking, Darcian conductivity can be measured in applying Darcy's law only provided that porous media are tightly fitting a container. Because of problems of bypassing, many real porous media cannot be subjected to such precise assessment, therefore, a great deal of ingenuity has been used to devise a variety of different permeameters. There are practical solutions, e.g., unsteady state permeametry, falling head permeametry that might be applied in analogy to certain resistance parameters that are customary in ultrasound/Doppler velocimetry of the uterine arteries.

FLOW THROUGH CAPILLARY ARRAYS
HAGEN – POISEUILLE law and KIRCHHOFF's rules

$$\dot{V}_{HP} = \frac{\Delta P}{L} \cdot \varphi \cdot k_{HP} \qquad\qquad k_{HP} = n \cdot \frac{\pi D^4}{128}$$

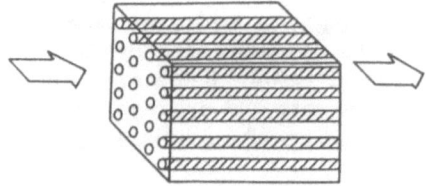

INTERVILLOUS PERFUSION AS FLOW IN POROUS MEDIA

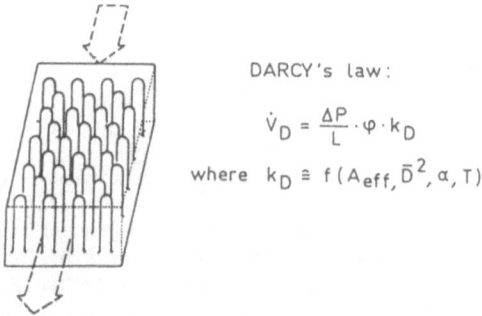

DARCY's law :

$$\dot{V}_D = \frac{\Delta P}{L} \cdot \varphi \cdot k_D$$

$$\text{where} \quad k_D \cong f(A_{eff}, \bar{D}^2, \alpha, T)$$

Figure 4.  Comparison of the perfusion of a material pierced by cylindrical conduits to the percolation of the void spaces between staggered rows of cylinders. The perfusion is defined by the Hagen-Poiseuille law and Kirchhoff's rule (parallel conductances add up to a total conductance). The percolation of the void spaces cannot simply be calculated, conductance can be measured empirically. These empirical measurements can be related to geometrical factors such as the effective cross sectional area, the square of the hydraulic diameter, empirical shape factors, and tortuosity (T).

It is conceivable that in the future "dead space" of delivered placentae might be estimated by various engineering methods which in principle, are applicable to placentological research (i.e., optical methods, imbibition methods, the mercury injection method after fixation, gas expansion methods, or density methods, (cf., Dullian, 1979).

If these methods are utilized after prior nuclear magnetic resonance measurement of the true placental volume $(V_V + V_D)$ in situ, an estimate of the porosity by determining fractional voidage $(\kappa = V_V/V_V + V_D)$ will be possible. Also, functional parameters, such as permeability and geometric conductivity, respectively, which are obviously a function of porosity, can be determined in principle by relating voidage to geometrical determinants (shape factor $\alpha$, tortuosity T) and to hydrodynamic parameters (such as hydraulic diameter, wetted surface) or to their respective analogues.

For this purpose, many empirical equations have been developed in hydrological literature, one of the most popular is based on the work of Carman and Kozeny (for details, see Dullian, 1979 and Scheidegger, 1970). In their honor, the Carman-Kozeny equation has been developed:

$$k_{C.K.} = \frac{\kappa_{eff} \cdot \bar{D}_H^2}{16 \, \alpha \, (L_{eff}/L)^2}$$

which is the basic form of all empirical modeling of porous bed geometry, differing only in methods of calculating the average hydraulic diameter $(\bar{D}_H)$ and the shape factor $(\alpha)$ and tortuosity $(L_{eff}/L)$, respectively (Dullian, 1979). A lucid example of the strategies employed in hydrology are the attempts to determine the hydraulic diameter by using the Carman-Kozeny equation. The procedure starts from the simple assumption that flow of fluids in porous media can be imagined with equal justification to either occur in a network of closed conduits or to occur around solid particles forming a spacial array. In either case, one need not pay any attention to the irregular way that pore sizes are interconnected. Conceptionally one can reduce a porous medium to one conduit which has an extremely complicated shape but, on average, a constant cross sectional area and which can be expressed as an equivalent hydraulic diameter $(D_H)$.

In analogy with established practices in hydraulics, it is equated to four times the ratio of void volumes $(m^3)$ and surface area $(m^2)$ (Dullian, 1979).

$$D_H \overset{\wedge}{=} \frac{4 \, V}{S_O} \, [m]$$

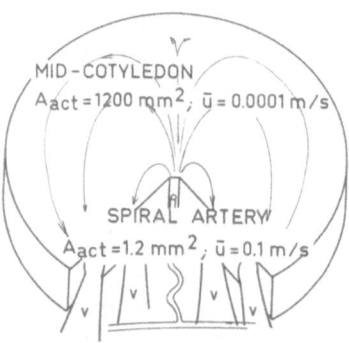

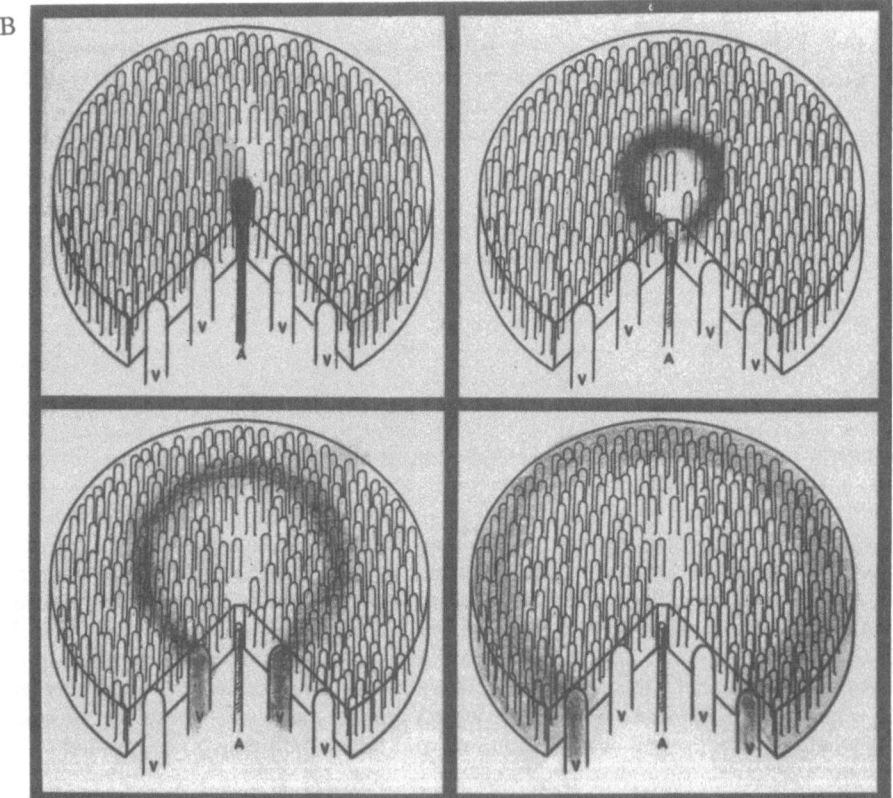

Figure 5. A) Schematic representation of an idealized primate cotyledon reduced to a chromatographic trough perfused from a single well (spiral artery) active area 1.2 mm² expanding into a wide bed and draining into multiple sinks (uterine veins). It follows from the law of continuity that the mean velocity (ū) at each cross section is inversely proportional to the active cross sectional area $A_{act}$ is assumed to be 1200 mm²; therefore the average velocity must be reduced to 0.001 m/s. B) These considerations offer an explanation for the spreading of angiographical contrast media as a diverging chromatographic front. For details, see text. Its position at various times after the initial spurt is shown schematically.

Table 1

Empirical Parameters for the Estimation of the Geometry and Hydraulics of "Porous Media"
as Applicable to the Intervillous Spaces of Multivillous Hemochorial Placentae
(See List of Symbols for Definition of Symbols and Letters)

| Parameter | Theoretical model (CARMEN-KOZENY Theory) | Possibility for experimental estimation in placentology |
|---|---|---|
| "Dead volume" $V_D$ | - | Total volume of trophoblast |
| Void volume = $V_V$ (intervillous space) | - | Subtraction of trophoblast volume from placental volume in vivo |
| Perfused void = connected void $V_C$ | - | Product of flow rate and mean passage time $V_C = \dot{V} \cdot \bar{t}$ |
| Effective voidage $\kappa_{eff} = \dfrac{V_C}{V_D + V_C}$ | - | Product of flow rate and mean passage time normalized by total placental volume |
| Darcian conductance of porous bed $(C_D)$ | $C_D = \dfrac{\kappa_{eff} \cdot D_H^2}{16\,\alpha\left(L_{eff}/L\right)^2}$ | 1) Ratio of flow-rate and driving pressure $C_D = \dot{V}/\Delta P$ <br> 2) Reciprocal value of empirical deceleration parameters in U.S. doppler velocimetry of uterine arteries |
| Wetted surface = connected void surface | $S_O = \sqrt{\dfrac{\kappa_{eff}^3}{\alpha_O \cdot (L_{eff}/L)^2 \cdot (1 - \kappa_{eff})^2 \cdot C_D}}$ <br> $= \dfrac{\kappa_{eff}}{1 - \kappa_{eff}}\sqrt{\dfrac{\kappa_{eff}}{5 \cdot C_D}}$ | Ratio of effective voidage and conductance |
| Equivalent channel diameter $D_H$ | $D_H = \dfrac{4\,\kappa_{eff}}{S_O\,(1 - \kappa_{eff})}$ | $D_H = \dfrac{\text{Void volume}}{\text{"Wetted surface"}}$ |
| Tortuosity correction | $T = \left(\dfrac{L_{eff}^2}{L}\right)$ | Histology |
| Empirical tortuosity - shape correction | $Y = 16\,\alpha\,\dfrac{L_{eff}^2}{L}$ <br> Approximation: $\pi/2$ | not possible |

There is much (and well founded) debate about this approach. For example, application of the procedure to estimate hydraulic diameter constant as a procedure to analyze all kinds of porous media (e.g., to those with highly variable porosities and pore diameters or of both) has widely been criticized (Dullian, 1979). Nevertheless, such concepts enjoy great popularity by workers assessing only one class of porous media. With this reservation, it might be justified to propose its use in placentology.

## Research Proposals for Future Strategies to Estimate Geometric Parameters in Concealed Porous Media

High porosity can be intuitively associated with high conductance, a high degree of void space proliferation with low conductance. However, it is extremely difficult, if not impossible, to quantify the geometrical details and their functional sequelae in actual porous media. It is even more difficult to quantify the geometry of pores than that of capillaries. In this respect, engineers and placentologists face very similar, at first glance, insurmountable problems. It should be stressed that in engineering research or practical work, the all important details on the geometric parameters of porous media are not known to any better precision than that obtainable in present day research on human placentae. However, in light of the pragmatic successes of defining certain indirect dynamic, geometric, and functional parameters, which can be measured and can be related to a sort of averaged geometry, it seems justified to present the pragmatic proposals of the Carman-Kozeny school of thought to the placentological community. Where lengths (as in diameters, perimeters, and distances), surface areas (i.e., the specific internal area for exchange and places wetted by flow, v.i.) and volumes (absolute and effective voidage, dead volumes, perfused volumes) are not measurable by any available method, derived analogues can be helpful for comparative purposes. It an attempt to translate the terminology developed in one applied science (hydrology) to another (medicine) a few of these indirect parameters (Table 1) will be interpreted. They were chosen on the basis of their physiological relevance, on the potential applicability for human placental research with presently available techniques or those (e.g., NMR, see Panigel et al., 1988) that will be available in the near future.

In many porous media, and most probably in certain placentae, the total voidage is made up of two distinct parts, namely the interconnected and the isolated pores (which are not perfused). Thus, the more important parameter from a functional point of view would be effective voidage ($\kappa_{eff}$), conducting porosity, defined as the sum of the volumina of all interconnected pores, divided by the total volume. Its direct estimation is impossible. For this reason, it is of interest that there are potentials to approximate the effective voidage by indirect means, namely flow analyses.

According to Dullian (1979), $\kappa_{eff}$ can be estimated by any measurement (or combination of such measurement, e.g., by indicator dilution method) that provides data on flow rate ($V = dV/dt$) and on mean transit times (t). The product of these two parameters that could be obtainable for example from the NMR tracer washout curves is equivalent to the perfused volume.

$$\dot{V} \cdot \overline{t} = V_{conn} \left[ m^3 \right]$$

By normalizing this entity with the total placental volume in situ, an analogue to $\kappa_{eff}$ in defined porous media can be approximated, which opens the possibility to estimate other parameters. This procedure is closely related to those already applied in experimental placental research, e.g., in determining a parameter called clearance by Moll (1972). It goes without saying that once an analogue to the effective voidage ($\kappa_{eff}$) could be determined, the effective fractional dead volume (1 - $\kappa_{eff}$) could be calculated (composed of true dead volume, the villous tree) and various subdivisions of functional dead volumes (non-perfused cotyledonal parts, intervillous spaces plugged by coagulae, fibrinoid, fibrin, and overt infarcts).

In all real porous systems and in placentae as well, the specific surface area (also called wetted surface, S) can be considered as the functionally most important variable. S is defined as the total surface of the interconnected pores, normalized by total volume. Since this surface can be assumed to be washed by the perfusate, it can be assumed to partake in exchange. According to the Carman-Kozeny equation (Scheidegger, 1960) $S_o$ can be approximated if $\kappa_{eff}$ and the Darcian conductance ($C_D$) are known. In essence, the Carman-Kozeny approach is based on the assumption that the wetted surface must be proportional to the ratio of effective voidage ($\kappa_{eff}$) and effective fractional "dead space" (1 - $\kappa_{eff}$), multiplied by the square root of the ratio $\kappa_{eff}$ over conductance. It is plausible that the wetted surface of a porous medium of unknown geometry should be somehow related to: 1) the effective void volume, and 2) the reciprocal of conductance.

In light of the availability of empirical "resistance parameters" from the deceleration of late systolic and early diastolic phase of ultrasound doppler measurements (Campbell, 1983; Klosa, 1983; Fendel, 1985), one can foresee that analogues to $S_o$ will be obtained in the future, based on an appropriate modification of the Carmen-Kozeny approach. $S_o$ data would greatly help in estimating other important functional parameters, for example, average hydraulic pore diameter as defined above. The approach is not a truly rigorous one but nevertheless provides some semiquantitative functional indicators, simply because in real porous media (and certainly in placentae) there is a very wide distribution of true pore diameters. Nevertheless, the application of suggested approximations in the differential diagnosis of various forms of placental hypoperfusion in patients might augment the diagnostic, functional, and prognostic potentials of each individual non-invasive method which has not become available.

## EPILOGUE

The present treatize aims at developing a hypothetical model of the hypoperfused placenta as a case of a Darcian system with functionally non-homogenous geometric conductivity. It embraces not just structural abnormalities with various forms of villous hypertrophy with the existence of additional dead volume, such as fibrinoid, coagulae, or infarcts in various forms of placental dysfunction, but also functional abnormalities of a rheological nature (see Appendix). It follows from the logic of Darcian fluid dynamics that clogged porous media provide ideal conditions for the manifestation and self perpetuation of blood viscidation in the intervillous space, leading to a disseminated blood standstill in the presence of finite pressure gradients (rheological occlusion).

Another analogy from human pathology might be worth mentioning, the human lung, an exchanger, perfused with low driving pressure (Fung and Sobin, 1972) but highly susceptible to non-homogenous perfusion, various forms of reversible stand still and heterophase effects (e.g., in hypostatical pneumonia). The complex techniques developed for differential diagnosis and therapy supervision of acute pulmonary disorders (Comroe, 1964; West, 1969) ought to be a further source of inspiration for the future development of the ideas presented here.

At present, these considerations are conjectural. There is, however, one classical experiment by the founder of contemporary clinical hemorheology that can be cited as support of the speculations presented. Fahraeus (1962) demonstrated in simple experiments with a fibrous porous medium (measuring the spontaneous spreading of blood in a paper filter) that highly aggregated blood of pre-eclamptic women showed clearly a deficient ability to move in the spaces of a fairly good experimental in vitro model of the hemochorial, multivillous placenta of primates.

## SUMMARY

There is increasing evidence that abnormal flow behavior of maternal blood complicates high risk pregnancies. Owing to a strongly exaggerated red cell aggregation and abnormally high hematocrit values (on the basis of normal standards for pregnant women) maternal blood in EPH-gestosis and small-for-date babies on the basis of oligohydramnion shows pathological blood thixotropy, i.e., has a tendency to lose its fluidity in a reversible fashion when subjected to very low shear stresses. In order to develop a conceptual frame work for analyzing blood flow in the intervillous spaces, the fluid dynamics of flow around baffles is developed and compared to Poiseuille in tubes. On the basis of this analysis, the maternal perfusion in hemochorial multivillous placentae is treated as flow in a porous media. The latter is governed by Darcy's law. Experimental concepts taken from the engineering sciences to analyze various dynamic parameters (Darcian conductance, effective voidage, and wetted surface) are discussed with the aim of a future in vivo analysis of pathological perfusion states in the placentae of patients with high risk pregnancies.

## ADDENDUM

Note added after the presentation at the Rolduc Conference: It is a pleasure to acknowledge the fact that the group of Dr. Philip A. Rice, Department of Chemical Engineering, State University of New York, Syracuse, New York, has pursued a similar concept to the one developed on hemorheological grounds by the present author, who was unaware of Dr. Rice's efforts.

## APPENDIX

### Fluid Dynamic and Hemorheological Phenomenology of the Individual Cotyledon

When dealing with the flow of anomalous fluids and complex hydrodynamic conditions (geometries, topologies, and driving forces), it is essential to define as closely as possible the local flow conditions as well as the rheological properties of the perfusate in order to predict the flow behavior. In the present context, this would require a macroscopic description of the cotyledonal maternal blood conduit on one hand, and on the other hand, of the characteristic suspension properties of the abnormal blood in pregnancy (and the more pronounced abnormalitiy in pathological cases). Neither task can be solved for space reasons, therefore marked simplifications are necessary.

As a first approximation, one can reduce the individual cotyledon to a fluid filled, covered trough, drained from an individual point source (single well flow) into multiple sinks (Figure 5), which the villous tree is submerged and acts similar to a diffusor. This is a flow situation dominated by strictly laminar flow and purely viscous energy dissipation (Moll and Freese, 1972). The so-called jet injection of arterial blood from the mouth of the spiral arteries into the center of the cotyledon (Borrell-jets as evidenced from studies of intra-arterially injected radio contrast media) most likely represents a strictly local and short lived exception to the rule of creeping flow in the placenta. Immediately after the narrow spurt of arterial blood has expanded from the mouth of the spiral artery into the wide intervillous space, local fluid velocities, Reynolds numbers (v.i.), and shear stresses vanish drastically over short distances. An initially fast but narrow jet with relatively high kinetic energy (coming from a conduit of small cross sectional area) expands rapidly and is slowed down as it moves into a conduit of very large cross sectional area, low velocity, and negligible kinetic energy. Here, fluid motion is driven by a small gradient of pressure between the villous free center of the cotyledon and the marginal veins (Figure 5).

## Flow Phenomena Are Related to Viscous Energy Dissipation and to Fluid Particle Inertia

Obviously, inertial energy is restricted to situations associated with strong acceleration and thence with rapid flow. Creeping flow is exclusively governed by frictional interactions between fluid elements and the wall of the conduits and thence only viscous energy dissipation needs to be considered:

$$Re = \frac{\bar{u} \cdot D \cdot \sigma}{\eta}$$

where $\bar{u}$ = average velocity, $\sigma$ = density, and $\eta$ = viscosity. The estimation of Reynolds number allows a classification of any type of flow by taking the ratio of inertial energy dissipation associated with flow ($\bar{u}$, D, $\sigma$) over the viscous energy dissipation ($\eta$). As any textbook of fluid dynamics teaches, extremely high (ReN > 1000) flow is associated with turbulence, sudden local changes in ReN give rise to complex, yet ordered secondary flows (e.g., smoke rings, eddies, recirculation zones). The ReN in primate and human placentae can be estimated to range between 0.1 and 1 (creeping flow), i.e., flow can be assumed to be exclusively associated with viscous interactions (Fung, 1969). Since deviations from simple laminar flow can be excluded, estimation of ReN allows you to refute the idea that the smoke ring analogue should actually occur in mammalian placentae.

In the phenomenological analysis of x-ray image of moving boluses of radiopaque contrast media in primate placentae the term "smoke ring flow" has been introduced. A similar phenomenon was also studied extensively in vitro by Lemtis (1967). At this point, an alternative analysis of the hydrodynamic situation in the intervillous spaces is given which can still explain the observed phenomena. It is probably more realistic to interpret the circular radiological images of the injected y-ray contrast as optical sections through an advancing front of dye. A three dimensional analogue to the passage of a dye bolus through a chromatographic column occurs, the point source of the dye particles feeds into expanding trajectories of fluid. These form a dome-like dye shell expanding excentrically in all directions much like a veil of mist. The slow motion of such a veil through a forest and around each tree with all its branches is a descriptive aerodynamic analogue for the fluid dynamic events associated with percolation of the villous tree by maternal blood. Obviously, dye particles (a representative indicator of blood element) travel on trajectories, which inevitably become retarded as they are proceeding more or less equally in all directions moving from the center of the cotyledon to the uterine veins.

The well known high conductance of the maternal placental bed (Moll and Bartels, 1971) is in major part caused by the large cross sectional area that the trajectories cross; many microscopic conduits of high conductance are being placed in parallel. This notwithstanding, transfer from the maternal to the fetal blood (and back) is greatly facilitated due to maximum area of exchange (S), high contact time (dt) and maternal blood mixing, minimum diffusion distances (x). Overall, this Darcian system maximizes exchange area (S) as well as concentration gradients (dCN/dx) for all species.

Therefore, from a rheological standpoint, all early phases of pregnancy are characterized by extremely favorable conditions for overall cotyledonal percolation of a highly porous Darcian system with high specific surface. Relatively few obstacles impede the flow of a Newtonian fluid under high pressure gradient. The maternal blood in its physiological dilution (caused by excess plasma volume) with hematocrit values around 0.33 guarantees ideal perfusion and exchange, and automatic perfect match of these two vital functions.

However, these advantages can be expected to occur only provided that the perfusate behaves as an Newtonian fluid, that is to say provided its apparent fluidity is independent of the incident shear forces so that at each point the flow velocity is directly proportional to the locally acting pressure gradient. Human blood, however, (a multiphase system and one of the most non-Newtonian fluids known) (Chien, 1975; Dintenfass, 1976; Schmid-Schönbein, 1982) exhibits such rheological anomalies as pseudoplasticity, shear thickening, and shear thinning. Most importantly, it shows various so-called heterophase effects (for a detailed discussion of all these phenomena) (Schmid-Schönbein, 1988). The best known heterophase effect, a separation of slowly moving red cells from the plasma, is caused by sedimentation of the slowly moving suspended phase under gravity. Sedimentation velocity, in turn, depends upon the degree of aggregation of red cells into primary rouleaux and secondary networks of clumps of rouleaux. Other phase separation phenomena of a more complex nature are axial migration of red cells and red cell aggregates at high shear and local increases and decreases in red cell volume fraction (hematocrit) under a variety of low flow conditions (Schmid-Schönbein, 1987)

The most important functional consequence is a pronounced, fully reversible decrease in apparent fluidity. Stagnating red cell plasma mixtures behave like a Bingham body below its yield point, i.e., can in the extreme case, have zero fluidity under the influence of finite shear stresses, a phenomenon known to cause total flow stop in the presence of finite pressure gradients. Such systems are subject to positive feed back where decrease in velocity leads to aggregate formation, in reducing apparent fluidity they further retard flow rate. Such positive feed back responses are established once the shear stresses fall below a critical threshold which are insufficient to disperse the aggregates in flow. This critical threshold, in turn, depends on the plasma protein composition and is increased by several 100% in a vast variety of diseased states, e.g., EPH gestosis - toxemia of pregnancy (Heilmann, 1977), where in addition the low albumin concentration accelerates red cell aggregate formation (Maeda, 1985).

Therefore, in late stages of pregnancy, characterized by an increasing villus proliferation and thrombotic deposition hydraulic problems in combination with abnormal blood thixotropy are likely to further hold up flow, impede exchange, and jeopardize homogeneity of the intervillous flow. One can predict from vast experience in sewage technology see (v.i.) the microfluid dynamic viscoelastic and heterophase effects (which are specific for creeping blood in highly non-uniform conduits) can rapidly but reversibly after $C_D$, $S_o$, and $\kappa_{eff}$).

For obvious reasons, ramdomly connected porous beds are far more prone to be the site of such heterophase effects, simply because of the much higher distribution of residence times and shear stresses when compared to tube systems.

There is extensive literature (Greeley and Stanley, 1952) on these phenomena in sewage technology, where various kinds of sieves are readily clogged by slowly moving sediments of soft, suspended phases. It is of historical interest that the term "sludge" (Knisely, 1947) was originally transferred from these well known phenomena to medicine when intravascular red cell aggregation was observed subjectively in vivo. Contemporary hemorheologists shun the term "blood sludging" but in the present context, it may serve to illustrate to a lay readership an important yet strange event caused by non-Newtonian suspensions of low stability. One is, therefore, safe in speculating that a densely crowded porous system such as it exists in the various forms of villus hypertrophy, complicated by the existence of additional dead volume (e.g., fibrinoid, coagulae, etc.) in various forms of placental dysfunction provides ideal conditions for the manifestation and self-perpetuation of the described blood viscidation in the intervillous space, leading to a disseminated blood standstill in the presence of finite pressure gradients (rheological occlusion).

## LIST OF SYMBOLS

| | |
|---|---|
| $\alpha$ | Shape factor for pores |
| $A_{tot}$ | Total cross sectional area of porous medium |
| $A_{act}$ | Cross sectional area of perfused porous container |
| $A_{eff}$ | Fractional cross sectional area of void ($A_{tot}/A_{act}$) |
| $\dot{\gamma}$ | Shear rate (velocity difference divided by distance of two fluid lamellae in flow: $m/s \cdot m = s^{-1)}$ |
| $C_D$ | Darcian conductance: ratio of flow rate and driving pressure in porous media |
| $C_{H.P.}$ | Poiseuillian conductance; Ratio of flow rate and driving pressure in tube flow |
| $D_H$ | Hydraulic pore diameter, a theoretical equivalent to a length parameter defined as the ratio of absolute void and wetted surface |
| $\varphi_{app}$ | Apparent blood fluidity $m^2/N \cdot s$ |
| $h$ | Height of a slit |
| $\kappa$ | Voidage: total volume of pores in porous medium normalized by total volume of porous bed (dimensionless) |
| $\kappa_{eff}$ | Effective = interconnected = perfused voidage (dimensionless) |
| $K_D$ | Darcian geometric conductivity, Syn: permeability of porous media |
| $K_{HP}$ | Poiseuillian geometric conductivity ($n \cdot \pi D^4/128\ L$): $m^3$ |
| $L$ | Length of pore or porous medium |
| $L_{eff}$ | Effective length due to tortuosity of void space |
| $L_{eff}/L$ | T (tortuosity of pores): $L \cdot \pi/2$ when dead volume is cylinder shaped |
| $S$ | Wetted surface = pore surface area participating in exchange |
| $S_o$ | Specific surface = surface per volume of void $S/V_v$ |
| $T$ | Tortuosity of void or pores ($L_{eff}/L$) |
| $\dot{V}$ | Flow rate ($m^3/s$) |
| $V_C$ | Connected void = perfused void |
| $V_D$ | Dead volume: volume of solid in porous medium |
| $V_V$ | Void volume: volume between solid in porous medium |
| $W$ | Width of a conduit |

## REFERENCES

Campbell, S., Griffin, D.R., Diaz-Recasens, J.M., Cohen-Overbeek, T.E., Wilson, K., and Teak, M.J. (1983) New doppler technique of assessing uteroplacental blood flow. *Lancet* , 675.

Chien, S. (1975) Biophysical behaviour of red cells in suspension. In: *The Red Blood Cell*, 2nd edition, Vol. II, (cd.)., D.McN. Surgenor, New York: Academic Press.

Comroe, J.H., Forster, R.E., Dubois, A.B., Biscoe, W.A., and Carlson, E., (eds.), (1964) *Die Lunge*. Stuttgart: Schattauer.

Davis, C.V., (ed.) (1952) Handbook of Applied Hydraulics, New York, Toronto, London: McGraw-Hill.

Dintenfass, L. (1976) *Rheology of Blood in Diagnostic and Preventive Medicine*, Butterworths.

Dullian, F.A.L. (1979) *Porous Media. Fluid Transport and Pore Structure*. New York, London, Toronto, Sydney, San Francisco: Academic Press.

Fahraeus, R. (1962) Eclampsia - disease of checked microcirculation. *Acta Obstet. Gynecol. Scand.* 41, 101-114.

Fendel, H., Pauen, A., and Jung, H. (1985) Fetal and uterine blood flow during labor. *Arch. Gynecol.* 237, 225.

Franke, H. (1971) *Lexikon der Physik* Vol. 7, Muenchen: Deutscher Taschenbuch-Verlag.

Freese, U.E. (1968) The uteroplacental vascular relationship in the human. *Am. J. Obstet. Gynecol.* 101, 8.

Fung, Y.C. (1969) *A First Course in Continuum Mechanics.* Englewood Cliffs, New Jersey, Prentice Hall.

Fung, Y.C. and Sobin, S. (1969) Theory of sheet flow in the lung alveoli. *J. Appl. Physiol.* 26, 472-488.

Fung, Y.C. and Sobin, S.S. (1972) Elasticity of the pulmonary alveolar sheet. *Circ Res.* 30, 451-469.

Greeley, S.G. and Stanley, W.E. (1952) Sewage treatment hydraulics. In: *Handbook of Applied Hydraulics,* (ed.), C.V. Davis, New York, Toronto, London: McGraw-Hill, pp. 1085-1120.

Happel, J. and Brenner, H. (1965) *Low Reynolds Number Hydrodynamics, with Special Application to Particulate Media.* Englewood Cliffs, New Jersery: Prentice Hall.

Heilmann, L., Mattheck, C., and Kurz, E. (1977) Rheological changes in the blood in normal and pathological pregnancies and their influence upon oxygen diffusion. *Arch. Gynaekol.* 223, 283.

Heilmann, L. (1981) *Haemorheologische Untersuchungen in der Schwangerschaft*. Erlangen: Perimed-Verlag.

Heilmann, L. and Buchan, P.C. (eds.) (1984) *Hemorheological Disorders in Obstetrics and Neonatology.* Stuttgart, New York: Schattauer.

Kaufmann, P., Luckhardt, M., and Leiser, R. (1988) Three-dimensional representation of the fetal vessel system in the human placenta. *Trophoblast Research* 3, 113-137.

Klosa, W. and Schillinger, H. (1983) Durchflussmessungen in der fetalen Aorta and Umbilicalvene mit dem gepulsten Dopplerverfahren. In: *Ultraschalldiagnostik 82*, (eds.), R.Ch. Otto and F.X. Jann, Stuttgart: Thieme.

Knisely, M.H., Bloch, E.H., Eliot, T.S., and Warner, L. (1947) Sludged blood. *Science* 106, 431-433.

Lemtis, H. (1967) Neue Befunde ueber die Blutzirkulation in den muetterlichen Strombahnen der menschlichen Plazenta. *Arch. Gynaek.* 204, 114-124.

Maeda, N. and Shiga, T. (1985) Inhibition and acceleration of erythrocyte aggregation induced by small macromolecules. *BBA* 843, 128-137.

Moll, W. and Bartels, H. (1971) Fetal- und Placentarkreislauf. In: *Physiologie des Kreislaufs*, Bd. I, (ed.), E. Bauereisen, Berlin: Spring, p. 425.

Moll, W. and Freese, U.E. (1972) Haemodynamik des intervilloesen Raumes der Primatenplacenta. In: *Perinatale Medizin*, Bd. III, (ed.), E. Saling and J.W. Dudenhausen, Stuttgart: Thieme, p. 680.

Moll, W. (1981) Physiologie der maternen plazentaren Durchblutung. In: *Die Plazenta des Menschen*, (eds.), V. Becker, Th. Schiebler, and S. Kubli, Stuttgart, New York: Thieme, pp. 172-193.

Murphy, J.F., Newcombe, R.G., O'Riodan, J., Coles, E.C., and Pearson, J.F. (1986) Relation of haemoglobin levels in first and second trimesters to outcome of pregnancy. *Lancet* , 992-995.

Muskat, M. (1949) *Physical Principles of Oil Production*, New York: McGraw-Hill.

Novak, J. (1984) Principles and theory of chromatography. In: *New Comprehensive Biochemistry, Vol. 8, Separation Methods*, (ed.), Z. Deyl, Amsterdam, New York, Oxford: Elsevier, pp. 1-27.

Pangiel, M., Coulam, C., Wolf, G., Zeleznik, A., Leone, F., and Podesta, C. (1988) Magnetic Resonance Imaging (MRI) of the placental circulation using gadolinium-DTPA as a paramagnetic marker in the rhesus monkey in vivo and the perfused human placenta in vitro. *Trophoblast Research* 3, 271-282.

Ramsey, M., Martin, C.B., and Donner, M.W. (1965) Radiographic studies of the venous drainage of the placenta in rhesus monkeys. *Obstet. Gynecol.* 25, 417.

Scheidegger, A.E. (ed.) (1960) *The Physics of Flow Through Porous Media*. New York: MacMillan Co.

Schmid-Schönbein, H. (1981) Factors promoting and preventing the fluidity of blood. In: *Microcirculation. Current Physiological, Medical and Surgical Concepts*. (eds.), R.M. Effros, H. Schmid-Schönbein, and J. Ditze, New York: Academic Press, pp. 249-269.

Schmid-Schönbein, H. (1982) Hemorheology and thrombosis. In: *The Thromboembolic Disorders*. (eds.), F.K. Beller, C.R.M. Prentice, and J. van De Loo, Stuttgart: Schauttauer, pp. 1-27.

Schmid-Schönbein, H. (1988) Fluid-dynamics and haemorheology in vivo: the interactions of haemodynamic parameters and haemorheological "properties" in determining the flow behaviour of blood in microvascular networks. In: *Clinical Blood Rheology*. (ed.), G.D.O Lowe, Boca Raton: CRC Press, Inc., in press.

West, J.B., Glazier, J.B., Hughes, J.M.B., and Maloney, J.E. (1969) Pulmonary capillary flow, diffusion, ventilation and gas exchange. *Ciba Foundation Symposium on Circulatory and Respiratory Mass Transport*, (eds.), G.E. Wolstenholme and J. Knight, London: Churchill, pp. 256-276.

Trophoblast Research 3:39-48, 1988

# IN VIVO ASPECT OF THE MATERNAL - TROPHOBLASTIC BORDER DURING THE FIRST TRIMESTER OF GESTATION

J.P. Schaaps[1,3] and J. Hustin[2]

[1]Department of Obstetrics and Gynecology
University of Liege
Bd de la Constitution, 81
B4020 Liege, Belgium

[2]Institute of Histopathology
Allée des Templiers 41
B6288 Loverval, Belgium

## INTRODUCTION

For the first time, ultrasonic investigation of pregnancy has permitted direct observation of the conceptus in vivo with safety to embryo and fetus. The information gathered thanks to this technique are of a morphological, dynamic, and biometric nature. During the first trimester, the gestational sac can be measured by ultrasound and the dating of the pregnancy can be assessed with a precision of about 3 days (Robinson, 1975). The development of a new generation of high frequency probes has improved the physical properties of the ultrasound beam and, consequently, the possibilities of ultrasonic investigation. This ultrasound study will examine the uterus and implantation site between 6 and 12 weeks of gestation.

**Ultrasonic Device**

The information provided by an ultrasonic system depends upon the electronic capacities, the probe characteristics, and the physical properties of the sound used. The definition of an ultrasonic beam is closely linked with the sound wave-length.

The shorter this wave-length is, the sharper the longitudinal definition is. The width of high frequency beam is smaller because the emitting wave can also be smaller. The problem which prevents increasing the frequency in ultrasound examination is the attenuation of the sound energy through the tissues. This attenuation is in direct relation to the frequency, i.e., if the frequency of the sound is high, the penetration in depth is strongly reduced. This physical dilemma has been also avoid off with the development of miniaturized contact probes. They permit the introduction of an ultrasonic device in the natural cavities or during surgery. Accordingly, the probe can be placed in contact with the organ to be explored. High frequencies can be used and the high level of attenuation does not to be taken into account. This study used a 7 MHz miniaturized linear array (4.5 cm

[3]To Whom Correspondence Should Be Addressed

length and 1.2 cm width) manufactured by Siemens AG on the Sonoline 8000 and SL systems.

The increase in the definition in the observation of the pregnancy during the first trimester has provided a sub-macroscopic approach to the embryonic development.

The gestational sac is detectable at 4 weeks of gestation as a small echogenic ring located outside the endometrium echos (Figure 1). That topographic distinction is very important in cases of suspected ectopic implantation. Moreover,the pseudo-gestational sac found sometimes in pathologic conditions is, in fact, due to a dilatation of the uterine cavity by glandular secretions or blood from the endometrium.

The components of the gestational sac are better defined:

a) the limit between the amniotic cavity and the extracoelomic space is clearly demonstrated like an excentric, inner, low echogenic ring containing the embryo (Figure 2).

b) the yolk sac is well defined in the extra embryonic coelom (Figure 3). The length of its pedicle can be quite different for each case. For this reason, the position of the yolk sac in the gestational sac is not an indication of the decidua basalis. The biometry of the yolk sac is the same between 6 to 9 weeks: 4 mm (Table 1).

c) The embryo is better defined when using a contact probe. Its biometry is more accurate, and the dynamic observation of its mobility is easier (Figure 4). The cardiac activity of the embryo can be detected when the embryonic heart begins to pulse (23rd day of life, 5.5 weeks of gestational age) (Figure 5). From 5.5 to 6.5 weeks, the cardiac pulsation is not a global contraction but rather a peristaltic-like pulsation transmitted all along the primary cardiac tube. The same observation has been made by Loeber et al. (1983) when they studied the ultrasonic appearance of the cardiac activity in guinea pig embryos.

Table 1

Diameter Of The Yolk Sac

---

(7 to 9 weeks)

N = 35

M = 4 mm    (Range : 3 - 5 mm)

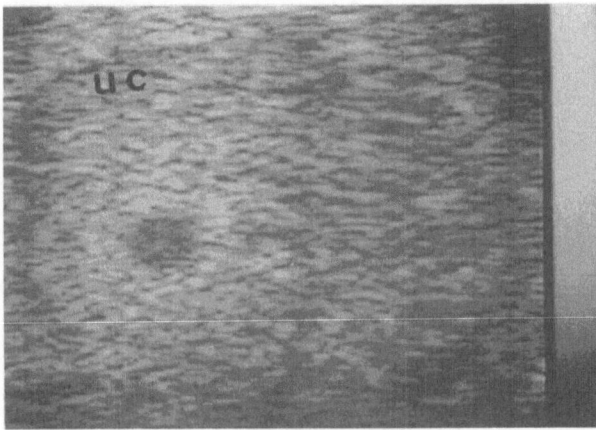

Figure 1. Intrauterine pregnancy at 4.5 weeks. The gestational sac is located outside the echos generated by the endometrium (u.c.).

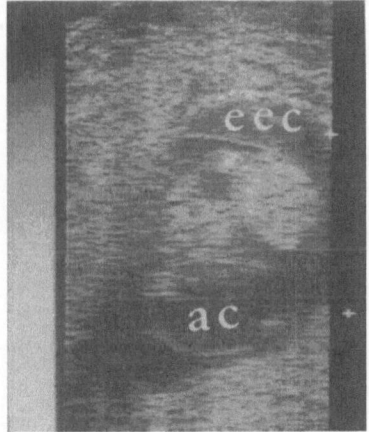

Figure 2. The gestational sac and its components: the extra-embryonic coeloma (e.e.c.) and the amniotic cavity (a.c.)

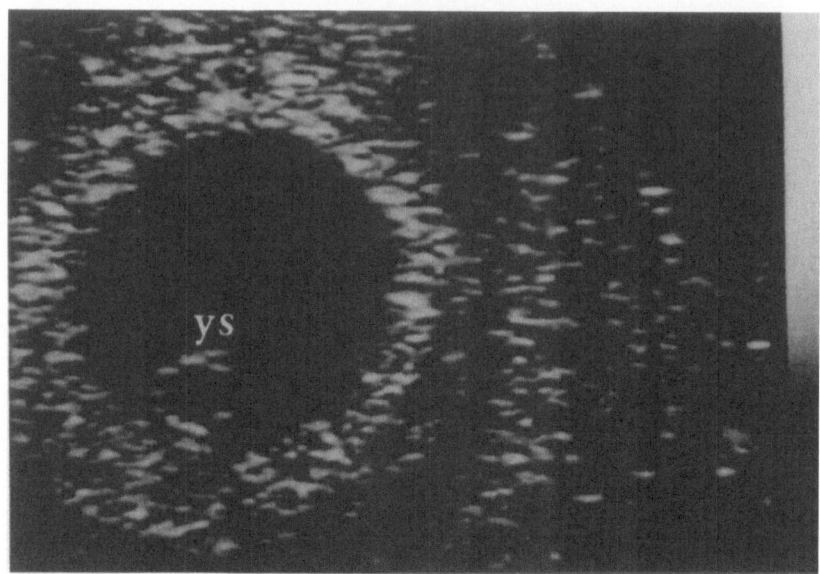

Figure 3.    The yolk sac (y.s.) conserves the same size all along its ultrasonographic observation from 6 to 10 weeks of gestation (4 mm).

The ring:    The limits of the gestational sac are described in ultrasonography like a continuous echodense ring well distinguished from the uterine echos.  Until now, the interest of the ultrasonographer has not been centered on the demarcation and interrelation between endometrium, myometrium and trophoblast, probably because of a lack of sufficient definition.    Contact ultrasonography is, in this respect, a powerful tool.

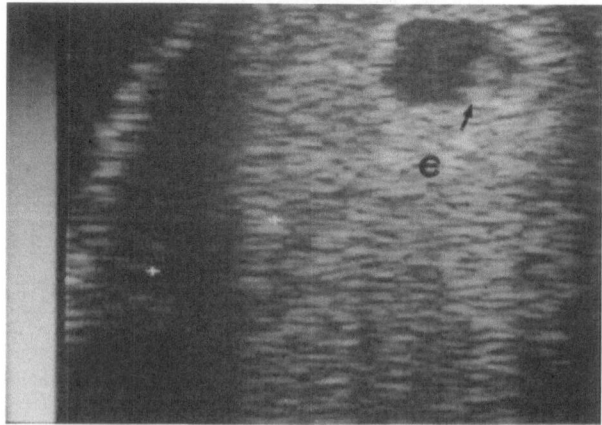

Figure 4. The embryo (e) can be detected at 5 weeks of gestation (3 mm of crown-rump length).

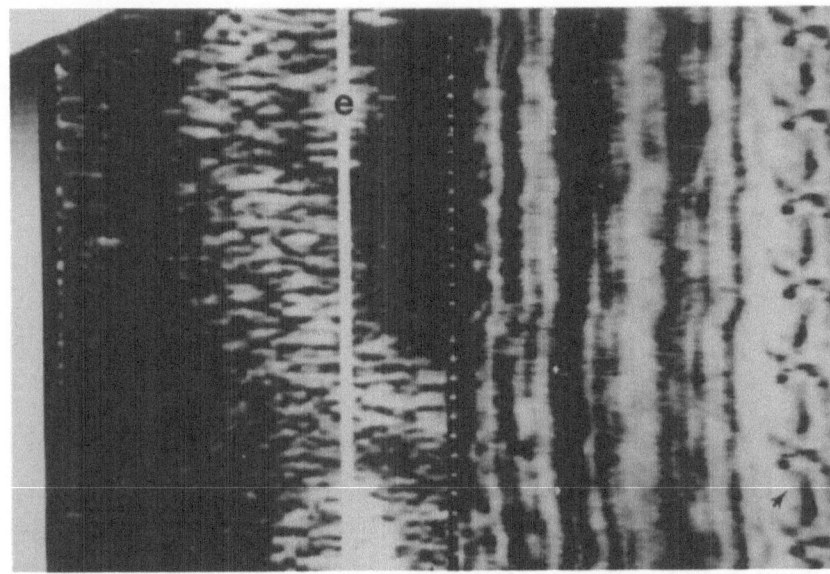

Figure 5. The heart activity can be observed when the cardiac tube begins to pulse (23rd day post conception; e:embryo; Arrow: T.M. mode of the cardiac activity).

## Ultrasonographic Appearance of the Trophoblast/Uterine Border When Using the Contact Probe Technique

The differences from the conventional ultrasound examinations remain at two levels: the trophoblastic area and the intramyometrial changes during the first trimester of pregnancy.

The trophoblastic ring is constituted by echos generated by the trophoblastic villi, the intervillous space, and the interface between the extravillous trophoblast and the decidua basalis. All those components generate echos of high intensity producing the picture of an echodense ring. When using a contact high frequency probe, this area seems to be "static", except sometimes for a small pulsation corresponding to the embryonic heart rate.

In the uterus, it is possible to detect maternal vessels in the myometrium. At the beginning of pregnancy (5 weeks) they can be detected relatively far from the gestational ring (> 1 cm) and at 6.5 weeks they are visualized close to the ring.

Inside these vessels it is possible to detect small moving echos synchronous with the maternal pulse (Figure 6). As pregnancy progresses, the vascular network becomes more and more conspicuous and grows nearer to the trophoblastic shell. However, uterine vessels do not reach the placental area, and it is impossible to define any particular movement in the trophoblastic echos during the first trimester of gestation. This observation was unexpected when we observed normal pregnancies. In older placentae (2nd and 3rd trimester) with conventional ultrasonography, no blood cell movement could be detected in the placenta. Surprisingly, when pregnancies with primary embryonic death or in cases of

Table 2

Ultrasound First Trimester Vaginal
Examination

---

N = 201

Normal pregnancies: 152

Embryonic deaths:      38
                                      } 24.3%
Blighted Ova:               11

blighted ova were observed, it was possible to detect blood cells movement in this area.

## MATERIALS AND METHODS

Two hundred and one patients have been examined prospectively with the contact probe between the 5th and the 12th week of gestation. All investigations were recorded on videotapes. Except for 12 patients, all were completely asymptomatic. The 12 remaining subjects presented only with discrete uterine bleeding and moderate lumbar pain.

## RESULTS

In this population, 38 primary embryonic deaths and 11 blighted ova (24.3% of the total number) were diagnosed (Table 2). The "symptomatic" population was equally distributed in both groups (5 patients with normal pregnancies and 7 with abnormal). In the absence of heart activity in primary embryonic death or the absence of embryo, amniotic cavity and yolk sac in cases of blighted ovum, the aspect of the gestational ring is quite different from that in normal pregnancies.

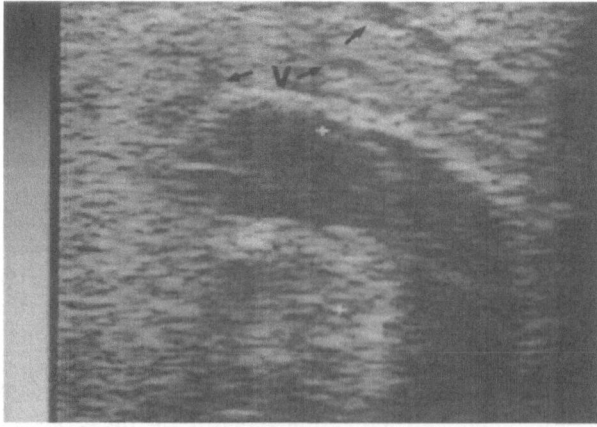

Figure 6. Intrauterine blood vessels (v) all around the trophoblastic ring.

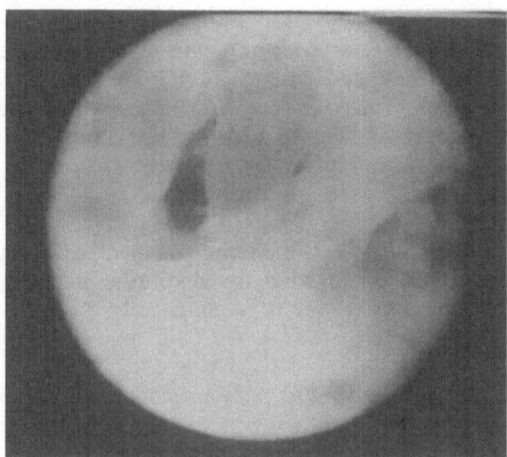

Figure 7. Hysteroscopic view in vivo of the intervillous space in a normal pregnancy, no washing.

Table 3

Ultrasonographic Signs

|  | Missed Abortions 38 |  | Normal 152 |  | Blighted Ova 11 |
|---|---|---|---|---|---|
| Intratropho-blastic circulation | 38 | p<0.001 | 9 | p<0.001 | 9 |

Uterine vessels are close to the gestational ring echos in both populations, but in the abnormal group it is possible to detect a slow turbulent movement in the trophoblast area.  In some cases, it is possible to define a communication between the uterine vessels and the trophoblastic region (Table 3).

The differences found between the two groups are certainly surprising. Indeed, the classical interpretation of the data concerning the uteroplacental blood flow claim that the maternal circulation is present in the intervillous space around the 29th day of life.  In contrast, the ultrasonographic observations suggest that a difference between normal and abnormal pregnancies can occur before any clinical sign is evident.  This difference consists in an ultrasonographic appearance of a turbulent flow in the intervillous space in missed abortion.

## DISCUSSION

These observations have to be linked to other types of information concerning the first trimester of pregnancy: the chorionic villi sampling (CVS). Since 1983, CVS was introduced into our antenatal diagnosis unit using the biopsy grip technique.  Under ultrasonographic control, small forceps were introduced through the cervix in the uterine cavity and guided into the trophoblastic area at the level of the decidua basalis. The sampling was performed between 9 and 11.5 weeks of gestation. When the grip was properly located, it was opened, closed again, and slowly pulled out of the uterus. We have always been amazed because samplings are white, bloodless. The quality of the sampling taken by a biopsy forceps was different from those obtained by suction through a catheter. In those cases, chorionic villi are mixed with maternal blood.

It was also surprising that the introduction of a biopsy forceps into the intervillous space was not accompanied by systemic bleeding, as the grip was effectively pushed into a region where it is classically claimed that an important maternal circulation was present.

Some other teams (Gustavii et al., 1984; Ghirardini, 1985) have developed a technique of CVS under direct visual control using a chorionoscope. It is a small optical system with a cutter for picking chorionic villi in the intervillous space. This manipulation does not require any washing to clearly distinguish and choose villi to be cut. We have performed such manipulations 10 times in order to observe the intervillous space in vivo using a small hysteroscope. The villi were demonstrated as whitish "worm-like" structures. It was often possible to see embryonic vessels within the villous core. They appeared as pinkish threads. Blood discoloration was not observed in the intervillous space (Figure 7).

Using this ultrasound technique, we had the impression that the maternal blood circulation was nonexistent in the intervillous space during the first trimester of normal gestation. In contrast, primary embryonic deaths or blighted ova showed a slow turbulent aspect in the trophoblastic area. When confronting data provided by CVS and hysteroscopy it is obvious that, during the first trimester, the intervillous space is bloodless and that the uteroplacental arteries are occluded during this period. The ultrasonic visualization of such small moving particules could be artifactual. In fact and in theory, red blood cells are under the resolution of the ultrasonic beam. It seems that such an observation can be possible when the retrodiffusion properties of the sound are taken into account.

The ultrasound examination offers a dynamic difference between normal and pathological pregnancies. Elsewhere, the endoscopic observations made on a large series by others (Gustavii, 1984; Ghirardini et al., 1985) confirm the fact that the intervillous space can be observed without any washing. A maternal reflex constriction of the arteries are not considered because there is a non-existence of nervous tissue at the level of the eruption in the intervillous space from the uterine cavity. All of these assertions seem to be supported by the results of an anatomical study of the trophoblastic bed which is reported.

## SUMMARY

Technological advances in ultrasound diagnosis have allowed internal contact examinations. The uterus and its content can be observed with a small linear 7 MHz probe inserted in the fundus of the vagina. The gestational sac can be located in the uterus from 4.5 weeks of gestation on. The cardiac activity can be detected when the heart begins to pulse (23rd day post conception), and the uterotrophoblastic border can be observed with better definition. In a prospective study, 201 patients have undergone a vaginal ultrasonic investigation between 6 and 12 weeks of gestation. In the normal cases, the uterine blood vessels are visualized all around the uterine border of the gestational sac. Moving echos generated by the red blood cells are distinguished in the maternal vessels but never in the thickness of the trophoblastic ring. In cases of missed abortions or of blighted ova, such a movement can be detected in the trophoblastic area and communications between maternal blood vessels and the intervillous space can be observed. For performing chorionic villi sampling (C.V.S.), the catheter, the needle, or the biopsy grip must be introduced into the intervillous space. All those samplings are relatively bloodless. When using the chorionoscopic method for sampling, it is possible to demonstrate in vivo that the intervillous space, during the first trimester of gestation, is normally free of maternal blood. In contrast, in cases of missed abortions, before any clinical signs appear, a maternal blood circulation is noted in the intervillous space. We can conclude that the human placenta is not hemochorial during the first trimester.

## REFERENCES

Ghirardini, G., Camurri, L., Guarlerzi, C., Fochi, F., Spreafico, L., and Agnelli, P. (1985) *Chorionic Villi Sampling by Means of a New Endoscopic Device: First Trimester Fetal Diagnostic,* (eds.), M. Fraccaro, B. Brambati, and G. Simoni, Springer Verlag: Berlin, Heidelberg, New York, Tokyo, p.54.

Gustavii, B., Chester, M.A., Edvall, H., Iasif, S., Kristofferson, V., Lofberg, L., Meneur, A. and Mitelman, F. (1984) First trimester diagnosis on chorionic villi obtained by direct vision technique. *Hum. Genet.* 65, 373-376.

Gustavii, B. (1983) First trimester chromosomal analysis of chorionic villi obtained by direct vision technique. *Lancet* 2, 507.

Hustin, J. and Schaaps, J.P. Echographic and anatomic studies of the materno-trophoblastic border during the first trimester of pregnancy. *Am. J. Obstet. Gynecol.,* in press.

Leroy, B. and Schaaps, J.-P. (1985) Echographie endovaginale *9th Congress SFAUMB,* Grenoble.

Loeber, C., Goldberg, S.J., Hendrix, M.J.C., and Sahn, D.J. (1983) Dynamic mammalian cardiogenesis investigated by high resolution ultrasound in guinea pigs. *Circulation* 68, 841-845.

Nordenskvold, F. and Gustavii, B. (1984) Direct vision chorionic villi biopsy for prenatal diagnosis in the first trimester. *J. Reprod. Med.* 29, 572-574.

Robinson, H.P. and Caines, J.S. (1977) Sonar evidence of early pregnancy failure in patients with twin conception. *Br. J. Obstet. Gynaecol.* 84, 22-25.

Robinson, H.P. (1975) The diagnosis of early pregnancy failure by sonar. *Br. J. Obstet. Gynaecol.* 82, 849-857.

Schaaps, J.P. (1983) *Gynecological Contact Ultrasonography: Laparoscopic and Vaginal Way. Ultraschall Diagnostik*, (ed.), R. Lutz, Georg Thieme Verlag, Stuttgard.

Schaaps, J.P. and Thoumsin, H.J. (1986) Vaginal ultrasonography of early pregnancies. *The Society of Perinatal Obstetricians*, p. 205.

Schaaps, J.P., Hustin, J., and Lambotte, R. (1985) Aspects echographiques de la circulation utero-trophoblastique. *Soir. Echo. Gyn. Obstet.* p. 39.

Schaaps, J.P. and Lambotte, R. (1985) *Ultrasonic Observation of Pregnancy During the First Trimester Using a Vaginal Approach. First Trimester Fetal Diagnosis*, (eds.), M. Fraccaro, G. Simoni, and B. Brambati, Springer Verlag: Berlin, pp. 78-79.

Schaaps, J.-P., Hustin, J., and Lambotte, R. (1986) *Vaginosonographische Aspekte der Uterus - Trophoblastzirkulation*, Popp L. W. (Hrsg.):Gynaekologische Endosonographie Ingo Klemke Verlag, Quickborn, pp. 127-132.

Trophoblast Research 3:49-60, 1988

# ANATOMICAL STUDIES OF THE UTERO-PLACENTAL VASCULARIZATION IN THE FIRST TRIMESTER OF PREGNANCY

Jean Hustin[1,3], Jean Pierre Schaaps[2] and René Lambotte[2]

[1]Institut de Morphologie Pathologique (IMPL)
B-6280 Loverval, Belgium

[2]Department of Obstetrics and Gynecology
University of Liege
B-4020 Liege, Belgium

## INTRODUCTION

The development of the placenta, the growth and organogenesis of the feto-placental unit have always attracted considerable interest (Boyd and Hamilton, 1971). The reciprocal, tolerant relationship between mother and offspring has puzzled generations of scientists who have devoted themselves to the comprehension of the physiology of gestation.

At this time, the second and third trimester are fairly well understood, from endocrinological, physiological, and biochemical points of view. It remains clear, however, that the development of the embryo and placenta during the first weeks has not been well examined due to the lack of sufficient material. Conclusions concerning this period have been obtained by extrapolations from second trimester measurements (Contractor, 1983).

Now when one reviews recent literature, it appears that the early placenta may differ from specimens at term. Contractor (1983) has recently reviewed major biochemical properties of the trophoblast and has stressed some evolutionary differences.

From an endocrinological point of view, the well known secretory peak of hCG in the first trimester correlates well with increased tissue values, while it appears that early trophoblast is capable of synthetizing prolactin, a property clearly lost after 12 weeks (Hustin, unpublished observations).

Anatomical studies of early placentae have never been numerous and have usually been published during an epoch when specimens were not easily available and were usually obtained in the fixed state. Moreover, the precise dating of pregnancy was often ill-defined (Wilkin, 1958; Martin, 1967; Thomas, 1968).

[3]To Whom Correspondence Should Be Addressed: J. Hustin, IMPL, Allée des Templiers 41, B-6280, Loverval (Gerpinnes), Belgium

The current dogma concerning implantation is that as soon as the blastocyst has implanted, a number of maternal sinusoids are opened by phagocytic activity of trophoblast and that some maternal blood enters the future intervillous space (IVS). Within a relatively short time, spiral arterioles of the myometrium are tapped and a true blood flow begins even at a reduced pressure, bringing nutrients and oxygen to the growing embryo (Wilkin, 1958; Thomas, 1968; Boyd and Hamilton, 1971; Kaufmann, 1981; Ramsey and Donner, 1980). As a consequence, the histological appearance of utero-placental arteries is considerably modified (Brosens et al., 1967; Pijnenborg et al., 1983). It is customary to speak of "pregnancy induced physiological changes", but it has always been extremely difficult to correlate these changes with first trimester uterine hemodynamics.

The growing number of voluntary terminations of pregnancy has allowed us to collect well preserved placentae from normal pregnancies with a precise gestational age defined by echographic biometry (Gaspard et al., 1980). Simultaneously, chorion villous sampling (CVS) has allowed us to "peep" at what was happening "in vivo". Preliminary results have thrown a different light on the events taking place during the first weeks of gestation, which is a crucial period of organogenesis (Thomas, 1968).

This study shall try to define clearly how we conceive early materno-fetal exchange judging by serial section and reconstruction techniques and also by perfusion and slice radiographs of hysterectomy specimens with pregnancy in situ.

Lastly, some preliminary data obtained from pathological cases will be discussed in which the pregnancy was not progressing normally and where interesting echographic findings were present (Schaaps, 1987).

## MATERIALS AND METHODS

The material was collected from 75 normal pregnancies (6-12 weeks) voluntarily interrupted either by aspiration or by curettage. As these specimens are usually lacerated, the information obtained is essentially incomplete and might be frought with artifact. To avoid some of these problems, five hysterectomies with pregnancy in situ were examined in detail.

In the first two cases, the pregnancies were respectively 7 and 9 weeks old. Histological study of serial sections from step blocks involving the implantation site was performed. Spatial reconstructions of maternal vessels were attempted. In the two other cases, the pregnancies were respectively 8 and 13 weeks old. Uterine arteries were cannulated. Perfusion with heparinated saline was initiated and quickly followed by barium sulfate suspension in neutral formalin. X-ray studies of slices and microradiographs of 50 mm sections were performed on these specimens together with standard histology. The last specimen was obtained from a hysterectomy at 21 weeks of gestation. It was perfused via uterine veins.

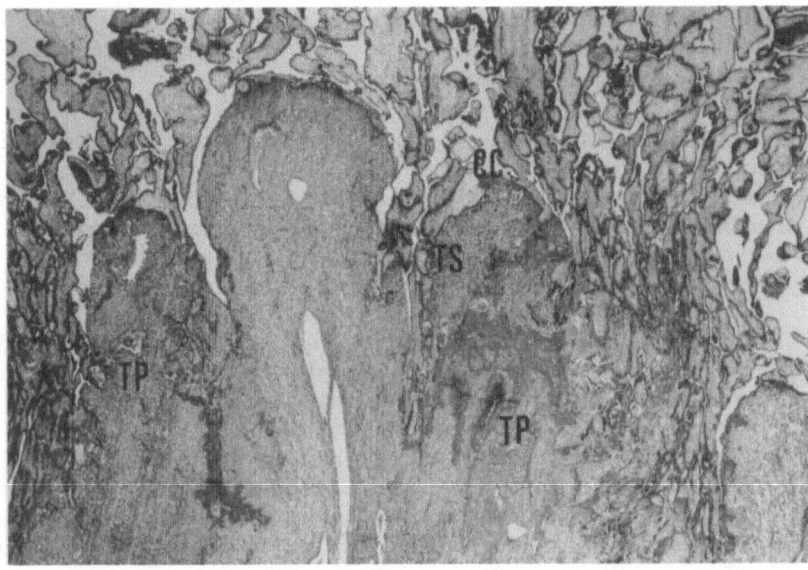

Figure 1. Eight week pregnancy. The trophoblastic shell (TS) is covered on both sides, with trophoblastic "bursts" which correspond to the cytotrophoblastic cell (CC) columns on the embryonic side and to the intravascular trophoblastic plugs (TP) on the maternal side. (HE X23)

## Pathological Cases

One specimen was included from a case in which a hysterectomy was performed for hydatidiform mole. In this instance, interest focused primarily on the implantation site. There was also a number of curettage specimens (7) from first trimester arrested pregnancies.

Spontaneous arrest of viability occurred during the interval between two contact echographic studies, the first one having demonstrated moving echos synchronous to the maternal heart rate in the intervillous space (Schaaps, 1987). Once again, the curetted specimens were fixed in neutral formalin and embedded after proper orientation was achieved.

Descriptions of regressive villous changes were not attempted. The study was directed to the materno-embryonic relationship at the insertion site.

## RESULTS

Disruption artifacts were of course present in curettage and aspiration products but they were usually clear cut.

The trophoblastic shell was continuous at the insertion site (Figure 1). On the site of reflected decidua, however, the layer was thin and soon enmeshed with fibrin, while villi on this side looked regressive.

The trophoblastic shell was, in fact, the union of all cytotrophoblastic cell columns. On the maternal side, the shell was bristling with spikes which entered arterial apertures. These spikes ended as isolated trophoblastic cells, which at 10 weeks, occupied the whole length of the artery. When compared with the serial sections performed on hysterectomy specimens, no obvious difference was found. Trophoblastic plugs extended to the deciduo-myometrial junction.

The distal openings of spiral arteries did not communicate with the IVS but instead, the vessel wall was disrupted and irregular, tortuous slits extended from the arterial wall and the trophoblastic shell (Figure 2).

The shell was pierced with small cavities where some maternal red blood cells were identified. Reconstruction of the course of spiral arteries demonstrated that they were extremely tortuous, coiled several times with openings between contiguous coils. They ran an horizontal length of 500-750 mm in the decidua (Figure 3).

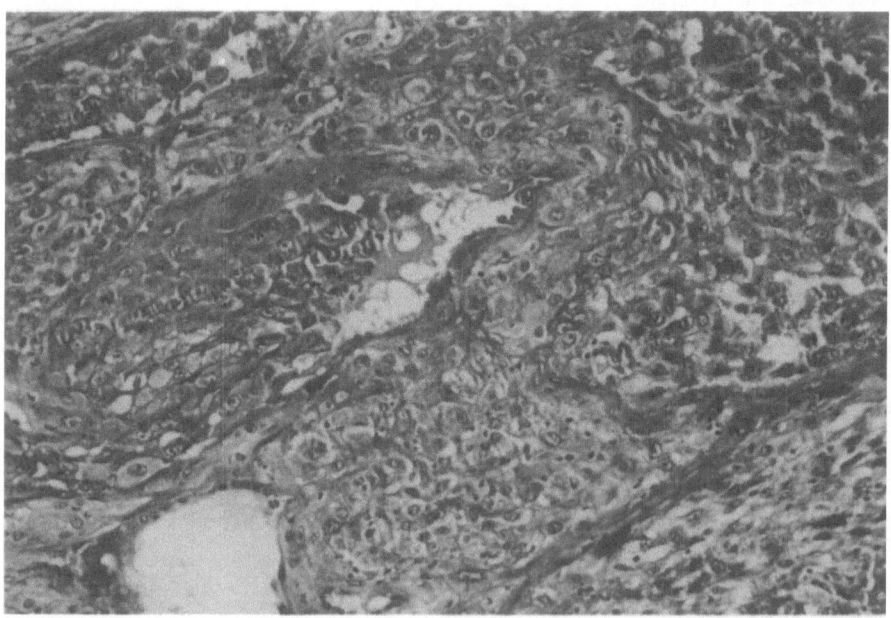

Figure 2. Eight week pregnancy. The tip of a spiral artery is occluded by trophoblast cells which communicate with the trophoblastic shell. Irregular slits extend from vessel wall to lacunae in the trophoblastic shell. (HE X79)

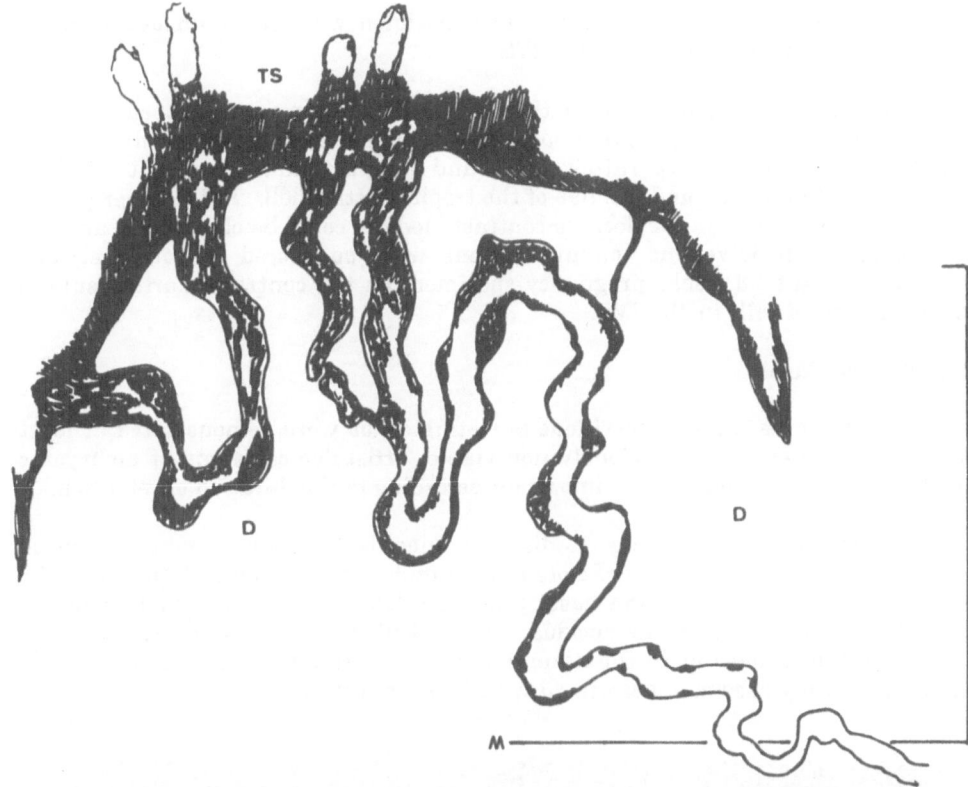

Figure 3. Reconstruction of the course of a spiral artery based on serial sections. Hysterectomy specimen with 9 weeks pregnancy. Apparent intradecidual horizontal length of the vessel is between 500-750 mm. TS: Trophoblastic Shell; D: Decidua; M: Myometrium.

The vascular lumen was completely occluded by trophoblast cells in many segments. As a rule trophoblastic plugs were not tight, and some fluid filtration was achieved.

The three hysterectomy specimens which had been injected with barium sulphate, demonstrated different patterns according to their gestational age and mode of injection. The specimen from the 8 week pregnancy was completely injected but no permeation of the IVS could be achieved. It was noteworthy that the periphery of the insertion site was very rich in vessels but even in 50 mm sections no contrast medium could be demonstrated in the placental area (Figures 4 and 5).

At 13 weeks (specimen II), the IVS was rapidly filled with barium sulphate, showing parallel vertical streaks but no circular orientation (Figure 6). Injection via uterine veins in a 21 weeks pregnancy specimen was totally unsuccessful, as regards retrograde penetration in the IVS.

Histological examination of these injected uteri was performed. In the eight week pregnancy, spiral arteries appeared somewhat distended. Trophoblastic plugs where rather loose and let particulate contrast medium percolate up to the slits and lacunae of the trophoblastic shell. In the inner part of the myometrium, close to the decidua contrast medium could be observed in arteries and veins. Arterio-venous communications were suspected in some sections (Figure 7). In the 13 weeks pregnancy specimen, on the contrary, barium sulfate readily encircled villi in the IVS.

## Pathological Cases

In all cases where intervillous pulsating echos were demonstrated at least once, the pregnancy was obviously non-viable. Histological signs of embryonic death were present, more or less important according to the duration of retention.

It was most fascinating to discover unequivocal signs of maternal blood penetration in the IVS in form of clots located under the chorionic plate (Figure 8). Most often, examination of the basal plate, disclosed an evident insufficiency of trophoblast penetration in the decidua. In particular, plugs were either scarce or did not extend as deep as in the normal cases. This finding was also observed in the hysterectomy specimen associated with hydatidiform mole.

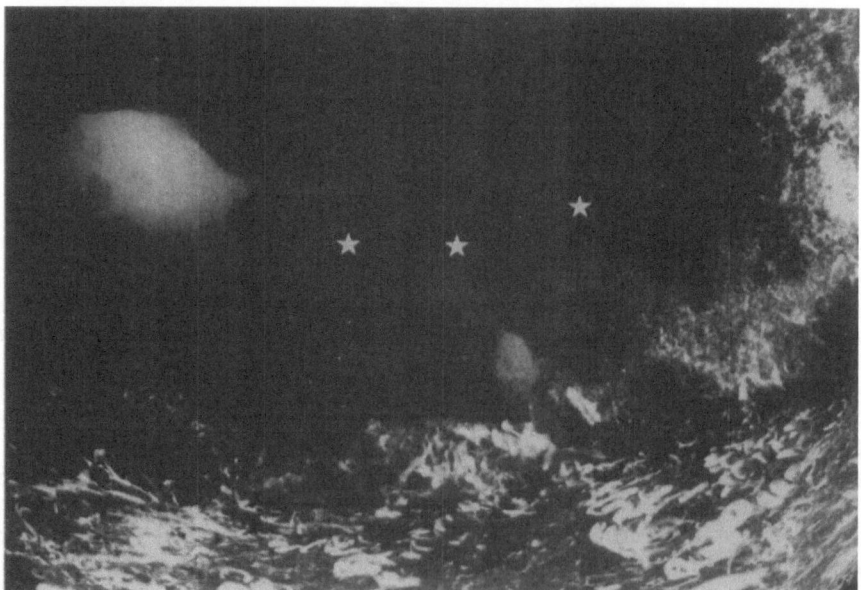

Figure 4. X-ray of a 1 cm thick slide from pregnant uterus (8 weeks) injected with barium sulphate. No contrast medium is observed in the whole thickness of the placental area.

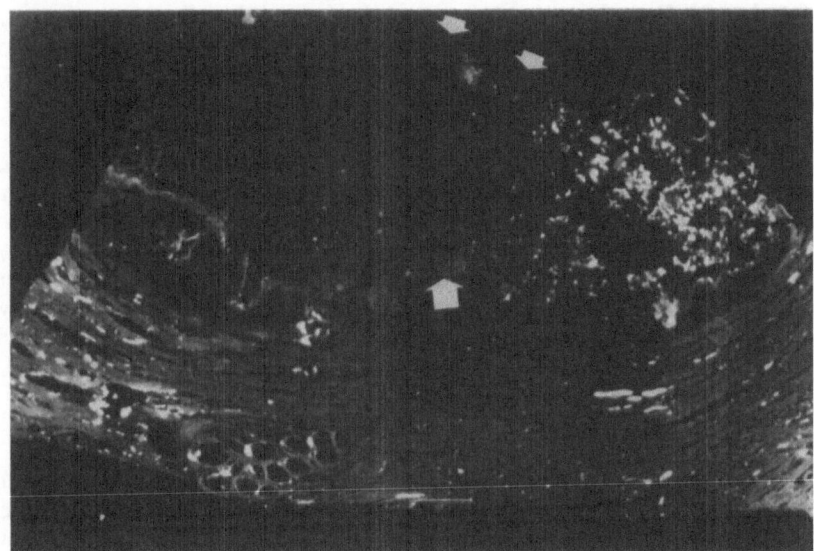

Figure 5. X-ray of a 50 mm section from the same specimen at the lateral side of the placenta. Decidual vessels are obvious, but there is no injection of the IVS (arrows). The density of decidual vessels laterally to the placenta is remarkable.

## DISCUSSION

The utero-placental vascularization theory, which we now define as "classical", states that maternal blood enters the intervillous space by limited seepage at day 11 or 12 (Kaufmann, 1981) and that true blood flow, originating from tapped utero-placental arteries, is obvious some time between days 14 and 15 (Wilkin, 1958) or during the seventh week (Thomas, 1968) or at day 22 (Martin, 1967) or days 29 through 40 (Kaufmann, 1981). Ramsey and Donner (1981) cast some doubts on the reality of a true effective and early maternal blood flow in the IVS and suggest that under normal conditions, free circulation could not be achieved before the 12th week. The fact that CVS can be readily performed under chorionoscopy without obvious blood leakage casts some doubt on the accuracy of this schedule.

With spatial reconstruction of spiral arteries, the tip of these vessels, which is eventually tapped by the growing trophoblast, can be seen not to be in direct connection with the IVS. Up to about 12 weeks, there is a continuous barrier, made of the trophoblastic shell (Larsen and Knoth, 1971) which thins progressively. This barrier is covered with spikes, the trophoblastic plugs on the maternal side, and the cytotrophoblastic cell columns of the fetal side.

The importance of intra-vascular trophoblastic plugs has been stressed by several authors. Ramsey and Donner (1981) stated that "...complete or partial plugs of trophoblasts ... will greatly impede free flow."

Boyd and Hamilton (1971) were impressed by the fact that "..It is remarkable that the cells (trophoblast) migrate against the arterial blood flow and pressure without being dislodged and without showing obvious histological signs of adhesion to one another ..".

Boe (1967) was very close to what we now think is more realistic. He described spaces within the cytrophoblastic shell and demonstrated that they were in continuity, forming a labyrinth which communicated at intervals with the IVS.

The current reconstruction studies support this view. It is suggested that until late in the first trimester, there is a barrier between the growing embryo and maternal tissues. This mechanism (trophoblastic plugs and shell) could act as a filter for maternal blood cells of which few ever reach the IVS. The IVS could, thus, be bathed by an almost a cellular fluid possibly composed of plasma and some uterine gland secretions.

That contrast medium perfusion of IVS was not obtained in a case of hysterectomy with a 9 week pregnancy in situ is significant. One may object that Kormano et al. (1974) were able to perfuse IVS in their 3 cases with intra-arterial perfusions. It must be stated, however, that those hysterectomies were performed from 12 to 16 weeks (second trimester).

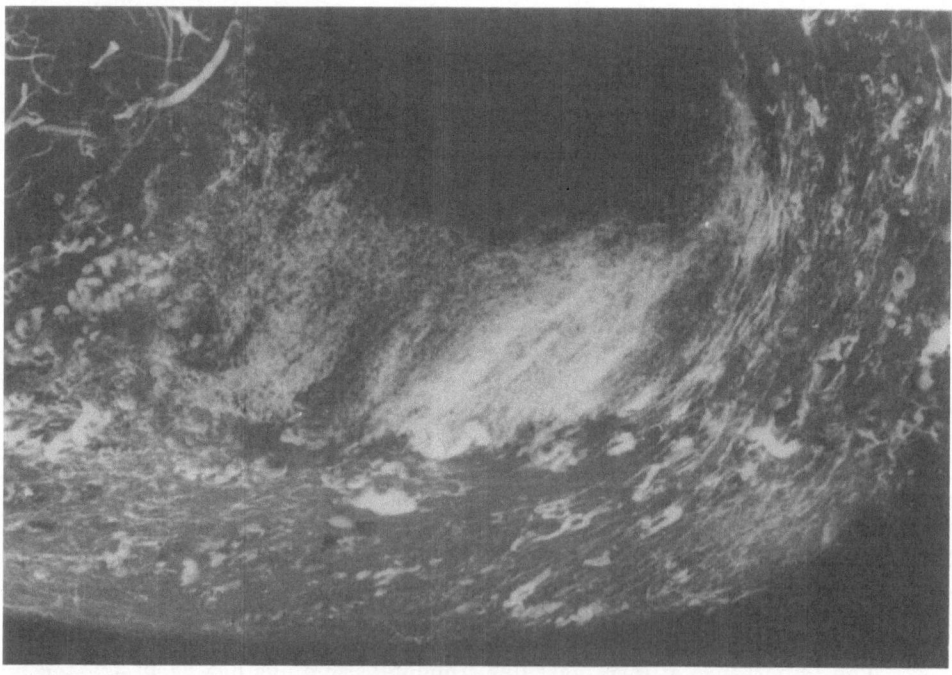

Figure 6. X-ray of a 1 cm thick slice of a 13 week pregnant uterus. IVS is readily demonstrated with parallel streaks of contrast medium.

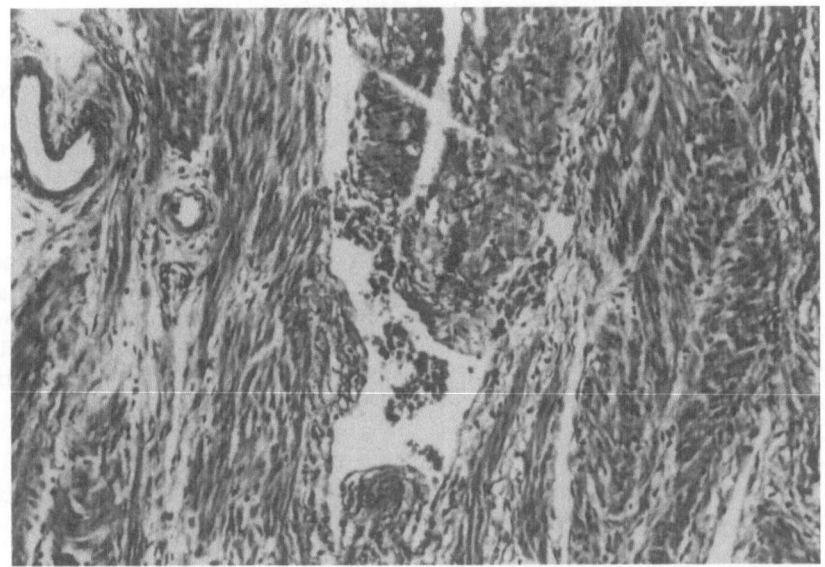

Figure 7. Eight week pregnant uterus injected with barium sulphate. In this section there is an obvious arterio-venous communication. (HE X79)

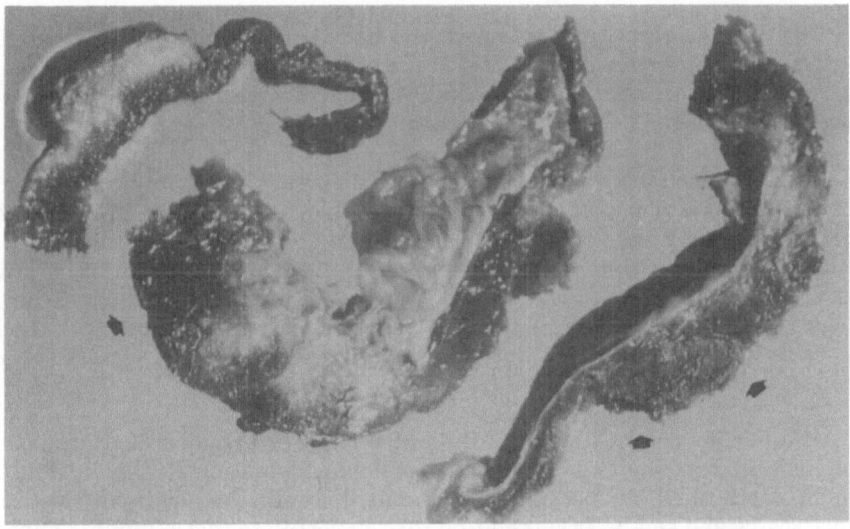

Figure 8. Curettings from a case of developmental arrest at 8 weeks of pregnancy. Conspicuous clots (arrows) fill the intervillous space.

In their description of IVS perfusion, Kormano et al. (1974) admitted that contrast medium permeation was irregular, a feature not unlike our second injected case, also belonging to the second trimester.

It must be remembered that Kormano et al. (1974) and this laboratory employed the same contrast medium (i.e., barium sulphate). This medium is in a fine particulate state, considerably smaller than blood cells. Perfusion of this type is by no means indicative of a real blood flow in vivo. No explanation can be offered for the lack of IVS perfusion via the venous route even later in the second trimester.

Another problem arises. If during the first 12 weeks, no perfusion of the IVS can be observed, what are the pathways for contrast medium elimination? Barium sulphate can be traced up to the end of spiral arteries. Therefore, one must consider the possibility of arterio-venous shunts. Only the existence of such functional shunts could explain why there is usually no significant blood pressure in the spiral arteries, and thus, why trophoblastic plugs are not dislodged for a time.

It appears that there is a critical moment, probably around 12 weeks, when abrupt changes take place in the materno-fetal relationship. A real circulation is then established in the intervillous space.

Amniotic fluid volume increases together with its prolactin content (Van Cauwenberge, in press). hCG (human chorionic gonadotropin) release decreases steadily while maternal serum hPL (human placental lactogen) becomes significant (Gaspard, 1980). PLAP (placental alkaline phosphatase) appears and probably reflects trophoblastic growth control (Risk and Johnson, 1985).

The decidua reflecta fuses with the decidua parietalis. The diameter of UPA (utero placental arteries) widens, the trophoblastic plugs become looser and looser. Isolated trophoblast cells slip toward myometrium. Embryonic organogenesis subsides. Fetal growth begins.

Turning now towards the pathology of the first trimester, it is to be noted that careful observation of spontaneous abortions or of currettings obtained from non-viable pregnancies also provide arguments in favor of our hypothesis. It has been shown that some time before the arrest of development, ultrasound studies disclosed what looked like pulsating echos in the IVS (Schaaps 1987). Gross and histological examinations often disclose maternal blood in the IVS, which is obviously not there by artifact but frequently appears as true clots sometimes entrapping a limited number of villi.

Another important finding is that very often in these cases (paradoxically also in hydatidiform mole) extravillous trophoblast invasion is limited and that the trophoblastic shell has become precociously discontinuous while intra-vascular plugs are scarce and small. It is tempting then to postulate that a number of arrests of evolution, (with or without spontaneous abortions) occur because of an insufficient trophoblastic barrier and thus because of a too early blood flow causing rapid overfilling of the IVS and eventual separation of the products of conception.

This pathological process could occur irrespective of any other ovular pathology but would probably be more frequent in cases where general trophoblastic hypoplasia exists, i.e., in cases associated with chromosome anomalies.

## SUMMARY

Anatomical studies were performed on 75 products of conception obtained from therapeutic abortions between 8 and 10 weeks, and 5 hysterectomies with pregnancy in situ. Results of histological and radiological examinations of the specimens tend to suggest that up to 12 weeks, there is no true blood flow in the intervillous space which is bathed by a clear fluid almost devoid of cells. Therefore, physiology and biochemistry of the feto-placental unit during the first trimester must be reconsidered. New pathogenic hypotheses concerning spontaneous abortions may also be suggested.

## REFERENCES

Boe, F. (1967) Studies on the human placenta. i. The cell islands in the young placenta. *Acta Obstet. Gynecol. Scand.* 47, 591-603.

Boyd, J.D. and Hamilton W.J. (1970) *The Human Placenta,* W. Heffer & Sons, Ltd., Cambridge.

Brosens, J., Robertson, W.B., and Dixon, H.S. (1967) The physiological response of the vessels of the placental bed to normal pregnancy. *J. Pathol. Bact.* 93, 569-579

Contractor, S.F. (1983) Metabolic and enzymatic activity of human trophoblast. In: *Biology of Trophoblast,* (eds)., Y.W. Loke and A. Whyte, Elsevier:Amsterdam, pp. 235-281.

Gaspard, U., Schaaps, J.P., Piront, F., Deville, J.L., Reuter, A.M., Vrindts-Gevaerts, Y., and Franchimont, P. (1980) Valeur pronostique des taux sériques maternels de la choriogonadotrophine et de sessubunitéslibres alpha et béta dans la menace d'avortement du premier trimestre. Corrélation avec l'examen ultrasonographique. *J. Gynecol. Obstet. Biol. Reprod.* 9, 62-66.

Gaspard, U. (1980) *Les hormones protéiques placentaires.* Masson: Paris.

Kaufmann, P. (1981) Entwicklung der Plazenta. In: *Die Plazenta des Menschen,* (eds.), V. Becker, T.H. Schiebler, and F. Kubli, Georg Thieme, Verlag:Stuttgart.

Kormano, M., Timonen, H., and Luukainen, T. (1974) Microangiographic observations on the uterine and material placental vasculature in early human pregnancy. *Am. J. Obstet. Gynecol.* 120, 8-13.

Larsen, J.F. and Knoth, M. (1971) Ultrastructure of the anchoring villi and trophoblastic shell in the second week of placentation. *Acta Obstet. Gynecol. Scand.* 50, 117-128.

Martin, C.B. (1967) The anatomy and circulation of the placenta. In: *Intra Uterine Development,* (ed.), A.C. Barnes, Lea Febiger:Philadelphia, pp. 35-57.

Pijnenborg, R., Bland, J.M., Robertson, W.B., and Brosens I. (1983) Utero-placental arterial changes related to interstitial trophoblast migration in early human pregnancy. *Placenta* 4, 397-414.

Ramsey, E.M. and Donner, M.W. (1980) *Placental Vasculature and Circulation.* Georg Thieme, Verlag:Stuttgart.

Risk, J.M. and Johnson, P.M. (1985) Antigen expression by human trophoblast and tumor cells: Models for gene regulation. In: *Contrib. Gynecol. Obstet., Vol. 14, Immunology and Immunopathology of Reproduction,* (eds.), V. Toder and A.E. Beer, Karger Basel, pp. 74-82.

Schaaps, J.P. (1988) Dynamic imaging of the utero-placental border in the first trimester of human prequancy. *Trophoblast Research* 3, 37-45.

Thomas, J.P. (1968) *Introduction to the Human Embryology.* Lea Febiger:Philadelphia.

Wilkin, P. (1958) Morphogenese. In: *Le Placenta Humain,* (ed.), Jean Snoeck, Mason, Paris.

Trophoblast Research 3:61-67, 1988

# THE UTERO-PLACENTAL VESSELS AT TERM - THE DISTRIBUTION AND EXTENT OF PHYSIOLOGICAL CHANGES

Ivo A. Brosens

Department of Obstetrics and Gynecology
University Hospital Gasthuisberg
Leuven, Belgium

## INTRODUCTION

The identification and characterization of the pathology for the uteroplacental vessels is obscured by the fact that these vessels, in the course of normal pregnancy, undergo extensive physiological changes (Brosens et al., 1967). It is self evident that to establish hemochorial placentation and then to provide a progressively increasing blood supply to the conceptus as pregnancy continues, the spiral arteries in the placental bed must first be opened and subsequently profoundly modified. The detailed work of many investigators (Harris and Ramsey, 1966; Brosens and Dixon, 1966; Hamilton and Boyd, 1960) has clarified the anatomy and morphology of the maternal vascular supply to the human placenta. This clear picture of the normal state of affairs is fundamental in discussing the acquired lesions of uterine blood vessels in abnormal placentation such as spontaneous abortion, ectopic pregnancy, antepartum hemorrhage, placenta accreta, preeclampsia, and intrauterine growth retardation.

This report examines the distribution, site, and number of uteroplacental arteries and the extent of their physiological changes at term. Data from previously published work (Brosens and Dixon, 1966; Brosens et al., 1972; Brosens and Renaer, 1972) are included for comparison.

## MATERIALS AND METHODS

### Specimens

The material includes 15 cesarean hysterectomy specimens including 3 specimens with the placenta at least partially in situ. In addition, several hundred placental biopsies taken at the time of cesarean section or per vaginam immediately following delivery have been examined.

The topography of the vessel changes was studied in the cesarean hysterectomy specimens. This large number of biopsies gave an excellent overall picture of the changes of the vessels in normal and abnormal pregnancy.

The study of the openings of uteroplacental arteries has been based on two uteri with the placenta in situ obtained by cesarean hysterectomy, one from a normal pregnancy and the other from a hypertensive pregnancy with severe intrauterine growth retardation. In both cases respectively, two fifths and one seventh of the specimen was cut in 8 micron sections which were examined at approximately 250 micron intervals.

The hysterectomy specimens, placental bed biopsies, and placentae were processed and examined by methods described previously. On large, histological sections cut in a step serial fashion, the individual arteries can be followed in their course through myometrium and decidua (Brosens and Dixon, 1966).

## Clinical Criteria

Throughout the study, normal pregnancies were defined as those which were not complicated by antepartum hemorrhage, preeclampsia, essential hypertension, intrauterine growth retardation, or diabetes mellitus. The clinical criteria for preeclampsia, essential hypertension, and intrauterine growth retardation have been described in previous papers. Clinical criteria for preeclampsia were a minimum blood pressure reading of 140/90 mm Hg twice $\geq 4$ hours apart associated with proteinuria of $\geq 500$ mg/l. Because much of this study was retrospective using archived material, the distinction between small for gestational age (SGA) and actual intrauterine growth retardation had not been made. Birthweight below the 10th centile for gestational age according to Lubchenco et al. (1963) was used as criterium for intrauterine growth retardation (Khong et al., 1986).

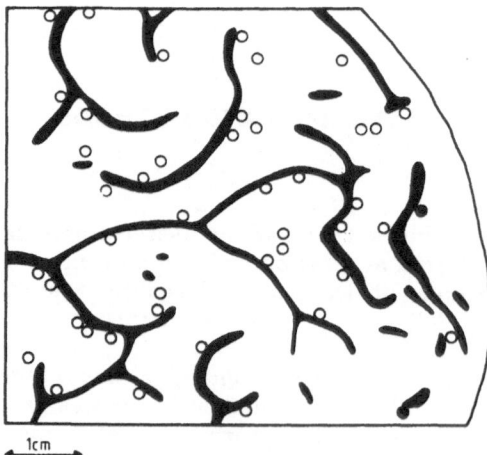

Figure 1. Plan of two-fifths of maternal surface of the placenta showing insertion of the septa and the openings of uteroplacental arteries with physiological changes (○) and with incomplete physiological changes (•) in a normal pregnancy.

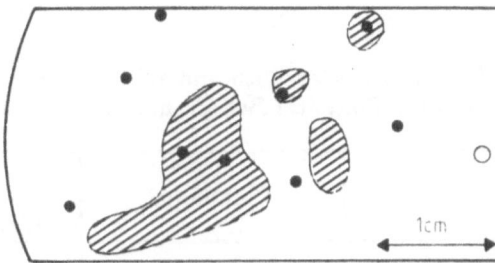

Figure 2. Segment of maternal surface of the placenta showing the areas of infarcted placenta (shaded area) and the openings of converted (○) and unconverted (●) uteroplacental arteries from a patient with severe pre-eclampsia and intrauterine growth retardation.

## RESULTS

### Distribution, Site, and Number of Openings of Uteroplacental Arteries

A diagram of the basal plate of the placenta from the normal pregnancy with indication of the site of placental septa and openings of spiral arteries is shown in Figure 1. The distribution of the arterial openings is irregular, and these openings occasionally tend to occur in groups of two or three. In this placenta, most of the arterial openings were found at the base or in the lower third of a septum. Forty-eight spiral arteries were counted in two fifths of the basal plate giving a total calculated number of 120 arterial openings for the entire placental bed. All arteries were found to communicate by only one opening with the intervillous space. The venous lakes in the decidua drain blood through multiple openings spread over the entire basal plate.

A diagram of the basal plate from the hypertensive pregnancy with severe intrauterine growth retardation is shown in Figure 2. The areas of placental infarcts and the related spiral artery openings are indicated. The calculated number of spiral arterial openings in this specimen was 72 for the entire placental bed.

### Physiological Changes

In the cesarean hysterectomy specimen from normal pregnancy and from the case with severe hypertension and intrauterine growth retardation respectively, 96% and 10% of the uteroplacental arteries demonstrated the presence of physiological changes (Table 1). In the hypertensive case, the few converted spiral arteries were situated in the center of the placental bed (Figure 2).

## Table 1

### Number of Spiral Arteries With and Without Physiological Changes in the Placental Bed From Single Placentae

|  | Normal Pregnancy | Severe Preeclampsia and Intrauterine Growth Retardation |
|---|---|---|
| Area examined | 32 cm² | 7 cm² |
| Number of spiral arteries | 45 | 10 |
| With physiological changes | 43 (96%) | 1 (10%) |
| Without physiological changes | 2 (4%) | 8 (90%) |

## DISCUSSION

At or near term, the spiral artery in its distal segment, as it opens into the intervillous space, bears little resemblance to any known vascular structure. There is complete absence of muscular and elastic tissue throughout the arterial wall, absence of a continuous endothelial lining, and the lumen is widely dilated and tortuous. The vessel wall is largely composed of fibrous tissue and remnants of fibrinoid deposition and large cells so characteristic of the early vessel changes associated with the original trophoblastic invasion of the vessel wall are found in the amorphous vessel wall.

As one follows the spiral artery proximally to the region of the myometrio-decidual junction and superficial myometrium, the arterial and venous structures become clearly distinguishable. The arteries are thick-walled structures with a caliber enormously greater than in the non-pregnant state. The endothelial lining is usually intact, the intima may show focal thickening and some fragments of elastica can be found. The internal elastic layer lamina and the smooth muscle layers of the media are totally or partially replaced by a thick layer of fibrinoid material containing some large cells identical with those described for the more distal portion of the artery.

In addition to the uteroplacental arteries small arteries or arterioles, can be seen which show none of the changes as described for the spiral arteries except for an apparent loss of elastic tissue. Placental bed trophoblastic cells are seen in the tissue around the uteroplacental arteries, the unchanged arterioles, and veins. In the unchanged basal arterioles, there is no evidence of trophoblast in the wall.

The veins traversing the decidual plate run more or less parallel to the basal plate and in the Nitabuch's layer show some of the features of the openings of the spiral arteries. Cytotrophoblast can be identified in the fibrinoid wall and the tips of placental villi can be found in the lumen. The veins in the deeper layer of the decidua and the myometrium do not show, apart from enlargement, the specific physiological changes of the arteries. Intimal cushions of fibrous tissue and smooth muscle are a common finding. Normal placentation results in the conversion of some 100 to 150 uteroplacental arteries that supply the maternal blood to the intervillous space (Figure 3) (Spanner, 1936; Boyd, 1956; Brosens and Dixon, 1966).

There is now good evidence that the transformation of the spiral arteries in the placental bed to uteroplacental arteries is achieved in two stages, the first occuring in the decidual segments during early placentation and the second occuring in the myometric segment during the second trimester of gestation (Pijnenborg et al., 1980).

Inadequate physiological change of the spiral arteries has now been demonstrated to be a significant characteristic of pregnancies complicated by hypertension where there is associated intrauterine fetal growth retardation and to some extent in intrauterine fetal growth retardation unassociated with maternal hypertension (Brosens et al., 1972; Sheppard and Bonnar, 1976; Brosens et al., 1977; De Wolf et al., 1980).

The exact evaluation of the extent of physiological changes in different clinical conditions of abnormal pregnancy on the basis of biopsies of the placental bed is hampered by a difficult sampling problem, but it has been confirmed recently that complete absence of physiological changes throughout the entire length of some spiral arteries can be seen in some cases of pre-eclampsia and intrauterine growth retardation (Khong et al., 1986). These findings point to a general defect in the mechanism of placentation during the first half of pregnancy resulting in partial or complete absence of physiological changes and probably also in a reduced number of uteroplacental arteries (Figure 4).

Recent application of the Doppler technique for assessing uteroplacental blood flow appears to be able to identify whether a normal or abnormal circulation to the placenta is developing (Campbell et al., 1983) and will help to clarify the mechanism of defective placentation in different clinical conditions.

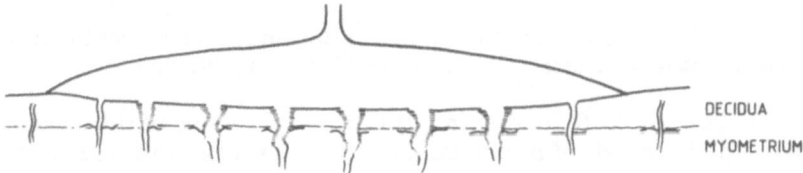

Figure 3. Diagrammatic representation of the extent and distribution of converted and unconverted uteroplacental arteries in the placental bed in normal pregnancy.

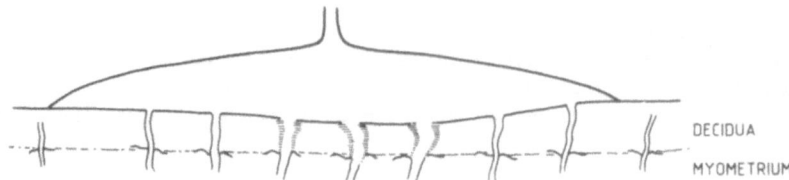

Figure 4. Diagrammatic representation of the extent and distribution of converted and unconverted uteroplacental arteries in pregnancy induced hypertension and intrauterine growth retardation.

## SUMMARY

The distribution of the uteroplacental vessels and the physiological changes they undergo are examined in 15 cesarean hysterectomy specimens including 3 specimens with the placenta at least partially in situ. The study of these specimens confirms the inadequate development of the uteroplacental vessels in hypertensive pregnancy complicated by fetal growth retardation and focusses the attention on the new finding of restricted physiological changes in the placental bed vessels of the decidua. These findings point to an inappropriate reaction between human invasive, migratory extravillous trophoblast, and uterine tissues.

## ACKNOWLEDGEMENTS

The author is grateful for the technical assistance of Mrs. Chantal VandenBosch and Mr. Luc Brullemans.

## REFERENCES

Boyd, J.D. (1956) Morphology and physiology of the uteroplacental circulation. In *Gestation, Transactions of the Second Conference,* (ed.), C.A. Villee, New York:The Josiah Macy Foundation, p. 132.

Brosens, I. and Dixon, H.G. (1966) Anatomy of the maternal side of the placenta. *J. Obstet. Gynaecol. Br.Cwlth.*73, 357-363.

Brosens, I., Robertson, W.B., and Dixon, H.G. (1967) The physiological response of the vessels of the placental bed to normal pregnancy. *J. Pathol. Bacteriol.* 93, 569-579.

Brosens, I. and Renaer, M. (1972) On the pathogenesis of placental infarcts in preeclampsia. *J. Obstet. Gynaecol. Br. Cwlth.* 79, 794-799.

Brosens, I., Robertson, W.B., and Dixon, H.G. (1972) The role of the spiral arteries in the pathogenesis of preeclampsia. *Obstet. Gynecol. Ann.* 1, 177-191.

Brosens, I., Dixon, H.G., and Robertson, W.B. (1977) Fetal growth retardation and the arteries of the placental bed. *Br. J. Obstet. Gynaecol.* 84, 656-663.

Campbell, S., Griffin, D.R., Pearce, J.M., Diaz-Recasens, J., Cohen-Overbeek, T.E., Willson, K., and Teague, M.J. (1983) New doppler technique for assessing uteroplacental blood flow. *Lancet* I, 676-677.

De Wolf, F., Brosens, I., and Renaer, M. (1980) Fetal growth retardation and the maternal arterial supply of the human placenta in the absence of sustained hypertension. *Br J. Obstet. Gynaecol.* 87, 678-685.

Hamilton, W.J. and Boyd, J.D. (1960) Development of the human placenta in the first three months of gestation. *J. Anat. (London)* 94, 297-340.

Harris, J.W.S. and Ramsey, E.M. (1966) The morphology of human uteroplacental vasculature. *Contrib. Embryol.* 38, 43-58.

Khong, T.Y., De Wolf, F., Robertson, W.B., and Brosens, I. (1986) Inadequate maternal vascular response to placentation in preeclampsia and intrauterine fetal growth retardation. *Bri J. Obstet. Gynaecol.* 93, 1049-1059.

Lubchenco, L.O., Hausman, C., Dressler, M., and Boyd, E. (1963) Intra-uterine growth as estimated from live-born birthweight data at 24 to 42 weeks of gestation. *Ped.* 32, 793-800.

Pijnenborg, R., Dixon, G., Robertson, W.B., and Brosens, I. (1980) Trophoblastic invasion of the human decidua from 8 to 18 weeks of pregnancy. *Placenta* 1, 3-19.

Sheppard, B.L. and Bonnar, J. (1976) The ultrastructure of the arterial supply of the human placenta in pregnancy complicated by fetal growth retardation. *Bri J. Obstet. Gynaecol.* 83, 948-959.

Spanner, R. (1936) Muetterlicher und kindlicher Kreislauf der menschlichen Placenta und seine Strombahnen. *Zschr. Anat. Entwickl. Gesch. (Berlin)* 105, 163-199.

Trophoblast Research 3:69-81, 1988

# THE MATERNAL BLOOD SUPPLY TO THE PLACENTA IN PREGNANCY COMPLICATED BY INTRAUTERINE FETAL GROWTH RETARDATION

Brian L. Sheppard and John Bonnar

Trinity College
Department of Obstetrics and Gynaecology
Sir Patrick Dun Research Centre
St. James's Hospital
Dublin 8, Ireland

## INTRODUCTION

Pathology of the placenta and utero-placental spiral arteries in hypertensive pregnancy has been recognized for many years. However, only during the last decade has serious attention been directed towards the study of uterine vascular pathology associated with intrauterine fetal growth retardation not only in pre-eclampsia but also in normotensive pregnancy. Although several factors are known to be associated with the etiology of intrauterine fetal growth retardation, no morphological explanation for this pregnancy complication had previously been forthcoming. Indeed, such a concept is still not accepted by all, and the relationship between uteroplacental vascular pathology, the extent of physiological adaptations of spiral arteries, hypertension in pregnancy, and intrauterine fetal growth retardation remains a subject of controversy.

In 1976, the uteroplacental vascular changes in 15 well documented cases of intrauterine growth retardation were reported by Sheppard and Bonnar (1976). This was the first description of a uteroplacental vasculopathy in normotensive intrauterine fetal growth retardation which contained many of the morphological features previously attributed to vascular lesions of the placental bed in pre-eclampsia. These observations were later confirmed in a subsequent, larger study (Sheppard and Bonnar, 1981). This report will review the present understanding of uteroplacental vascular changes in intrauterine fetal growth retardation and compare the uteroplacental vasculature in 15 normotensive and 15 hypertensive pregnancies complicated by intrauterine fetal growth retardation.

## PATIENTS AND METHODS

Thirty placental bed biopsies, each of which contained at least one spiral artery, and placentae were obtained at cesarean section from pregnancies complicated by severe intrauterine fetal growth retardation (birth weight below the 10th centile - Figure 1). Ten of the pregnancies were complicated by pre-eclampsia, 5 by essential hypertension with superimposed pre-eclampsia, and 15 remained normotensive throughout.

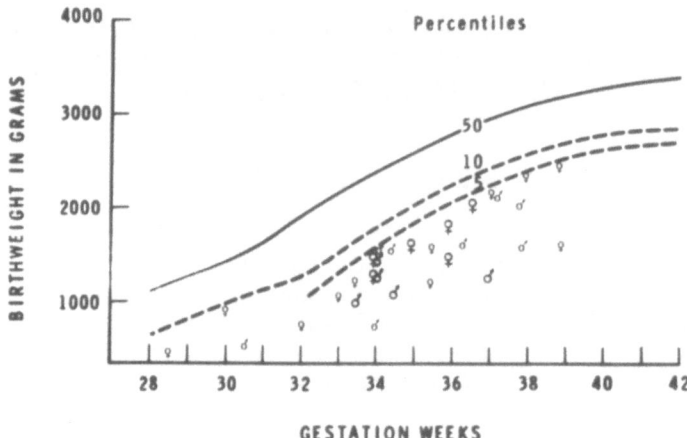

Figure 1. Birthweight of the infants for the pregnancies included in the study.


        The wedge-shaped biopsies were taken under direct vision, following removal of the placenta, at cesarean section and placed immediately into fixative (cacodylate buffered glutaraldehyde). Each biopsy was divided into two, one half being prepared for examination by light microscopy and the other by electron microscopy in methods previously described (Sheppard and Bonnar, 1974).

### RESULTS

        During the examination of uteroplacental spiral arteries special emphasis was placed on: (1) the extent of physiological changes of pregnancy and (2) the morphological features and frequency of vascular lesions, both in the myometrium and the decidua of the placental bed (Figure 2).

| | PHYS. CHANGES | | LESIONS | |
|---|---|---|---|---|
| | Present | Absent | Decidua | Myometrium |
| Normotensive (n = 15) | 2 | 13 | 12 | 4 |
| Pre-eclampsia (n = 10) | 1 | 9 | 10 | 8 |
| Essential hypertension & pre-eclampsia (n = 5) | 0 | 5 | 5 | 4 |

Figure 2. Summary of the morphological features of the placental bed spiral arteries in the pregnancies complicated by intrauterine fetal growth retardation, included in this study.

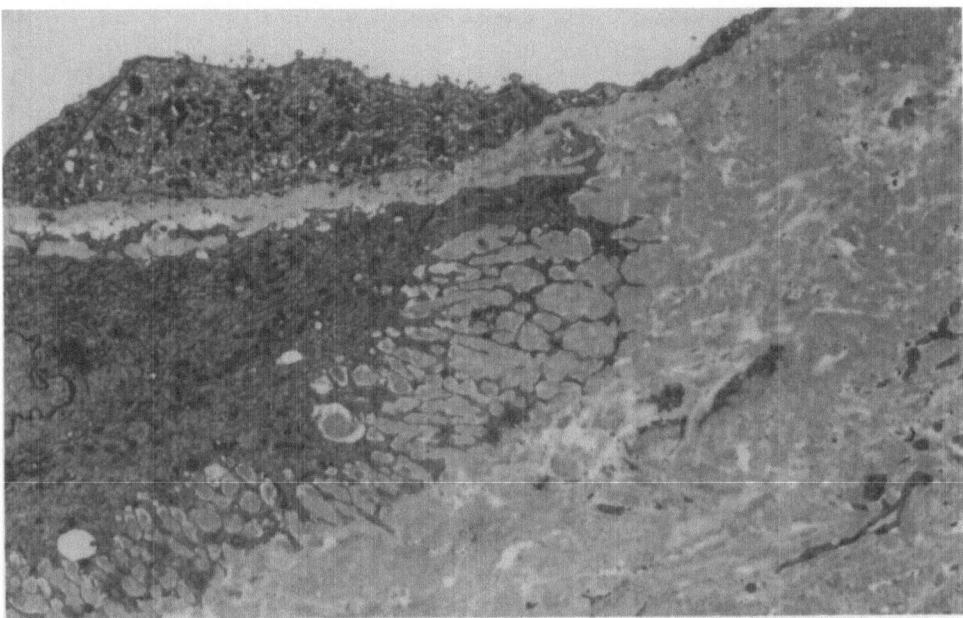

Figure 3. An electron micrograph of part of the wall of a decidual spiral artery. Trophoblast cells are seen within the media of the vessel surrounded by an amorphous matrix containing fibrin. (X4000)

## Physiological Changes

The physiological changes of pregnancy were seen in decidual segments of spiral arteries from all biopsies from the placental bed and the basal plate of the delivered placenta. By electron microscopy, the musculo-elastic content of the vessel media was seen to be replaced by trophoblast cells surrounded by an amorphous matrix containing fibrin (Figure 3).

In 13 of 15 normotensive, 9 of 10 pre-eclampsia, and all 5 essential hypertension with superimposed pre-eclampsia, the physiological changes of pregnancy were restricted to the decidual segments and not observed in the spiral arteries of the myometrium (Figure 4). In one pregnancy complicated by pre-eclampsia, these physiological changes were found only in the superficial layer of the myometrium.

## Arterial Lesions

Vascular lesions were observed in the decidua of the placental bed from 12 to 15 normotensive, and all 15 hypertensive pregnancies. These lesions in decidual spiral arteries from both the normotensive and hypertensive pregnancies complicated by intrauterine growth retardation exhibited extensive fibrin deposition and accumulation of lipid-laden cells in the media (Figures 5 and 6).

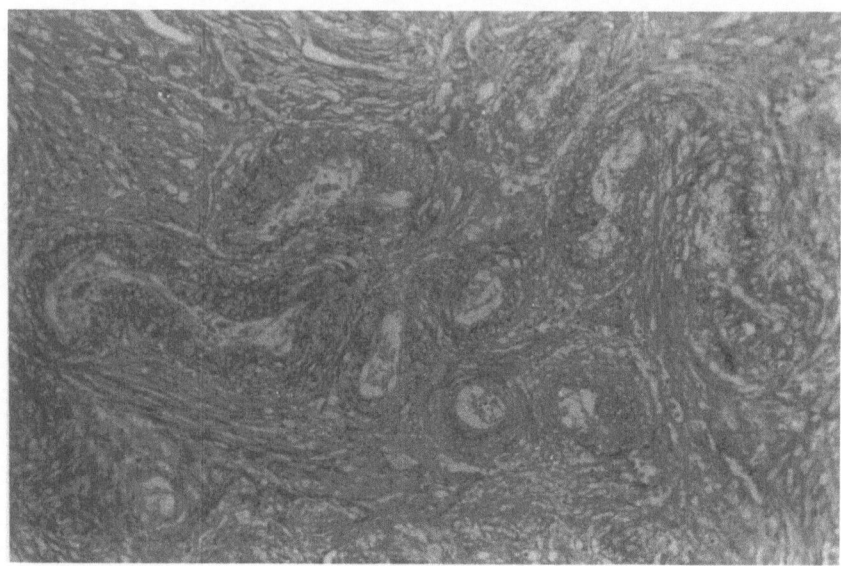

Figure 4. Spiral arteries of the placental bed myometrium in a normotensive pregnancy complicated by severe fetal growth retardation. The vessels have not undergone the physiological changes of pregnancy. (X150)

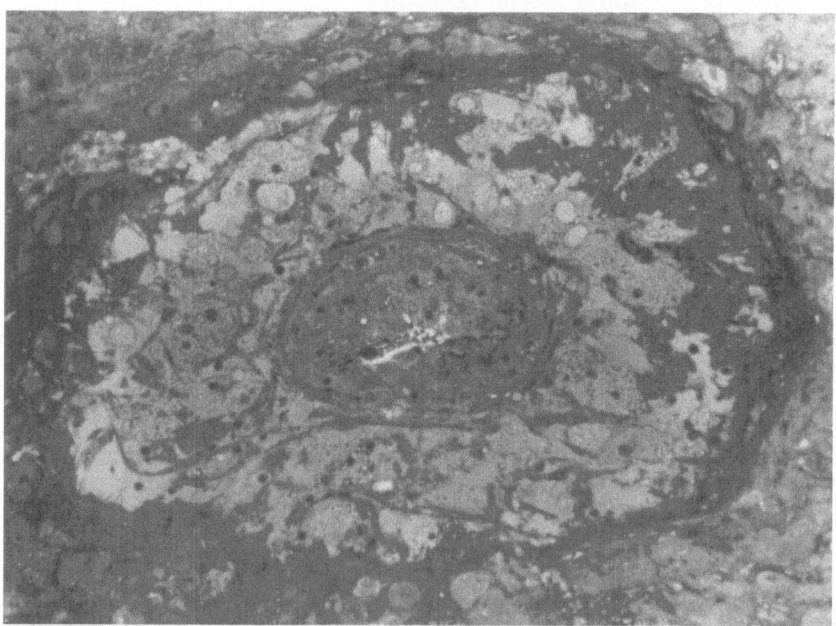

Figure 5. A uteroplacental spiral artery in the decidua of a normotensive pregnancy complicated by severe intrauterine fetal growth retardation. Numerous lipid-containing cells and fibrin are seen within the vessel wall. (X200)

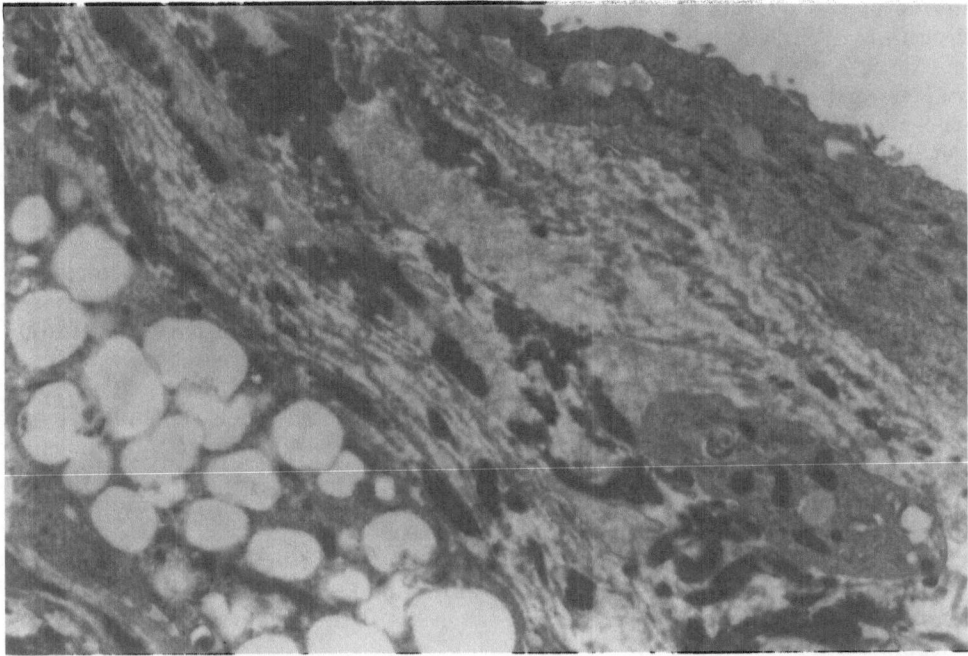

Figure 6. Electron micrograph of part of a lesion within a decidual spiral artery in normotensive pregnancy complicated by intrauterine fetal growth retardation. Lipid is seen within the endothelium and within cells of the media surrounded by amorphous material containing fibrin. (X9000)

In 8 of the 10 pregnancies complicated by pre-eclampsia and intrauterine fetal growth retardation, lesions were found in the myometrial segments of spiral arteries. These lesions contained large amounts of fibrin and numerous cells packed with lipid - the features of "acute atherosis" (Figures 7 and 8). In 4 of the 5 pregnancies where the pre-eclampsia was superimposed on essential hypertension lesions of intimal smooth muscle hyperplasia with fibrin and lipid deposition in the media were encountered in myometrial spiral arteries (Figure 9).

In 4 of the 15 normotensive pregnancies resulting in the delivery of a severely growth retarded baby, lesions were observed in myometrial spiral arteries. Again, as in the hypertensive pregnancies, the principal features of these lesions were fibrin and lipid containing cells (Figure 10). Although the vessels exhibiting these lesions were surrounded by myometrial smooth muscle, they were clearly only in the distal segments of the vessels on the myometrial side of the decidual-myometrial junction.

## DISCUSSION

In pregnancy, maternal blood is supplied to the intervillous space of the placenta by way of the uterine spiral arteries and the growth and health of the fetus is dependent on an increasing supply of blood reaching the intervillous space as pregnancy progresses. It is now well recognized that physiological adaptations of uterine spiral arteries are an essential requirement to facilitate this increased blood flow. A relationship has been shown between the severity of fetal growth retardation and the degree of placental infarction (Little, 1960; Fox, 1963; Wigglesworth, 1969), between decidual spiral arterial lesions and ultrastructural abnormalities of placental villi in pregnancies complicated by intrauterine fetal growth retardation (Sheppard and Bonnar, 1980a) and between birth weight and pathological changes in vessels of the placental bed (Sheppard and Bonnar, 1980b; McFadyen et al., 1986).

In normal pregnancy the uteroplacental spiral arteries undergo structural modifications both in the decidua and myometrium of the placental bed. These have been described as "physiological changes" of pregnancy (Brosens et al., 1967) and have been described in detail both by light and electron microscopy (De Wolf et al., 1973; Sheppard and Bonnar, 1974). In the myometrium the musculo-elastic tissue of the media of the vessel wall is replaced by trophoblast cells surrounded by a thick layer of fibrinoid. In the decidua, similar changes are observed in the media of the vessel although in the distal segments where the vessel enters the intervillous space of the placenta, senescent trophoblast cells may be a common finding in the fibrinoid layer. An incomplete lining of trophoblast replaces much of the endothelium in these vessels and mural thrombosis is a common feature; although this may add to the thickness of the vessel wall - and thereby reduce the size of the lumen - it does not appear to have an effect on the fetal outcome of the pregnancy (Sheppard and Bonnar, 1974).

A failure of physiological changes to extend into the myometrial spiral arteries has been reported in pre-eclampsia and essential hypertension with superimposed pre-eclampsia irrespective of the birthweight of the baby at delivery

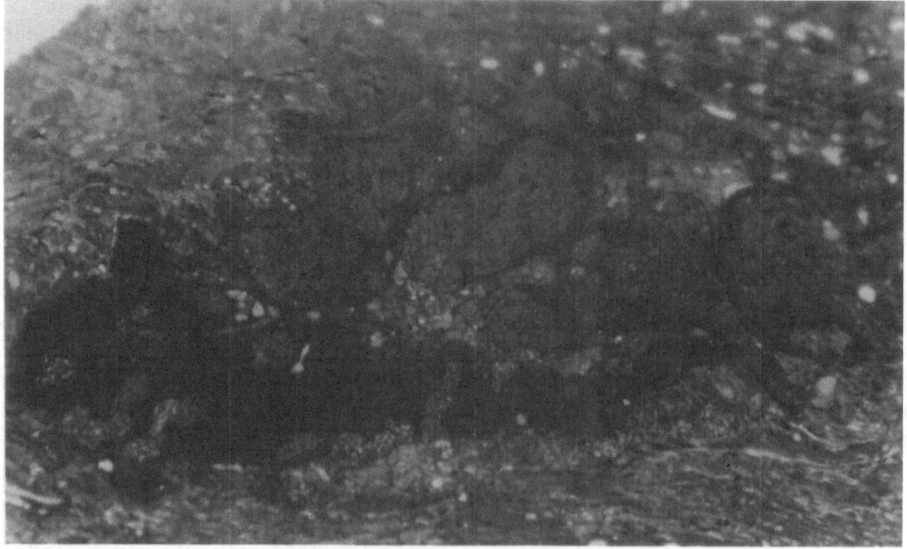

Figure 7. A myometrial spiral artery in pre-eclampsia complicated by intrauterine fetal growth retardation the lesion "acute atherosis". Large numbers of lipid containing cells and fibrin are observed within the vessel wall. (X250)

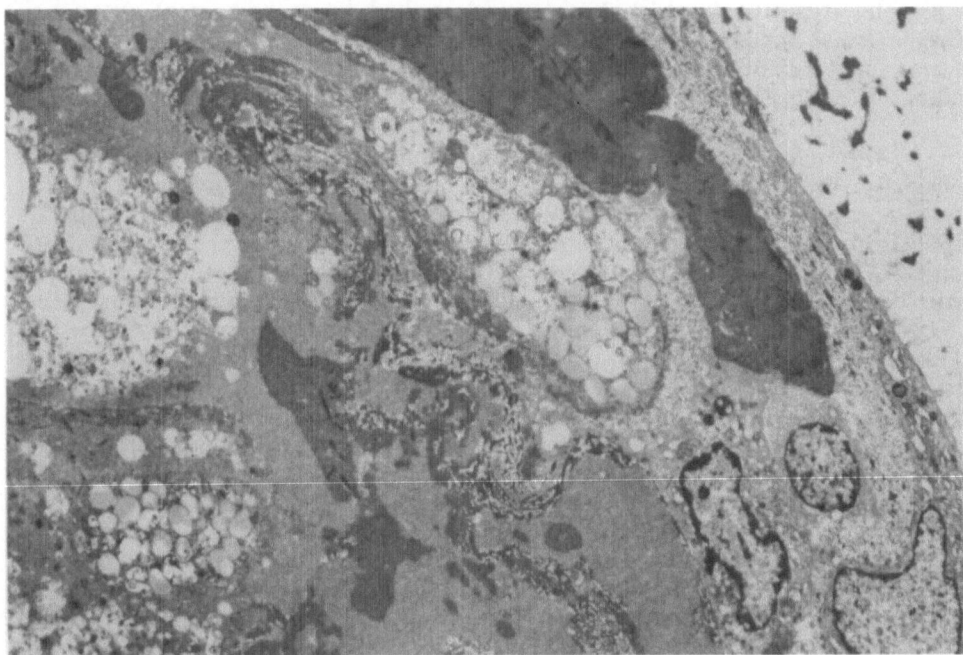

Figure 8. Electron micrograph of part of the wall of a myometrial spiral artery in pre-eclampsia exhibiting the lesion "acute atherosis". Lipid containing cells and fibrin are evident within the media below the endothelium. (X5000)


(Brosens et al., 1972). Our results, and those of others, also show a lack of progression of the physiological changes in spiral arteries beyond the decidual-myometrial junction in pregnancies complicated by intrauterine fetal growth retardation not only in pre-eclampsia but very often in normotensive pregnancy (Sheppard and Bonnar, 1976, 1981; Brosens et al., 1977; De Wolf et al., 1980; Gerretsen et al., 1981; McFadyen et al., 1986). Although it has been suggested that the reduced blood flow through the placenta and myometrium in pregnancies complicated by maternal hypertension and fetal growth retardation (Browne and Veall, 1953; Kaeaer et al., 1980; Campbell et al., 1983) may be due to the failure of complete trophoblast invasion to affect the physiological changes of pregnancy, little is known of the function of endovascular trophoblast which invades uteroplacental spiral arteries in pregnancy. Trophoblast cells lining decidual spiral arteries are known to have a reduced capacity for fibrinolysis, even in normal pregnancy (Sheppard and Bonnar, 1976) and placentae from pregnancies complicated by fetal growth retardation, but without hypertension, have an increased ability to inhibit urokinase-induced fibrinolysis when compared with normal placentae (Elder and Myatt, 1976). Trophoblast cells from pregnancies complicated by intrauterine fetal growth retardation also have a greatly reduced ability to produce prostacyclin compared to trophoblast in normal pregnancy (Jogee et al., 1983). Prostacyclin is a potent vasodilator and platelet anti-aggregator; a localized decidual decrease in production by the intravascular trophoblast could result in the increased platelet aggregation and fibrin deposition seen in the uteroplacental vasculature in intrauterine fetal growth retardation. An increase of platelet deposition, which has been described in early normal pregnancy (Sheppard and Bonnar, 1974), would account for the shortened life span of platelets in pregnancy complicated by intrauterine fetal growth retardation (Wallenburg and van Kessell, 1979).

Although decreased prostacyclin production and increased fibrin deposition may be etiological factors in the thrombotic occlusion of the uteroplacental circulation which impairs fetal growth, other factors may also be involved in pregnancies complicated by intrauterine fetal growth retardation. In 1950, Zeek and Assali introduced the term "acute atherosis" to describe lesions which Hertig (1945) found in the spiral arteries of patients with hypertensive albuminuric toxemia of pregnancy. The lesion is characterized by fibrinoid necrosis often affecting the whole thickness of the vessel wall and the accumulation of lipophages in the damaged wall of the spiral arteries. It was later suggested that this lesion only occured in pre-eclampsia in vessels which had not undergone the physiological changes of pregnancy (Brosens et al., 1967). The lesions in uteroplacental decidual vessels in normotensive intrauterine fetal growth retardation described by ourselves (Sheppard and Bonnar, 1976, 1981) and by others (De Wolf et al., 1980) exhibit many of the features of the lesion "acute atherosis". Although some of the lipid containing cells are difficult to identify within these lesions due to the lipid changes in senscent trophoblast which have been described in decidual spiral arteries, even in normal pregnancy (Boyd and Hamilton, 1970), the fact cannot be ruled out that the lesion "acute atherosis" may be occurring in normotensive intrauterine fetal growth retardation in decidual spiral arteries which have not undergone the physiological changes of pregnancy.

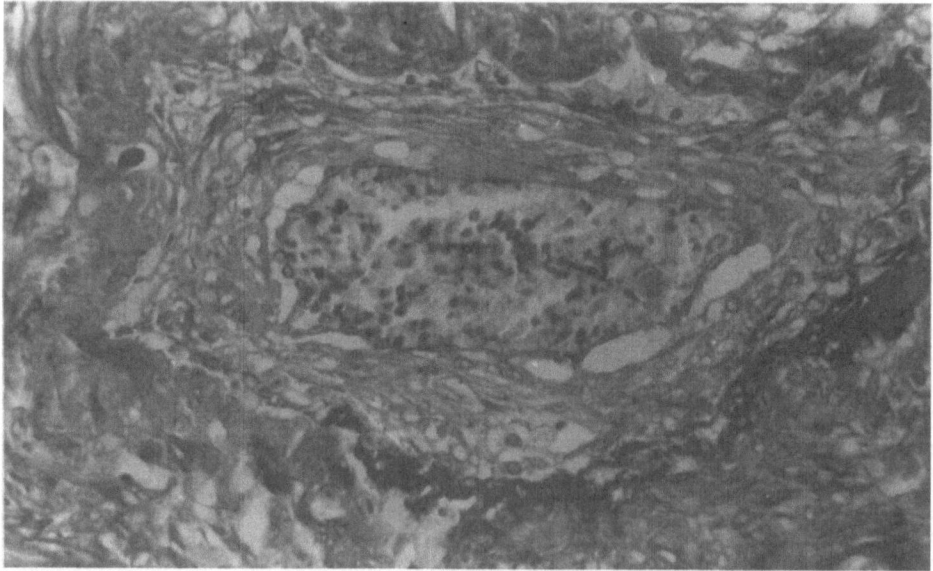

Figure 9. A myometrial spiral artery in the placental bed in essential hypertension with superimposed pre-eclampsia resulting in the delivery of a growth retarded infant. The lesion exhibits intimal smooth muscle hyperplasia with lipid loaded cells and fibrin within the media of the vessel wall. (X200)

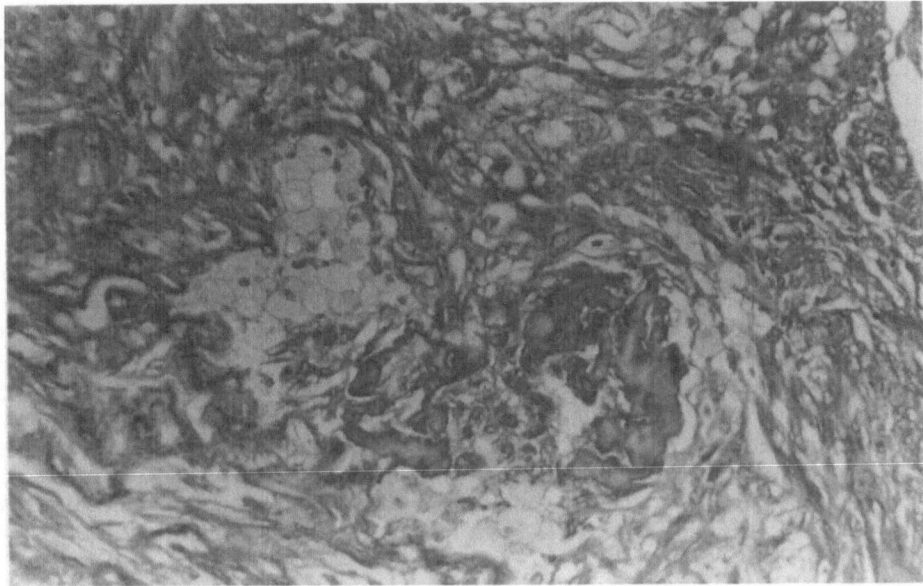

Figure 10. A lesion within a uteroplacental spiral artery of the placental bed myometrium in a normotensive pregnancy resulting in severe intrauterine fetal growth retardation. Fibrin and lipid containing cells are the major features of the

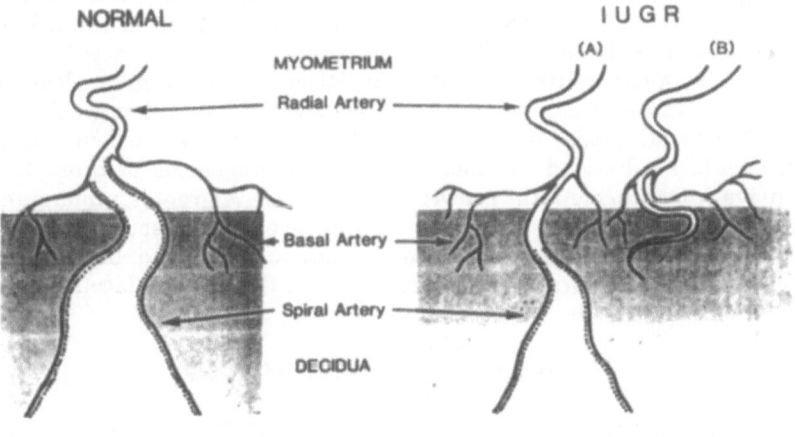

Figure 11. Diagram of the arterial supply to the placenta. In normal pregnancies, the decidual and myometrial segments of the spiral arteries are enlarged by physiological changes whereas in intrauterine fetal growth retardation (IUGR) there may be: (A) a failure of the morphological adaptions to extend beyond the decidual segments of the vessel or possibly, (B) a complete failure of the vessels to be "opened-up" to the intervillous space of the placenta in early pregnancy.

The pathogenesis of uteroplacental lesions in normotensive intrauterine fetal growth retardation is still unclear. Although the lesions appear morphologically similar to those seen in pre-eclampsia it is possible that the lesion seen in fetal growth retardation is analogous to but not identical with "acute atherosis". In intrauterine fetal growth retardation, as in pre-eclampsia, much of the vasculopathy in the maternal supply line to the placenta seen in late pregnancy is most likely due to a failure of adequate placentation in early pregnancy. In normal pregnancy between 120 to 150 spiral arteries supply the placenta at term (Brosens and Dixon, 1966). A recent study has shown a complete absence of physiological changes throughout the entire length of some spiral arteries in pre-eclampsia and intrauterine fetal growth retardation (Khong et al., 1986). In intrauterine fetal growth retardation, many of the vessels observed in the myometrium without physiological changes may in fact represent spiral arteries which were never "opened-up" to the intervillous space of the placenta in early pregnancy (Figure 11). This would result in, not only smaller, narrower vessels restricted to decidual adaptations, but also a reduced number of vessels supplying the placenta in intrauterine fetal growth retardation. The reason for failure of trophoblast invasion to effect complete physiological adaptations of placental bed spiral arteries in some pregnancies still remains to be elucidated in further studies.

## SUMMARY

During the past ten years, several studies have been directed towards the examination of uteroplacental vasculature in intrauterine fetal growth retardation in attempt to find a morphological explanation for this pregnancy complication. These findings and those of others have shown arestriction ofthe physiological changes of pregnancy to the decidual segments of spiral arteries in hypertensive, and to a lesser extent in normotensive, pregnancies resulting in the delivery of a growth retarded infant. Although the pathogenesis of uteroplacental lesions in normotensive intrauterine fetal growth retardation still remains unclear, many of the lesions seen in the decidual spiral arteries show the morphological features of the lesion "acute atherosis" previously attributed only to pre-eclampsia. Further research should be directed to elucidating the pathogenesis of these lesions in normotensive intrauterine fetal growth retardation. A greater understanding of the complex relationship between uteroplacental vascular changes in complications of pregnancy is required if advances are to be made in any therapeutic control to improve the maternal blood flowto the placenta preventing impairment of fetal growth.

## ACKNOWLEDGEMENTS

We are grateful for the technical assistance of Miss Marie Jordan. Part of this study was supported by the Friends of the Rotunda Hospital.

## REFERENCES

Boyd, J.D. and Hamilton, W.J. (1970) *The Human Placenta*, Heffer and Sons, Cambridge, p. 262.

Brosens, I. and Dixon, H.G. (1966)  The anatomy of the maternal side of the placenta. *J. Obstet. Gynecol. Br. Cmwlth*. 73, 357-363.

Brosens, I., Robertson, W.B., and Dixon, H.G. (1967) The physiological response of the vessels of the placental bed to normal pregnancy. *J. Pathol. Bact*. 93, 569-579.

Brosens, I., Robertson, W.B., and Dixon, H.G. (1972) The role of the spiral arteries in the pathogenesis of the pre-eclampsia. In: *Obstetrics and Gynecology Annual*, (ed.), R.M. Wynn, Appleton-Century-Crofts, New York, p. 177.

Brosens, I., Dixon, H.G., and Robertson, W.B. (1977) Fetal growth retardation and the arteries of the placental bed. *J. Obstet. Gynecol*. 84, 656-663.

Browne, J.C.M. and Veall, N. (1953)  The maternal placental blood flow in normotensiveand hypertensive women. *J. Obstet. Gynaecol. Br. Emp*. 60, 241-247.

Campbell, S., Diaz-Recasens, J., Griffin, D.R., Cohen-Overbeek, T.E., Pearce, J.M., Wilson, K., and Teague, M.J. (1983)  New Doppler technique for assessing uteroplacental blood flow. *Lancet* i, 675-677.

De Wolf, F., De Wolf-Peeters, C., and Brosens, I. (1973) Ultrastructure of the spiral arteries on the human placental bed at the end of the normal pregnancy. *Am. J. Obstet. Gynecol*. 117, 833-848.

De Wolf, F., Brosens, I., and Renear, M. (1980)  Fetal growth retardation and the maternal arterial supply of the human placenta in the absence of sustained hypertension. *Br. J. Obstet. Gynaecol*. 87, 678-685.

Elder, M.G. and Myatt, L. (1976)  Coagulation and fibrinolysis in pregnancies complicated by fetal growth retardation. *Br. J. Obstet. Gynaecol*. 83, 355-360.

Fox, H. (1963) White infarcts of the placentas. *J. Obstet. Gynaecol. Br. Cmwlth* 70, 980-991.

Gerretsen, G., Huisjes, H.J., and Elema, J.D. (1981)  Morphological changes of the spiral arteries in the placental bed in relation to pre-eclampsia and fetal growth retardation. *Br. J. Obstet. Gynaecol*. 88, 876-881.

Hertig, A.T. (1945)  Vascular pathology in the hypertensive albuminuric toxemias of pregnancy. *Clinics* 4, 602-613.

Joggee, M., Myatt, L., and Elder, M.G. (1983)  Decreased prostacyclin production by placental cells in culture from pregnancies complicated by fetal growth retardation. *Br. J. Obstet. Gynaecol*. 90, 247-250.

Kaeaer, K., Jouppila, P., Kuikka, J., Luotola, H., Toivanen, J., and Rekonen, A (1980)  Intervillous blood flow in normal and complcated late pregnancy measured by intravenous [133]Xe method. *Acta Obstet. Gynecol. Scand.* 59, 7-10.

Khong, T.Y., De Wolf, F., Robertson, W.B., and Brosens, I. (1986)  Inadequate maternal vascular response to placentation in pregnanciescomplicated by pre-eclampsia and by small-for-gestational age infants. *Br. J. Obstet. Gynaecol.* 93, 1049-1059.

Little, W.A. (1960) Placental infarction. *Obstet. Gynecol.* 15, 109-130.

McFadyen, I.R., Price, A.B., and Geirsson, R.T. (1986)   The relation of birthweight to histological appearances in vessels of the placental bed. *Br. J. Obstet. Gynaecol.* 93, 476-481.

Robertson, W.B., Brosens, I., and Dixon, H.G. (1967)  The pathological response of the vessels of the placental bed to hypertensive pregnancy. *J. Pathol. Bact.* 93, 581-592.

Sheppard, B.L. and Bonnar, J. (1974) The ultrastructure of the arterial supply of the human placenta in early and late pregnancy. *J. Obstet. Gynaecol. Br. Cmwlth.* 81, 497-511.

Sheppard, B.L. and Bonnar, J. (1976a)  The ultrastructure of the arterial supply of the human placenta in pregnancy complicated by fetal growth retardation. *Br. J. Obstet. Gynaecol.* 83, 948-959.

Sheppard, B.L. and Bonnar, J. (1976b)  Fibrinolysis in decidual spiral arteries in late pregnancy. *Thromb. Haem.* 39, 751-758.

Sheppard, B.L. and Bonnar, J. (1980a)  Uteroplacental arteries and hypertensive pregnancy.   In: *Pregnancy Hypertension.*, Proceedings of the First Congress of the International Society for the Study of Hypertension in Pregnancy, (eds.), J. Bonnar, I. MacGillivray, and M. Symonds, MTP Press Ltd., Lancaster, pp. 213-219.

Sheppard, B.L. and Bonnar, J. (1980b)  Ultrastructural abnormalities of placental villi in placentae from pregnancies complicated by intrauterine fetal growth retardation: their relationship to decidual spiral arterial lesions. *Placenta* 1, 145-146.

Sheppard, B.L. and Bonnar, J. (1981)  An ultrastructural study of utero-placental spiral arteries in hypertensive and normotensive pregnancy and fetal growth retardation. *Br. J. Obstet. Gynaecol.* 88, 695-705.

Wallenburg, H.C.S. and van Kessell, P.H. (1979)   Platelet life span in pregnancies resulting in small-for-gestational age infants. *Am. J. Obstet. Gynecol.* 134, 739-742.

Wigglesworth, J.S. (1969)  Vascular anatomy of the human placenta and its significance for placental pathology. *J. Obstet. Gynaecol. Br. Cmwlth.* 76, 979-989.

Zeek, P.M. and Assali, N.S. (1950) Vascular changes in the decidua associated with eclamptogenetic toxemia of pregnancy. *Am. J. Clin. Pathol.* 20, 1096-1105.

Trophoblast Research 3:83-96, 1988

# BLOOD FLOW REGULATION IN THE UTEROPLACENTAL ARTERIES

Waldemar Moll, Andrzej Nienartowicz, Herbert Hees,
Karl-Heinz Wrobel, and Andreas Lenz

Institut für Physiologie
Institut für Anatomie
Universität Regensburg
8400 Regensburg, FR Germany

## INTRODUCTION

The uteroplacental arterial system is rather similar in various species (see Lundgren, 1957; Reynolds, 1963; Moll and Künzel, 1971; Egund and Carter, 1974; Del Campo and Ginther, 1972). As shown for man and guinea pig in Figure 1, the uterine artery and the ovarian artery provide a dual arterial supply. From their anastomosis, the uterine arcade, segmental parametrial (mesometrial) off-shoots arise, divide in one or several branches and enter the uterus. These branches are short and barely accessible in the human but long and easily accessible in rodents. Inside the uterine wall the arteries form a network of arcuate (circumferential) arteries which gives rise to the coiled arteries, i.e., the radial arteries (in the strict sense) in the myometrium and the spiral arteries in the endometrium, part of which supply the placenta. There are differences in the extent to which the various components are involved in the control of uteroplacental blood flow; the basic anatomical pattern, however, is the same in the different species.

As shown by measurements of the intra-arterial pressure profile in pregnant animals of various species with a hemochorial placenta, a major part of the blood pressure fall, that is a major part of the limiting resistance to the placental blood flow exists in these uteroplacental arteries. Intra-arterial pressures are close to venous pressures at the entry into the placenta (Girard et al., 1971; Moll and Künzel, 1971, 1973; Moll et al., 1974). Thus, uteroplacental blood flow is controlled to a large extent by the flow resistance of the uteroplacental arteries. In species with a hemochorial placenta, uteroplacental blood flow control means control of the resistance of the uteroplacental arteries.

As reviewed at the Cambridge symposium (Moll, 1985), adjustment of the placental blood flow to fetal growth is adequate during normal pregnancy. Thus, there is clear evidence that the resistance of the uteroplacental arteries is effectively and precisely controlled. The controlling mechanism is an extraordinary one. None of the known vasoactive factors is able to produce, by smooth muscle relaxation, dilatation of placental vessels of a comparable degree which develops during the course of pregnancy (Bell, 1974; Rankin and McLaughlin, 1979). The common vasodilators usually reduce placental blood flow

(Rankin et al., 1979), presumably by redistributing uteroplacental blood flow in favor of the myometrium. A non-muscular mechanism of dilatation operates (Moll and Götz, 1985). During pregnancy the uteroplacental arteries undergo drastic structural changes. These changes were studied thoroughly in the human spiral arteries and called the physiological changes of the placental arteries by Brosens et al. (1967). These physiological changes comprise structural widening with breakdown of elastic tissue and degeneration of the arterial wall. In the hamster (Pijnenborg et al., 1974; Carpenter, 1982) and in the guinea pig (Albert, 1967; Moll et al., 1983; Hees et al., 1984), similar changes were described for the segmental mesometrial arteries. In addition, massive growth which precedes degeneration was demonstrated in the guinea pig. The complex process of structural widening is obviously the crucial event in the adjustment of uteroplacental blood flow to the requirement of fetal growth and development. Control of uteroplacental blood flow means control of the structural widening of the uteroplacental arteries.

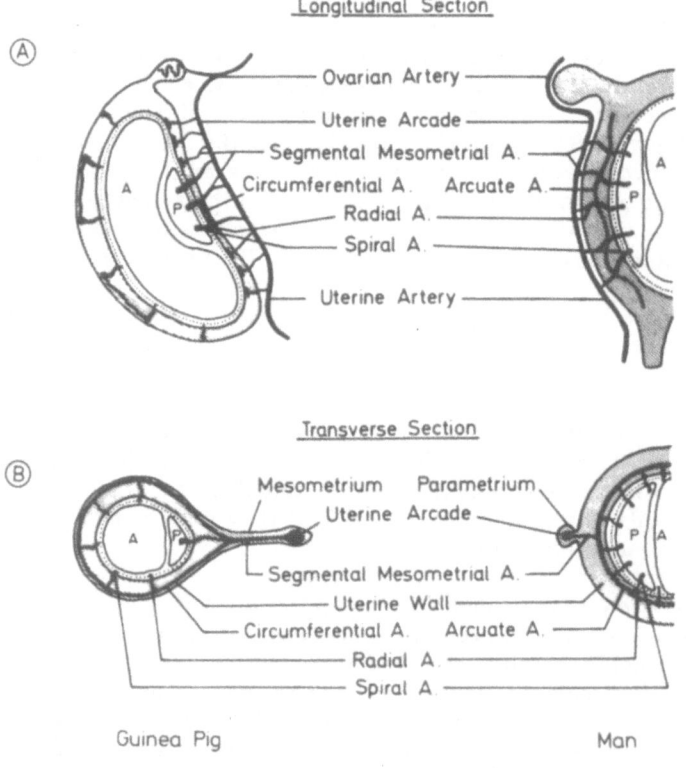

Figure 1. Schematic representation of the arterial uteroplacental system in guinea pig and in man illustrating the homology of the two systems. A) Longitudinal section. B) Transversal section. The dotted line indicates the decidua.

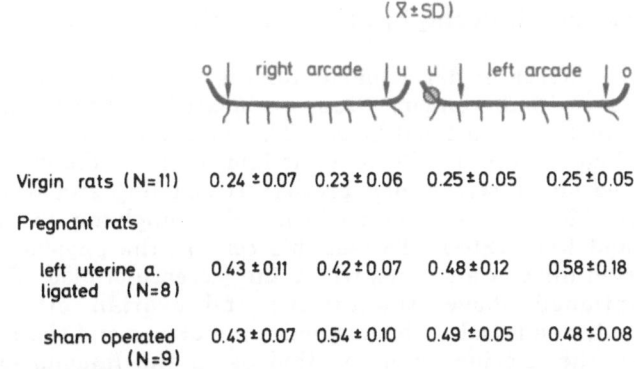

| | right arcade | | left arcade | |
|---|---|---|---|---|
| Virgin rats (N=11) | $0.24 \pm 0.07$ | $0.23 \pm 0.06$ | $0.25 \pm 0.05$ | $0.25 \pm 0.05$ |
| Pregnant rats | | | | |
| left uterine a. ligated (N=8) | $0.43 \pm 0.11$ | $0.42 \pm 0.07$ | $0.48 \pm 0.12$ | $0.58 \pm 0.18$ |
| sham operated (N=9) | $0.43 \pm 0.07$ | $0.54 \pm 0.10$ | $0.49 \pm 0.05$ | $0.48 \pm 0.08$ |

Figure 2. Internal diameter and wall thickness of the uterine arcade in virgin rats, in pregnant rats (day 21) after ligating the left uterine artery on day 8, and in sham operated pregnant rats (day 21). The schematic diagram indicates the uterine arcades with the uterine arteries (u) and the ovarian arteries (o). The arrows indicate the point of measurement. N = number of animals used. There was no significant difference between the diameters of the right intact and the left ligated arcade. The hatched circle indicates the site of ligation.

The controlling mechanism of such structural widening is not yet known. Three possible regulators are to be considered:

1. Increase in blood flow velocity caused by implantation
2. Invading trophoblast
3. Estrogens or other humoral factors

For each of the three possible regulators, a consistent theory of placental blood flow control can be proposed and tested:

### Control of the Structural Widening by Blood Flow Velocity

During the course of development for the placental vascular bed, local peripheral resistance in the endometrium is replaced by the highly conductive trophoblastic channels for maternal blood. This means increased blood flow and increased wall shear stress on the endothelium of the uteroplacental arterial system. Increased shear stress may provoke remodeling and widening of the arteries (Rodbard, 1975) as is observed in arteries supplying an arterio-venous fistula (Schoop and Rau, 1958). To test this concept the physiological changes should be evaluated under conditions, where the increase of blood flow velocity is absent. As mentioned above, the uterine and ovarian arteries form an anastomosis, the uterine arcade, which supplies the uterus and the placenta like a manifold. When the uterine artery is tied as in the famous experiment of Wigglesworth (1964), blood flow velocity remains near zero at the cervical end of the arcade during pregnancy. In the rat, the uterine arcade is readily accessible, and the internal diameter at the cervical end developing after ligation can be measured to test the velocity concept.

## Control of the Structural Widening by Blood Flow Velocity

During the course of development for the placental vascular bed, local peripheral resistance in the endometrium is replaced by the highly conductive trophoblastic channels for maternal blood. This means increased blood flow and increased wall shear stress on the endothelium of the uteroplacental arterial system. Increased shear stress may provoke remodeling and widening of the arteries (Rodbard, 1975) as is observed in arteries supplying an arterio-venous fistula (Schoop and Rau, 1958). To test this concept the physiological changes should be evaluated under conditions, where the increase of blood flow velocity is absent. As mentioned above, the uterine and ovarian arteries form an anastomosis, the uterine arcade, which supplies the uterus and the placenta like a manifold. When the uterine artery is tied as in the famous experiment of Wigglesworth (1964), blood flow velocity remains near zero at the cervical end of the arcade during pregnancy. In the rat, the uterine arcade is readily accessible, and the internal diameter at the cervical end developing after ligation can be measured to test the velocity concept.

## Control of the Structural Widening by Invading Trophoblast

Trophoblast-like cells were found in the walls of arteries with structural widening. In man, intra-arterial cytotrophoblast was found in the spiral arteries (Harris and Ramsey, 1966; Brosens et al., 1967); trophoblastic giant cells were found in the mesometrial arteries of the hamster (Carpenter, 1982). The histological pictures suggest that invading trophoblast transforms the musculoelastic tissue in a fiberless, non-elastic structure whereby the artery looses its resistance to strain. This intriguing, perceptual concept, even when convincing by its simplicity, is not proved in the strict sense, since the correlation between the appearance of trophoblastic-like cells and physiological changes is no proof for a causal relationship. To test the concept more vigorously, the timing of events needs to be studied. Time comparisons can exclude a causal relationship in the sense that later events can never be the causes for former events. In order to determine whether structural widening or trophoblast invasion comes first, it appears necessary to study the timing of the trophoblast invasion in the distal portions of the segmental mesometrial arteries of the guinea pig since, for these arteries, the time course of the structural widening and growth is known quantatively (Moll et al., 1983).

## Control of Structural Widening by Humoral Factors

A likely hypothesis for the control of the structural widening is the concept that the control occurs by humoral factors possibly produced by the fetal-placental unit in proportion to the fetal-placental mass. A model for such a factor and possibly the factor itself is estradiol. Greiss and Marshton (1965) have reported a 40 percent increase in the uterine blood flow of ewes in the last third of pregnancy following the systemic infusion of exogenous estrogen. Rosenfeld and associates (1975) showed that estradiol induces vasodilatation in placental cotyledons of the ewe throughout pregnancy. Estradiol can even produce arterial changes which have some of the characteristics of the physiological changes. In guinea pigs, a single injection of a medium long acting estrogen (estradiol benzoate) provokes typical structural widening (Moll and Götz, 1985) and stimulates DNA synthesis (Makinoda and Moll, 1986). To test the concept of humoral control by estradiol, the structural widening during long term application of estradiol simulating continuous release of estradiol by the placenta should be studied.

In the present study, three concepts for triggering and control of the structural widening are tested by measurements of internal arterial diameters (Nienartowicz) and $^{3}$H-thymidine incorporation (Lenz) and by light and electron microscopic studies (Hees and Wrobel). The experiments were performed in rats and guinea pigs.

## MATERIALS AND METHODS

### Animals

Virgin guinea pigs and Sprague-Dawley rats were obtained from Dr. Ivanovas, Kisslegg, Allgäu, FRG. Estrous cycle in the guinea pigs was followed by

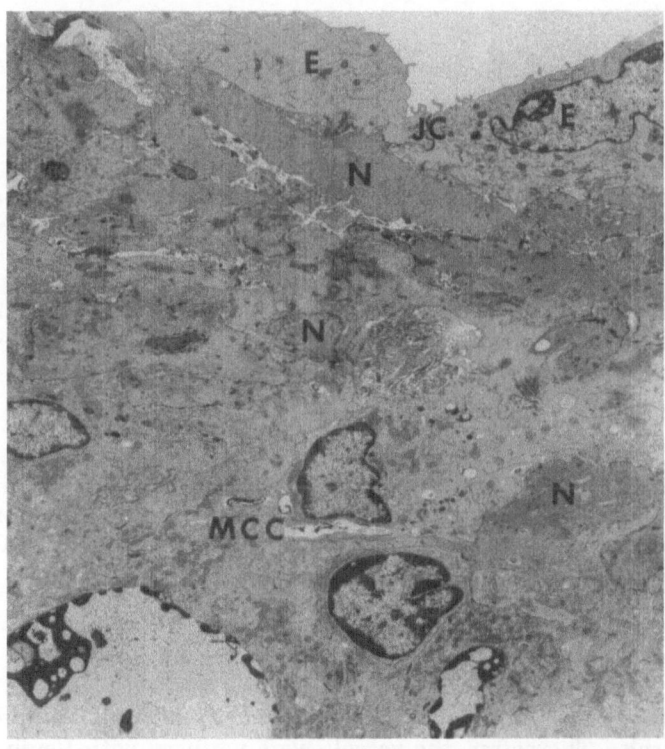

Figure 3. Complex of mononuclear cells in the media of a segmental mesometrial artery of a pregnant guinea pig (9th week). The wall shows degenerated and destroyed areas. Note the normal continuous endothelial lining. E = endothelial cells, JC = junctional complex, N = necrosis, MCC = medial cell complex. X4000.

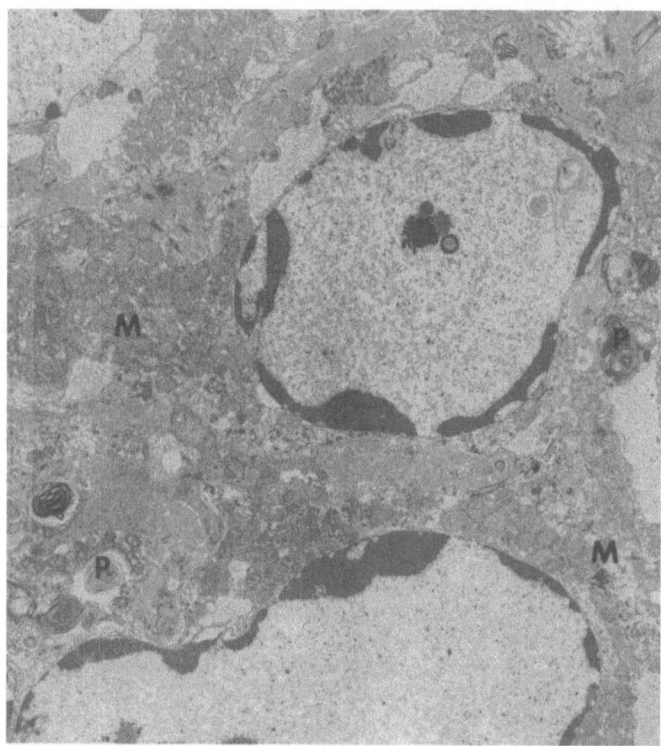

Figure 4. Giant cell in the media of a segmental mesometrial artery of a guinea pig (9th week of pregnancy). M = mitochondria, P = signs of phagocytosis. X7300.


daily vaginal inspection. The first day of the last rupture of the vagina was taken as day 0 of pregnancy. In rats, vaginal smears were taken. The day, when sperm was found in the vagina, was noted as day 1 of pregnancy.

## Anesthesia

For perfusion fixation of organs and for the excision of arteries, the animals were anaesthetized with diazepam (10 mg i.m.) and pentobarbital (30 mg/kg i.p.). The animals were ventilated using a Starling pump. Ovariectomy was performed under halothane anesthesia.

### Perfusion Fixation and Electron Microscope Studies

A catheter was inserted into the aorta via the left ventricle. A colloidal procaine solution (1 g/l) with polyvinylpyrolidone (25 g/l) was injected in order to dilate the vessels. Thereafter, the vessels were perfused with Bouin solution for light microscopy and with solution according to Karnovski (1965) for electron microscopy. For electron microscopy, the tissues were embedded in ERL 4206. The studies were performed on 4 virgin and 4 pregnant animals at each week of pregnancy.

## Microscopic Measurements for Diameters and Wall Thickness

These measurements were performed as described previously (Moll and Götz, 1985). Briefly, the arteries were excised from the fat-free mesometrium and cannulated using glass capillaries. The arteries were placed in $Ca^{2+}$-free Tyrode's solution containing papaverine (40 mg/l) and held at physiological temperature, pH and $pCO_2$. The arteries were filled with blood or gas in order to contrast the lumen. The arteries were closed at the distal end with a small clamp, and the intraarterial pressure was adjusted to 60 mm Hg. Measurements were made with a screw ocular micrometer.

$^3$H-thymidine incorporation as a measure of DNA synthesis was measured as described by Makinoda and Moll (1986). The excised arteries were incubated in culture medium containing $^3$H-thymidine (specific activity: 2 TBq/mmol; radioactive concentration: 185 KBq/ml). After 4 hours, the arteries were extracted with perchloric acid. The remaining radioactivity was measured and related to arterial length.

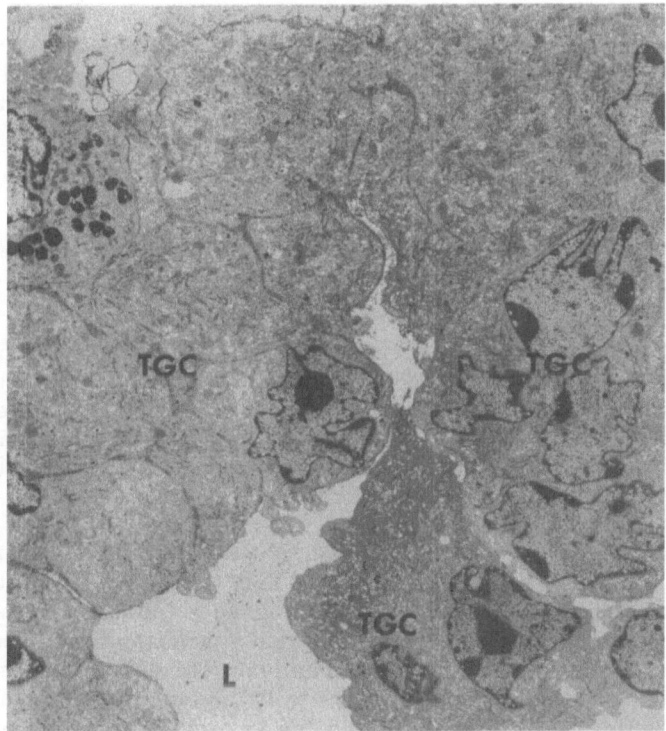

Figure 5. Apparent trophoblastic giant cells in the endothelium of a segmental mesometrial artery in the ninth week of pregnancy. L = lumen, TGC = apparent trophoblastic giant cell. X4000.

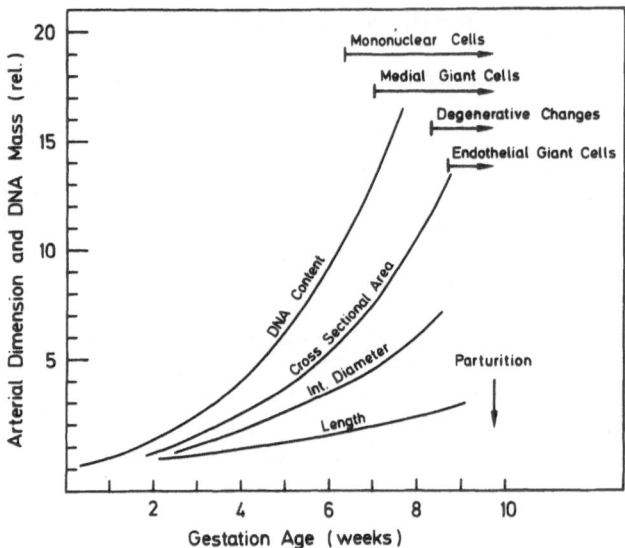

Figure 6. The timing of the appearance of mononuclear cells, degenerative changes and giant cells in the endothelium (horizontal arrows) compared to the time course of DNA content, cross sectional area, internal diameter, and length of preuterine segmental mesometrial arteries of guinea pigs during pregnancy. The lines are fitted curves of experimental data obtained by Moll et al. (1983) with the initial value as unity. The curves show the ratio of the data observed in pregnant animals over those observed in virgin animals. Degenerative changes and giant cells appear after most of the widening and the growth have already occurred.

## RESULTS AND DISCUSSION

### Widening of the Rat Arcade During Changed Blood Flow

In order to observe effects of altered blood flow on the physiological changes, the left uterine artery of the rat was tied on day 8. It is known that fetal growth is normal under these conditions (Barr and Brent, 1970). It is to be expected that, after ligation, blood flow velocity falls towards zero at the cervical end of the arcade (at the site of occlusion). For these conditions of drastically reduced blood flow velocity, the left and right cervical ends of the arcade were compared. The present data (Figure 2) do not show any significant difference between the left end (ligated cervical) and the right one (intact). The ligated left cervical end reached about the same internal diameter as the intact cervical end. Obviously, a drastic reduction in blood flow velocity did not prevent the pregnancy induced arterial widening. Interesting enough, the ovarian end of the ligated arcade appeared to be wider than the one of a non-ligated arcade in a control animal. The difference was at the limit of statistical significance. There appears to be a compensatory reaction to the ligation. While this reaction is in line with the concept of diameter control by blood flow velocity, it may also be explained by a humoral factor. Thus, conclusive evidence could not be found that the local shear stress on the arterial wall triggers and controls the normal structural widening of the uteroplacental arteries.

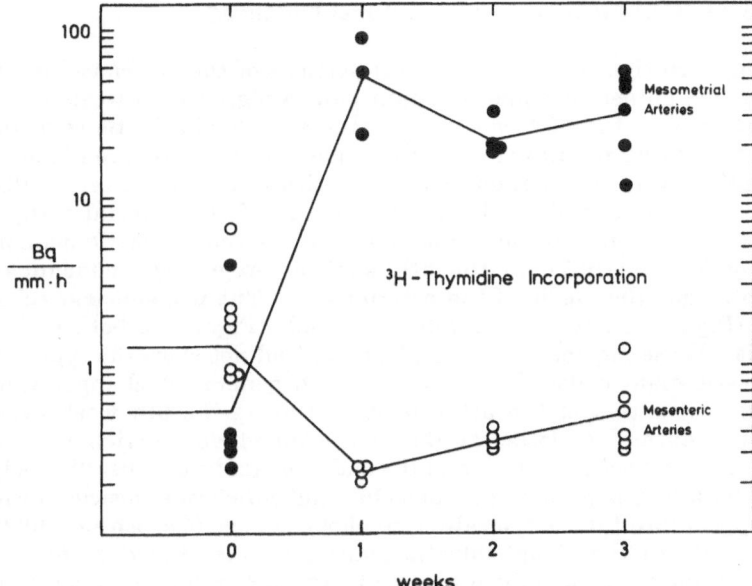

Figure 7. $^3$H-thymidine incorporation of segmental mesometrial arteries and mesenteric arteries of nonpregnant ovariectomized guinea pigs after daily injection of 7-11 µg estradiol benzoate. The open and closed circles indicate the means obtained in single animals. The number of animals used is equal to the number of closed circles.

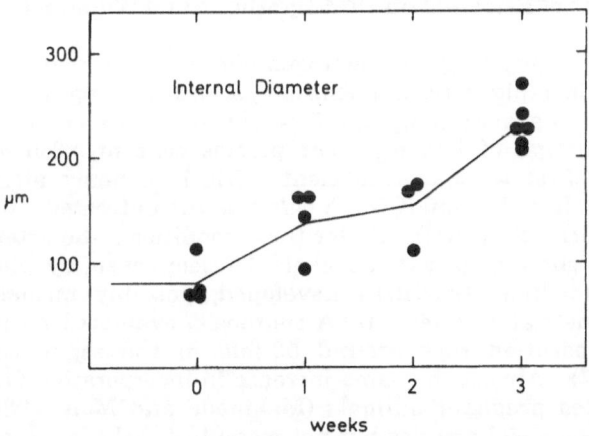

Figure 8. Internal diameter of segmental mesometrial arteries of ovariectomized guinea pigs during a 3 week treatment with estradiol benzoate (7-11 µg daily). The open and closed circles indicate the means obtained in single animals. The number of animals used is equal to the number of closed circles.

## Timing of Giant Cell Invasion and Structural Widening

Using perfusion fixation, the distal portions of the segmental mesometrial arteries of virgin guinea pigs and pregnant guinea pigs of each week of pregnancy from the 1st until to the 10th week were studied.  Trophoblastic cells which are described to be large multinucleated cells (giant cells) with prominent nucleoli and abundant cysternal endoplasmatic reticulum (Carpenter, 1982) were examined.  The sections showed massive growth of the arterial wall, signs of structural dilatation, and, in mid-pregnancy, dissolution of elastic membranes as described by Albert (1967). In the 5th week of pregnancy, mononuclear cells appeared to invade the media of the arterial wall.  The mononuclear cells formed aggregates (Figure 3) and occasionally giant cells (Figure 4), both with signs of phagocytosis.  These medial giant cells, however, did not show the typical features of trophoblastic giant cells.  In the 8th week, degenerative changes were found resulting in destruction of the arterial wall  During the 9th week even in the presence of a normal endothelial lining continued destruction was observed (Figure 3).  Giant cells were not seen in the endothelium before the 9th week (Figure 5).  These cells had a prominent nucleolus and numerous vesicles providing a sieve-like appearance that is typical for trophoblast cells (Carpenter, 1982).  Thus, there was evidence that trophoblastic giant cells also invaded the segmental mesometrial arteries of the guinea pigs as it was shown for the hamster by Ward Orsini (1954), Pijnenborg et al. (1974) and Carpenter (1982).  However, the endothelial, trophoblast-like giant cells were not seen before a stage of pregnancy where the physiological changes of the studied mesometrial arteries were almost fully developed (Figure 6).  This was even true for the giant cells found in the media. On the basis of this distinct sequential pattern, it was concluded for the mesometrial arteries of the guinea pig, that the physiological changes were neither triggered nor controlled by trophoblast giant cells.  Trophoblast cells were unlikely to be the regulators of the physiological changes of the segmental mesometrial arteries of guinea pigs (cf. Moll, Hees, and Wrobel, *Placenta*, in press).

## Long Term Effects of Estradiol on DNA Synthesis and Widening

In order to study long term estrogen effects on the segmental mesometrial arteries of the guinea pig, estradiol benzoate, a medium long acting estradiol, was injected s.c. into the neck daily for 3 weeks in nonpregnant, ovariectomized guinea pigs in dosages of 7-11 µg.  The plasma concentration of estradiol was measured in the first week of treatment.  Within 6 hours after injection, the concentration rose from 5 pg/ml (SD = 5 pg/ml) in the untreated animal to a level of about 60 pg/ml (SD = 25 pg/ml).  Under these conditions, the arteries of estrogen-treated animals showed growth as could be seen even by visual inspection.  Sometimes, tumor-like structures developed, possibly formed by confluent segmental mesometrial arteries.  DNA synthesis, evaluated on the basis of [3]H-thymidine incorporation rose around 50-fold in the segmental mesometrial arteries (Figure 7).  Almost the same increase in incorporation (40-fold) has been found in untreated pregnant animals (Makinoda and Moll, 1986).  Interesting enough, only mesometrial arteries but not mesenteric arteries responded this way.  DNA content (not shown) increased 2-3 times in the segmental mesometrial arteries.  Obviously, estradiol or one of its metabolites stimulated proliferation and widening of the arterial wall as it was observed during pregnancy.  There was a steady increase in internal diameter (Figure 8). The diameter at the end of the 3 week treatment was 2-3 times the initial diameter which meant a 10-100 times increase in vascular conductance. In pregnant animals, the internal diameter increased also 2 times during the course of 3 weeks (Moll et al. 1983). Thus long term increases in the plasma concentration of estradiol may well provoke proliferation and widening, i.e., typical physiological changes in the uteroplacental arteries. These experiments demonstrated that the structural widening may be provoked by humoral factors that were produced by the fetoplacental unit.

## Conclusions

The present data indicate that, in the segmental mesometrial arteries of rodents studied, neither increased flow rate nor invasion of trophoblastic giant cells trigger and control the structural widening. On the other hand, estradiol appeared to be able to provoke structural widening and growth of the segmental mesometrial arteries. Thus, the physiological changes in the uteroplacental arteries and placental blood flow were likely to be controlled by humoral factors. It is tempting to speculate that such factors were produced by the fetoplacental unit in proportion to its mass so that placental blood flow was adjusted to fetoplacental growth. However, further studies are needed to confirm this concept in rodents and to test it in primates.

### SUMMARY

As shown by measurements of the intravascular pressure profile, the uteroplacental arteries are the site of the limiting resistance to placental blood flow in species with a hemochorial placenta. During the course of pregnancy, the flow resistance of the uteroplacental arteries is decreased by structural widening of the lumen associated with growth and degeneration of the arterial wall (the physiological changes of the uteroplacental arteries), so that maternal placental flow is adjusted to fetal growth. As controlling factors of the physiological changes intra-arterial blood flow velocity, invading trophoblastic giant cells and humoral factors are likely candidates.

In order to test possible factors for control, (1) arterial widening of the uterine arcade during pregnancy was studied in the rat under conditions of reduced blood flow velocity, (2) the timing of trophoblastic giant cell invasion was compared with that of structural widening and growth of the distal portions of the segmental mesometrial arteries of guinea pigs, and (3) on the same arteries, it was tested whether long term treatment with estradiol might induce physiological changes. It was found that the physiological changes tested proceeded normally even under conditions of reduced blood flow velocity, appeared earlier than the trophoblast invasion and might be induced by long term estradiol treatment. It was concluded that neither increased local blood flow velocity nor invading trophoblastic giant cells were primarily responsible for the physiological changes in the mesometrial arteries of the species studied. The structural widening and placental blood flow were likely to be controlled by estradiol or other humoral factors.

## ACKNOWLEDGEMENTS

We are indebted to R. Götz, S. Klappstein, and R. Ludwig for their most expert technical help.

## REFERENCES

Albert, E.N. (1967) The effect of pregnancy on the elastic membranes of mesometrial arteries in the guinea pig. *Am. J. Anat.* 120, 611-621.

Barr, M. and Brent, R.L. (1970) The relation of the uterine vasculature to fetal growth and the uterine position effect in rats. *Teratology* 3, 251-260.

Bell, C. (1974) Control of uterine blood flow in pregnancy. *Medical Biology* 52, 219-228.

Brosens, I., Robertson, B., and Dixon, H.G. (1967) The physiological response of the vessels of the placental bed to normal pregnancy *J. Pathol. Bacteriol.* 93, 569-579.

Carpenter, S.J. (1982) Trophoblast invasion and alteration of mesometrial arteries in the pregnant hamster: Light and electron microscopic observations *Placenta* 3, 219-242.

Del Campo, C. and Ginther, O.J. (1972) Vascular anatomy of the uterus and ovaries and the unilateral luteolytic effect of the uterus: Guinea pigs, rats, hamsters, and rabbits. *Am. J. Vet. Res.* 33, 2561-2578.

Egund, N. and Carter, A.M. (1974) Uterine and placental circulation in the guinea pig: An angiographic study. *J. Reprod. Fert.* 40, 401-410.

Girard, H., Brun, J.-L., and Muffat-Joly, M. (1971) An angiographic study of the sensitivity to epinephrine of the uterine arteries of the guinea pig: A comparison with angiotensin. *J. Obstet. Gynecol.* 111, 687-691.

Greiss, F.C. and Marston, E.L. (1965) The uterine vascular bed: Effect of estrogens during ovine pregnancy. *Am. J. Obstet. Gynecol.* 95, 720-722.

Harris, J.W.S. and Ramsey, E.M. (1966) The morphology of human uteroplacental vasculature. *Carn. Inst. Contrib. Embryol.* 38, 43-58.

Hees, H., Moll, W., and Wrobel, K.H. (1984) Veränderungen an den Radialarterien des Meerschweinchens während der Gravidität. *Verh. Anat. Ges.* 78, 235-237.

Karnovsky, J. (1965) A formaldehyde-glutaraldehyde fixative of high osmolarity for use in electron microscopy. *J. Cell Biol.* 27, 137A-138A.

Lundgren, N. (1957) Studies on the vasculature of the corpus of the human uterus. *Acta Obstet. Gynecol. Scand.* 36, 13-19.

Makinoda, S. and Moll, W. (1986) DNA synthesis in mesometrial arteries in guinea pigs during oestrous cycle, pregnancy and under treatment with oestradiol benzoate. *Placenta* 7, 189-198.

Moll, W. and Kuenzel, W. (1971) Blood pressures in the uterine vascular system of anaesthetized pregnant guinea pigs. *Pflügers Arch.* 330, 310-322.

Moll, W. and Kuenzel, W. (1973) The blood pressure in arteries entering the placentae of guinea pigs, rats, rabbits, and sheep. *Pflügers Arch.* 338, 125-131.

Moll, W., Kuenzel, W., Stolte, L.A.M., Kleinhout, J., de Jong, P.A., and Veth, A.F.L. (1974) The blood pressure in the decidual part of the uteroplacental arteries (spiral arteries) of the rhesus monkey. *Pflügers Arch.* 346, 291-297.

Moll, W., Espach, A., and Wrobel, K.H. (1983) Growth of mesometrial arteries in guinea pigs during pregnancy. *Placenta* 4, 111-124.

Moll, W. (1985) Physiological aspects of placental ontogeny and phylogeny. *Placenta* 6, 141-154.

Moll, W. and Götz, R. (1985) Pressure-diameter curves of mesometrial arteries of guinea pigs demonstrate a non-muscular, oestrogen-inducible mechanism of lumen regulation. *Pflügers Arch.* 404, 332-336.

Pijnenborg, R., Robertson, W.B., and Brosens, I. (1974) The arterial migration of trophoblast in the uterus of the golden hamster, Mesocricetus auratus. *J. Reprod. Fert.* 40, 269-280

Rankin, J.H.G. and McLaughlin, M.K. (1979) The regulation of placental blood flows. *J. Develop. Physiol.* 1, 3-30

Rankin, J.H.G., Phenetton, T.M., Anderson, D.F., and Bersenbrugge, A.D. (1979) Effect of prostaglandin I on ovine placental vasculature *J. Develop. Physiol.* 1, 151-160.

Reynolds, M. (1963) Maternal blood flow in the uterus and placenta. In: *Handbook of Physiology*, Section 2: Circulation, Vol.II, (eds.), W.F. Hamilton and P. Dow.

Rosenfeld, C.R., Morris, F.H., Battaglia, F.C., Makowski, E.L., and Meschia, G. (1975) Effect of estradiol-17 on blood flow to reproductive and nonreproductive tissues in pregnant ewes. *Am. J. Obstet. Gynecol.* 124, 618-629.

Schoop, W. and Rau, G. (1958) Uber die Ursachen der Arterienveränderungen bei arteriovenösen *Fisteln. Zeitschrift Kreislaufforsch.* 47, 503-510.

Ward Orsini, M. (1954) The trophoblastic giant cells and endo-vascular cells associated with pregnancy in the hamster, Cricetus auratus. *Am. J. Anat.* 94, 273-321.

Wigglesworth, J.S. (1964) Experimental growth retardation in the foetal rat. *J. Pathol. Bact.* 88, 1-13.

**Trophoblast Research 3:97-110, 1988**

# MORPHOLOGICAL STUDIES OF LACUNAR FORMATION IN THE EARLY RABBIT PLACENTA

Rudolf Leiser[1] and Henning M. Beier

Department of Anatomy and Reproductive Biology
RWTH University Aachen
Melatener Strasse 211
D-5100 Aachen, FR Germany

## INTRODUCTION

Lacunae are maternal blood vessels, bordered by trophoblast cells, which begin to develop during late implantation. They are typical of hemochorial placentation. As shown in this comparative study by high resolution light microscopy and SEM micrographs of vessel casts, lacunae are formed from the preimplantational endometrial vasculature by the loss of vessel walls and partly by changing of the vessel's architecture.

This rather complex morphological process is susceptible to pathological deviations, which may be responsible for the fact that less than 50% of human fertilized eggs survive the time of blastocyst implantation (Lauritsen, 1982; Beier, 1984). However, since lacunar formation at these early stages cannot be adequately studied in the human, the rabbit serves as a model for this research. The rabbit and the human share hemochorial placentation, and to a certain extent, a similar endocrine background in early pregnancy (Beier et al., 1983; Fischer et al., 1985). This comparative study focuses on the morphological aspects only.

## MATERIALS AND METHODS

Fourteen nulliparous rabbits (mixed breeds) were mated and then studied between 7 d 16 h - 10 d post coitum (p.c.).

Pretreatment of the rabbits with 0.1 mg phentolamine i.m. (Regitin R, Ciba: Basel, Switzerland) to reduce vasoconstriction, and with 5000 I.E. sodium heparin as an anticoagulant (Thrombophob R: Nordmark-Werke, GmbH, Hamburg, FRG) was performed via injection into the lateral ear vein. The animals were anesthesized with sodium pentobarbital i.v. (Nembutal R, 24 mg/kg body weight). Later, an overdose of the same drug was used to kill the rabbits at the beginning of perfusion (see below).

For histology using semithin sections, after laparotomy, only a short perfusion of the uterus (10 sec) was used at a pressure of 80-100 mm Hg with 0.1 M phosphate/saccharose buffer (pH 7.4, 400 mosm, 37°C) through the abdominal aorta.

[1]To Whom Correspondence Should Be Addressed: Department of Animal Anatomy, University of Bern, Postfach 2735, CH-3001 Bern, Switzerland

Perfusion fixation, lasting 5 minutes, followed through one uterus only, using 2.2% glutaraldehyde in 0.1 M phosphate buffer (pH 7.4, 400 mosm, 20°C). Smaller specimens from the implantation sites were then fixed by immersion in the same solution for 2 hours at 20°C. Postfixation took place in 0.1 M phosphate buffered 2% $OsO_4$ for one hour at 4°C. Following dehydration in a graded series of ethanol, the material was embedded in Araldite. Semithin sections were stained using the Richardson's method with methylene blue.

For vessel casting, the contralateral uterus of the uterus duplex was isolated during the initial fixation by clamps, and the above described short perfusion with a buffer was prolonged through the uterine artery until the outflow through the uterine veins was free of blood. Afterwards the preparation was cooled to 5°C by rinsing with the same solution. As plastic components Batson No. 17 corrosion compound ® (Polysciences) was mixed with Sevritron ® (33:12), which were cooled and freshly prepared immediately before injecting into the rinsed uterine artery. Then the injected organ was excised and placed in a water bath at 20°C for 0.5 hours, followed by 80°C for 4 hours to allow for the plastic to harden.

Corrosion of the specimens was accomplished by alternating immersion in 40% KOH and distilled water at 60°C. To obtain suitable pieces for mounting, large pieces of the casts were embedded in 20% warm gelatin (50°C) and frozen to -5°C for cutting with a knife, or frozen in liquid nitrogen for cracking. After thawing, gelatin was removed by a second corrosion procedure. From the cut or cracked air dried casts, suitable specimens were selected by means of stereo microscopy, which were mounted on stubs, sputter-coated with gold and examined with the scanning electron microscope. For further technical details see Leiser and Kohler (1983), Leiser (1985), and Dantzer et al. (this volume).

## RESULTS

The subepithelial vascular plexus in the rabbit mesometrial endometrium at 7 d 16 h p.c. represents the latest "preimplantational" stage (Figures 1 and 2). This plexus shows no signs of lacunar development at this time, because the mesometrial definitive process of implantation with subsequent development of the chorioallantoic placenta does not start before 8 d p.c. (Larsen, 1961; for comparative review histology and vessel terminology see Mossman, 1926; Amoroso, 1952; Tsutsumi, 1962; Hafez and Tsutsumi, 1966; Carter, 1975). This plexus is located as a 0.7 mm thick layer in the upper third of the two mesometrial preplacental folds and connects the stem arterioles to the arcuate venules (Figure 8). The subepithelial plexus consists of numerous capillary loops with relatively wide arches (Figure 2). The arterial limbs of these loops are sparse; they are short (0.2 mm) but large in diameter (25 μm). In contrast, the venous limbs are numerous, long, (0.7 mm) and thin (10 μm). These venous limbs are found perpendicular to the surface of the preplacental fold (Figures 2 and 8). As part of the interglandular tissue, the venous limbs reflect the same orientation as the straight gland tubes, which are demonstrated histologically in Figure 1. Shown in detail on the casts, the capillary loops have a rather smooth surface with indistinct bulges and constrictions. Their arterial limbs are marked by clearly visible impressions of the endothelial nuclei oriented along the vessel axis, whereas in the venous limbs some shallow endothelial imprints may occasionally be observed (Figure 2).

The subepithelial vascular plexus of day 9 p.c. becomes distinctly involved in the implantation process at the mesometrial placental folds of the endometrium. As demonstrated by the casts (Figure 3), the outermost capillary loops are enlarged to 30 to 50 μm, and locally may show some extravasation of plastic. This is a typical indication of lacunar formation, observable by vessel casts. Such vessel dilatations (surface sinuses: Mossman, 1926), located in the neighborhood of the trophoblast, are called arterial prelacunae because of their development on the arterial side of the future lacunar system and their histologically visible vessel wall debris (Figure 8; compare also Figure 5). More distant from the trophoblast, at the subepithelial capillary plexus, distinct coilings and constrictions appear, which affect this vascular layer as a whole, being compressed to the same size (0.7 mm) as observed on day 7 d 16 h p.c. (see above; Figure 3).

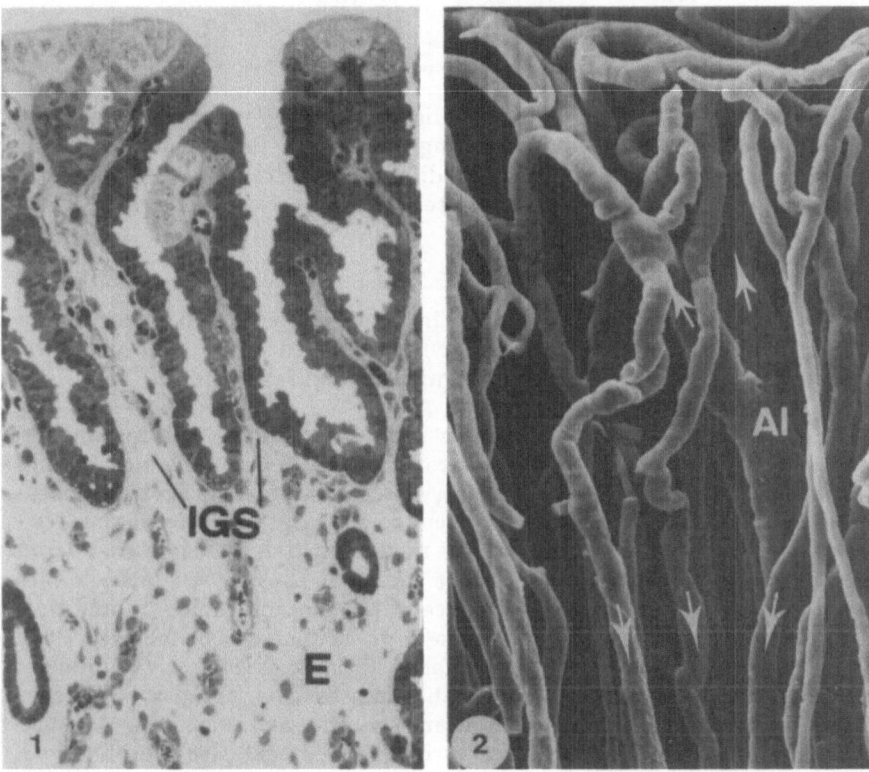

Figures 1 and 2. Correlative micrographs of histology and vessel casts from the mesometrially located endometrial fold of 7 d 16 h p.c. Typical for the preimplantational stage, the vasculature of the interglandular septa (IGS) is oriented strictly parallel to the gland tubes and forms wide subepithelial loops. An arteriole, characterized by endothelial impressions (AI), ramifies into a few thick arterial capillary limbs (upper arrows) which differ from the more numerous, thinner venous limbs (lower arrows). In Figure 1, stromal edema (E) and patches of clear epithelium forming a symplasma indicate the beginning of trophoblast contact. X130.

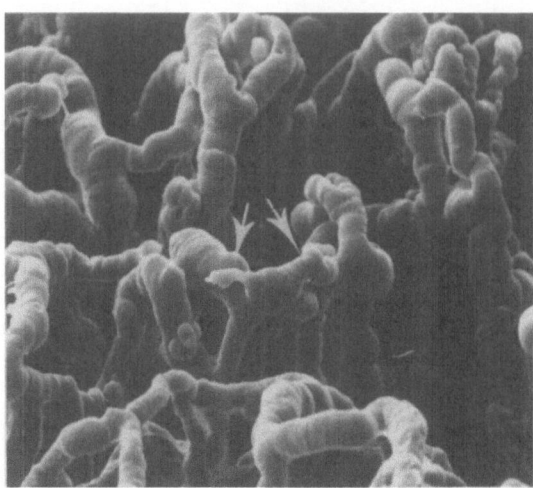

Figure 3.  A vessel cast of the subepithelial capillary plexus in the mesometrial endometrium on day 9 p.c.  The beginning of lacunar  formation is indicated by coiling and constrictions as well as by dilated parts of capillary loops.  Some extravasation of plastic on these dilated parts (arrows) refers to the first discontinuities in the vessel wall. X130.

The subepithelial capillary plexus, from day 9 to 10 p.c., becomes thoroughly transformed by chorionic processes, which extend some 300 µm into the endometrium.  Three zones can be distinguished (Figures 5 and 8):

1) At the base of these chorionic processes, Zone 1, the former arterial prelacunae on top of the capillary loops (compare day 9 p.c.) have now changed to real trophoblast-bordered arterial lacunae, which lack any debris of uterine tissue. As visible on the casts (Figure 4), these lacunae are large and have diameters of up to 150 µm. With a ratio of 1:3, they are less numerous than their precursors from the capillary loops.  This correlates with the fact that these large lacunae form by fusing into a network, covering the surface of the placental fold.  In addition, the stages of transition from capillary loops to large lacunae can be followed clearly in the fine structure of the vessel cast surface, shown in Figure 4.  Capillaries are characterized by a few scattered endothelial impressions, prelacunae by a grainy roughness derived from disintegrating uterine tissue, and lacunae by trophoblast-effected crinkles as well as circular constrictions (compare also Figure 5).

2) Situated between the intermediate parts of these chorionic processes, Zone 2 (Figures 5 and 8), are small capillary-type lacunae (trophoblastic tubules: Mossman, 1926), which are visible from day 9 to 10 p.c.  They have about the same vessel diameter as the former venous limbs of subepithelial capillaries (10-20 µm), have a similar orientation perpendicular to the surface of placental fold, and are nearly as numerous (compare Figures 2 and 6).  Therefore, the mode of development of the small capillary lacunae seems to be by growth of the chorionic processes along the venous limbs.  However, this original pattern of growth soon becomes obscure, probably as a result of trophoblast-mediated coiling, wrinkling, and branching of the vessels (Figure 5).  This development as a whole leads to the

appearance of a labyrinthine lacunal system, as conspicuously demonstrated on the vessel cast in Figure 6.

     3) The upper part of the chorionic processes at day 10 p.c. is characterized as Zone 3 (Figures 5 and 8). It represents a similar initial stage of lacunar formation, as first observed at day 9 p.c., but by now it has dislocated itself along with the edge of the trophoblast, advancing into the endometrium. Venous prelacunae develop from the venous limbs of subepithelial capillaries and/or endometrial venules by disintegration and dissolution of the vessel wall, increasing the vessel diameter up to 120 µm. Additional disintegration and degeneration of the adjacent decidual cells favor fusion of the venous prelacunae also (Figure 5). Therefore, a venous prelacunal system develops, which oriented roughly across the feto-maternal axis, collects many small capillary lacunae from the placental labyrinth. However, it gives rise to only a few moderately enlarged stem venules (diameter up to 100 µm), directed towards the venous sinus plexus (Mossman, 1926), as seen in Figures 7 and 8.

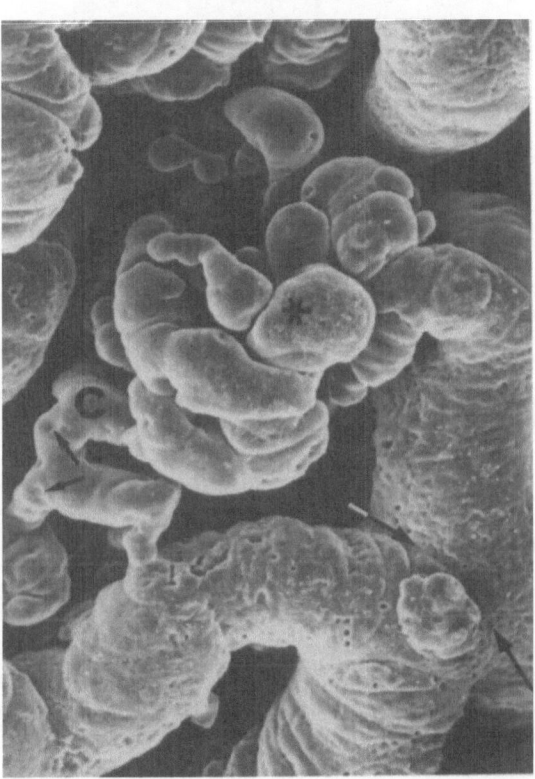

Figure 4. Formation of a network of large maternal lacunae viewed from the fetal side of the cast at 9 d 12 h p.c. The transition is well documented from capillary loops (C) with endothelial nuclear impressions (small arrows), to dilated prelacunae showing the grainy roughness of the disintegrating vessel wall(*), and then to large lacunae being characterized by crinkles and circular constrictions from trophoblast. The large arrows point to a possible fusion between two large lacunae. Note the small but distinct imprints from erythrocytes marginally located in the vessels. X250.

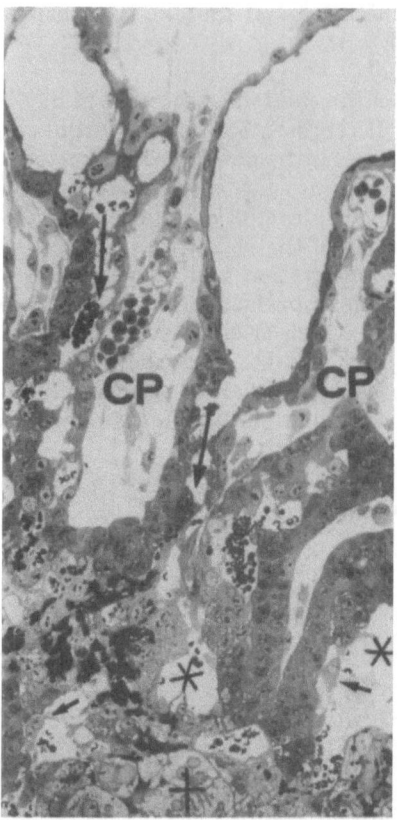

Figure 5. Histological micrograph of lacunal formation on day 10 p.c. Two large arterial lacunae (top) being separated by chorionic processes (CP), continue in small capillary-type lacunae (long arrows) and venous prelacunae (*). On the edge of the chorionic processes, these prelacunae, characterized by enclosed endothelial debris (short arrows), are surrounded by degenerating uterine tissue such as decidual cells (+). Note the scattered aggregations of extravasated blood close to the venous lacunae in the lower left corner. X130.

When crossing the advancing edge of the trophoblast, the few arterioles change by a similar phenomenon of prelacunar formation, as do the venules. The arterial prelacunae and lacunae, however, become more dilated (Figure 8).

## DISCUSSION

### Methodological Aspects

A combination of corresponding semithin section histology and micro-corrosion vessel casting with scanning electron microscopic analysis proved useful in studying the importance of microvasculature in lacunar formation. Semithin sections are convenient for recognizing arterioles, capillaries, venules and lacunae by their defined location in the endometrium, form, size, and vessel wall composition.   In addition, these histological procedures demonstrate the relationship of these vessels to the surrounding structures such as connective tissue and epithelium of the endometrial surface and glands.   In contrast, vessel casting lacks the corroded natural vascular environment, but impresses one by providing a clear three-dimensional replica of the general vascular architecture.   A clear distinction of the different parts of endometrial blood vessels also is possible in the casts by the different patterns and forms of imprints by endothelial or trophoblastic cell profiles.   Measurements of the diameters for the various vessel casts  are reliable because there is only a negligible difference between semithin sections and vessel casts caused by shrinkage (Kaufmann et al., 1985). The technique of vessel casting injected immediately before prelacunar formation also produces plastic leakage from vessel dilatations.   Although this extravasation may appear mainly as an artifact, and possibly can be avoided by injecting the resin smoothly at the lowest possible pressure (cf. rat: Rogers and Gannon, 1981), it is useful for the

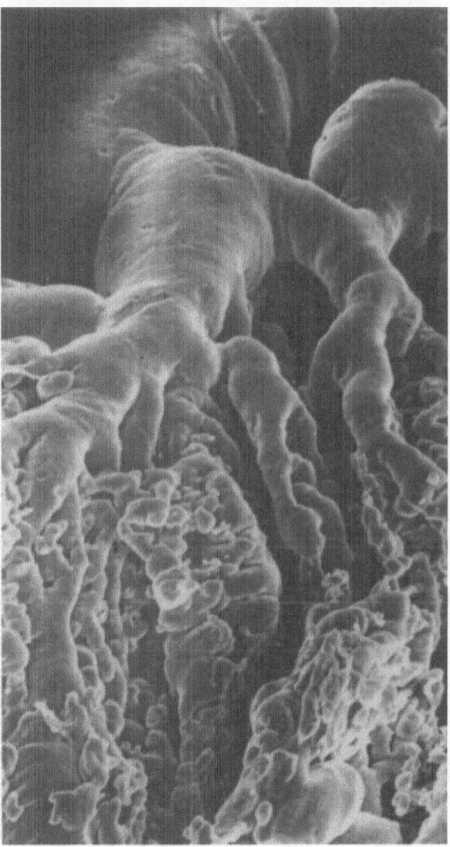

Figure 6.  Vessel cast corresponding to Figure 5.  Numerous small capillary-type lacunae ramify from the network of large lacunae (top).  Additional outgrowths and branchings of these small lacunae contribute to the complex labyrinthine lacunar system. X200.

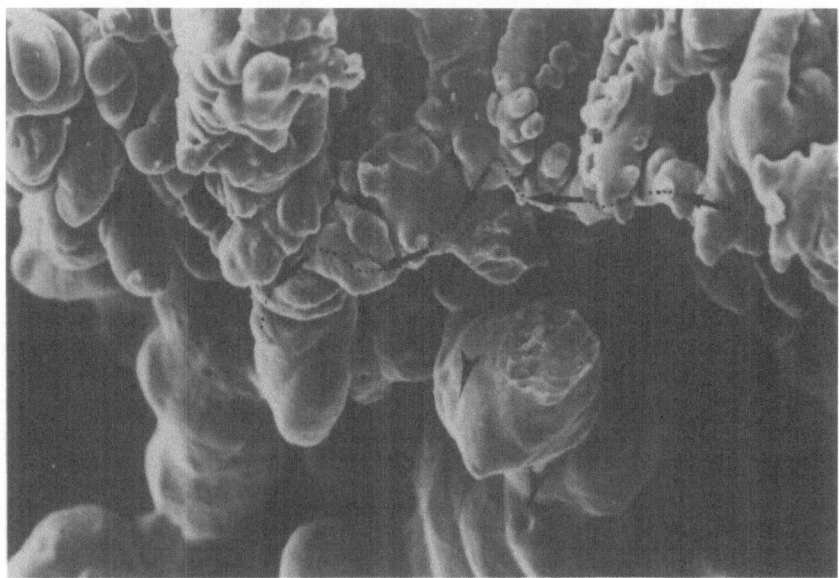

Figure 7. Vessel cast corresponding to the edge of chorionic processes in Figure 5. Numerous small capillary-type lacunae of the labyrinth (top) are collected by a complex system of fused venous prelacunae (arrows). A few stem venules, characterized by occasional endothelial impressions (arrowheads), continue from the prelacunal system to the venous sinus plexus not visible here. X350.

current interpretation and serves as the first distinct indication for localizing the "implantation reaction" in vessel casts.

## Selected Structural Phenomena of Lacunar Formation

The development of allantochorionic lacunar formation starts from the mesometrially located subepithelial capillary plexus. There are no distinct structural changes visible on vessel casts until about day 9 p.c., as suggested by Nakamura and Ninomiya (1979) and confirmed in this study. This period is defined as preimplantational (Figure 8), but lacunar development has already begun in the rabbit in a preparative and sustaining way by 6 d 12 h p.c. This so-called "uterine vascular response" is triggered by the presence of blastocysts in the uterus (Hoffman and Davies, 1971; Hoos and Hoffmann, 1980). This response involves morphological phenomena such as thickening of the layer of subepithelial capillary plexus (Hafez and Tsutsumi, 1966), stromal edema resulting from increased capillary permeability and, among others, the decidual cell reaction and degeneration (Finn, 1977; Hoos and Hoffman, 1980).

The coiling of the capillary limbs in the subepithelial plexus is observed by Hafez and Tsutsumi (1966) to be "slightly tortuous" and indicates a clear change from the preimplantational to implantational vascular architecture (Figure 8). Reduced stromal consistency, which is influenced by edema and decidualization, may allow for these morphological changes (see above).

However, the vessel wall with its distinct impressions of endothelial nuclei appear uninjured. The vessel dilatation first is noted at the outermost part of the subepithelial capillary loops (Figure 8). In addition to the influence from the edema and decidualization, this dilatation develops at the beginning of vessel wall disintegration, which is induced by the nearby chorion or invasiveness of the trophoblast, respectively (Larsen, 1961; Denker, 1980; Steven, 1983). In the early stage of this disintegration, the cast surface appears coarse and irregular, whereas in the late stages it is rather grainy. Vessel disruption may be a phenomenon equal to that of the vessel dilatation, but it is more conspicuous because of the artificial extravasation of plastic in the casts. Nakamura and Ninomiya (1978) described similar extravasations in the periplacental fold which, however in this study, was never seen as a site of a such implantation-dependent vessel reaction. Some natural extravasation of maternal blood may occur by the degeneration of the vessel wall and the disintegration of stroma in the placental fold, as is visible histologically in Figure 5, and as stated by Mossman (1926) and Hafez and Tsutsumi (1966). This phenomenon, however, requires further research.

Fusion of vessels form prelacunae, which are defined by a lytic vessel wall as well as the adjacent decidual stroma disintegrating and degenerating. Vessel fusion in this stage of development was not observed in the current morphological study, since it must be a very rapid process in vivo, probably controlled by blood flow dynamics. However, a strong suggestion of existing vessel fusion is proved by the fact that the network of large arterial lacunae distinctly originates from subepithelial capillary loops, being three times more numerous and with many fewer anastomoses.

Lacunae are vessels deformed by the total replacement of the lytic surroundings of maternal tissue to the chorion or the trophoblast, respectively. This vessel type, as a final step in the process of allantochorionic lacunar formation from the extremes of former subepithelial capillary loops to the network of large lacunae, appears first at about 9 d 12 h p.c. in the rabbit. In the casts, these lacunae during initial development, are rather smooth, but soon, because of the enormous shaping capacities of trophoblast (Larsen, 1961, 1962; Wynn and Davies, 1965; Denker, 1980), crinkles and constrictions develop. How the trophoblast and the decidual cell reaction, among other influences, may be involved in the detail of lacunar formation will be dealt with in another communication from the author's laboratory.

## Zonation of Lacunar Formation

The phenomena of lacunar formation are very distinct and rather easy to trace during the initial stages. They appear rather complex during zonation of the placenta. This zonation begins after 9 d 12 h p.c., when growth of the chorionic processes invades into the endometrium by passing the level of the large lacunae network, following the arterial and venous limbs of the subepithelial capillaries (Figure 8). These capillary limbs, continue to remain as numerous as earlier, change to lacunae by coiling, dilatation (disruption), and fusion as also observed in the extremes of capillary loops. There is a difference, however, in that the few arterial limbs which run into the network of large arterial lacunae, probably by high blood pressure, become more dilated than the venous ones; the latter vessels must compete for space and may remain narrow. Therefore these spaces are typically small (capillary-type) lacunae. Soon, these small lacunae lose their original rather smooth image on the casts, becoming shaped by trophoblast projections and new vessel branchings (unpublished data) into a very complex so-called placental labyrinth (Larsen, 1962). By the formation of this labyrinth, the network of large lacunae - zone 1 - becomes clearly distinguished from the system of small lacunae - zone 2 (Figure 8).

At the edge of advancing chorion, a zone 3 can first be defined about day 10 p.c. As part of the "intermediate region" between fetal and maternal tissue (Duval, 1889; Larsen, 1962), this zone will permanently give rise to lacunar formation (Figure 8). On its endometrially oriented side or front, the venous limbs of former subepithelial capillary plexus progressively transform to venous prelacunae showing the above described phenomena of lacunar formation. Even fusion may be very conspicuous here. It causes the development of a complex system of venous prelacunae from which only a few of the former vessels of the capillary plexus, as so-called stem venules, remain and connect this prelacunar system to the more centrally located venous sinus plexus. Behind this zone 3, venous prelacunae have changed into numerous small lacunae, which run out from the labyrinth and are collected by the system of venous prelacunae.

The 3-zone-pattern of the lacunar system in early rabbit placentation, established at day 10 p.c., remains the basic placental structure throughout pregnancy as evident from the histological figures of Mossman (1926). The labyrinth, inducing the system of small lacunae, however, will grow most and will provide, on the basis of its immense vascular surface, for the increasing needs in metabolic transport of the placenta (Amoroso, 1952).

### Lacunar Formation Related to Blood Pressure and Flow

Maternal blood permanently circulates through the lacunar system, when it is developing from the preimplantational subepithelial capillary plexus. It probably influences the channeling, as well as the shaping of vessels, partly by its pressure and flow characteristics (Carter, 1975). Because there are only a few arterioles irrigating the subepithelial capillary loops (Figure 8), the relatively high blood pressure helps, by dilatation and fusion, to change these loops into the voluminous system of the large arterial lacunar network (zone 1). Later the small capillary lacunae in formation (zone 2) do not dilate, since the blood pressure may not exceed the pressure from the numerous chorionic processes that flank these lacunae. In the zone of venous prelacunae (zone 3) the vessels are dilated, but some are obstructed and dislodged. This controversy may be a consequence of low (venous) blood pressure inducing almost a stagnation of blood as well as of the "softening" of the surrounding uterine tissue being in the state of decidual reaction and disintegration (Hoos and Hoffman, 1980; Garris and Dar, 1985). However, from this obstructed zone there is, and must be, outflow of blood towards the plexus of venous sinuses. A link is formed by a few so-called stem venules only. From these relatively small stem venules to this voluminous plexus the blood flow, according to the law of Hagen-Poiseuille, is accelerated (Carter, 1975; Faber and Thornburg, 1983). Therefore, this flow may affect, in addition, a rechanneling of vessels into the zone of venous prelacunae (Figure 8).

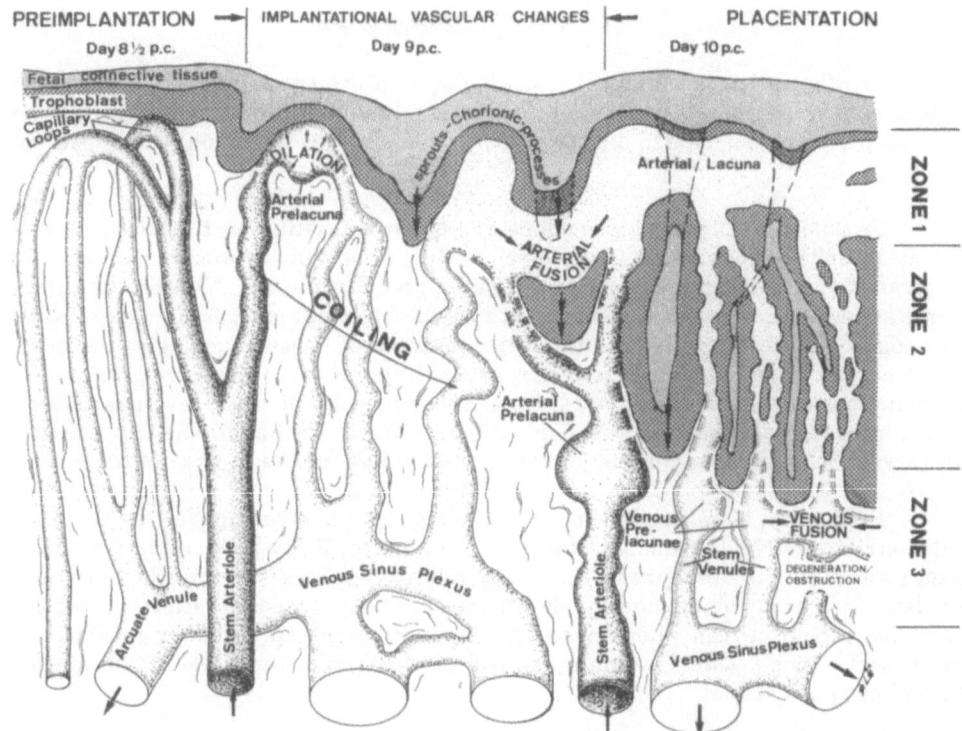

Figure 8. Scheme of developing lacunar formation from the subepithelial capillary plexus of the mesometrially located endometrial fold (visualized from left to right). This vascular system is preimplantational and remains until 8 d 12 h p.c. Coiling, dilation, and fusion of the vessel are the first vascular signs of lacunar formation, appearing during implantation at about day 9 p.c. By the growth of the chorionic processes into the endometrium these phenomena become more distinct and divide the lacunar formation in three zones, typical for placentation from day 10 p.c. onwards.

        Dead blastocysts of approximately day 9 age, blackened by surrounding clotted blood, were observed frequently during collection of material in this study. Occasionally, during this time even careful handling and perfusion of intact and fresh postmortum implantation sites could not prevent massive hemorrhage of maternal blood into the uterine cavity. Therefore, the shaping force of blood pressure and flow seems to be well equilibrated during lacunar formation, so as not to trigger too much extravasation of blood, which could possibly be deleterious to the implanting blastocyst. This consequence, leading to embryonic loss in the rabbit, needs to be studied in more detail. Nevertheless, this observation brings one back to the phenomenon in the human, where embryonic loss during implantation is a crucial problem, as initially mentioned in this study (Lauritsen, 1982; Grudzinskas and Nysenbaum, 1985).

## SUMMARY

The formation of maternal blood lacunae in the chorioallantoic placenta of rabbit, shown by correlative semithin section histology and scanning electron microscopy of vessel casts, develops from the preimplantational subepithelial capillary plexus.

First signs of lacunar development appear as coiling on the limbs and as dilatation of the loops of this capillary plexus, when chorionic sprouts begin to penetrate the endometrial surface at 8 d 12 h post coitum (p.c.). Vessel dilatations, surrounded by a degenerative and lytic wall on about day 9 p.c., are called prelacunae. They normally fuse to form a network of vessels lacking any uterine tissue called large arterial lacunae, representing zone 1. Some vessels in the prelacunar stage may disrupt resulting subsequently in blood extravasations, which occasionally can be sufficiently extensive to harm the implanting blastocyst. This observation may be related to embryonic loss in the human.

From day 10 p.c., chorionic processes, by penetrating deeper into the endometrium, follow the limbs of the subepithelial capillary plexus and transform them as a whole into a labyrinth of small capillary-type lacunae, zone 2. In front of this labyrinth or at the advancing edge of the chorion, a zone 3 of lacunar formation develops, including the phenomena of vascular coiling, prelacunar dilatations, and vessel fusion. Zone 3 remains as the permanent form of lacunar formation throughout placentation.

## ACKNOWLEDGEMENTS

We thank Ms. Gisela Bujotzek for her excellent technical assistance. This research was supported by a grant from the Deutsche Forschungsgemeinschaft program on "Biologie und Klinik der Reproduktion", and by a grant from the Stifterverband für die deutsche Wissenschaft to H.M.B.

## REFERENCES

Amoroso, E.C. (1952) Placentation. In: *Marshall's Physiology of Reproduction*, (ed.), A.S. Parkes, Vol. 2, Chpt. XV, London: Longmans, Green.

Beier, H.M. (1984) Physiologische und endokrinologische Grundlagen der Implantation. In: *Praktikum der extrakorporalen Befruchtung*, (ed.), D. Krebs, Muenchen, Wien, Baltimore: Urban and Schwarzenberg, pp. 166-194.

Beier, H.M., Beier-Hellwig, K., and Delbos, R. (1983) Hormones and proteins involved in uterine preparation for implantation. In: *Fertilization of the Human Egg In Vitro, Biological Basis and Clinical Application*, (eds.), H.M. Beier, and R. Lindner, Berlin, Heidelberg, New York, Tokyo: Springer, pp. 307-327.

Carter, A.M. (1975) Placental circulation. In: *Comparative Placentation. Essays in Structure and Function*, (ed.), D.H. Steven, London, New York, San Francisco: Academic Press, pp. 108-160.

Dantzer, V., Leiser, R., Kaufmann, P., and Luckhardt, M. (1988) Comparative morphological aspects of placental vascularization. *Trophoblast Research* 3, 235-260.

Denker, H.-W. (1980) Embryo implantation and trophoblast invasion. In: *Cell Movement and Neoplasia,* (ed.), M. de Brabander, Oxford, New York: Pergamon Press, pp. 151-162.

Duval, M. (1889) Le placenta des rongeurs: le placenta du lapin. *J. Anat. et Physiol.* 25, 309-342.

Faber, J.J., and Thornburg, K.L. (1983) *Placental Physiology. Structure and Function of Fetomaternal Exchange.* New York: Raven Press.

Finn, C.A. (1977) The implantation reaction. In: *Biology of the Uterus,* (ed.) R.M. Wynn, chpt. 9, New York, London: Plenum Press, pp. 245-308.

Fischer, B., Winterhager, E., Busch, L.C., and Beier, H.M. (1985) Die Pseudograviditaet des Kaninchens als reproduktionsbiologisches Modell. *Fertilitaet* 1, 101-109.

Garris, D.R., and Dar, M.S. (1985) Decidua-associated changes in guinea pig uterine blood flow and volume: Relation to uterine norepinephrine concentration. *Anat. Rec.* 211, 410-413.

Grudzinskas, J.G., and Nysenbaum, A.M. (1985) Failure of human pregnancy after implantation. In: *In Vitro Fertilization and Embryo Transfer*, (eds.) M. Seppala and R.G. Edwards, Ann. New York Acad. Sci. 442. New York: New York Acad. Sci, pp. 38-44.

Hafez, E.S.E., and Tsutsumi, Y. (1966) Changes in endometrial vascularity during implantation and pregnancy in the rabbit. *Am. J. Anat.* 118, 249-282.

Hoffman, L.H. and Davies, J. (1971) Production of the maternal placenta in rabbits following aspiration of conceptuses. *J. Repr. Fert.* 26, 255-257.

Hoos, P.G., and Hoffman, L.H. (1980) Temporal aspects of rabbit uterine vascular and decidual responses to blastocyst stimulation. *Biol. Reprod.* 23, 453-459.

Kaufmann, P., Bruns, U., Leiser, R., Luckhardt, M., Winterhager, E. (1985) The fetal vascularisation of term human placental villi. II. Intermediate and terminal villi. *Anat. Embryol.* 173, 203-214.

Larsen, J.F. (1961) Electron microscopy of the implantation site in the rabbit. *Am. J. Anat.* 109, 319-334.

Larsen, J.F. (1962) Electron microscopy of the chorioallantoic placenta of the rabbit. I. The placental labyrinth and the multi-nucleated giant cells of the intermediate zone. *J. Ultrastr. Res.* 7, 535-549.

Lauritsen, J.G. (1982) The cytogenetics of spontaneous abortion. *Res. Reprod.* 14, 3.

Leiser, R. (1985) Fetal vasculature of the human placenta: Scanning electron microscopy of microvascular casts. *Contr. Gynecol. Obstet.* 13, 27-31.

Leiser, R., and Kohler, T. (1983) the blood vessels of the cat girdle placenta. Observations on corrosion casts, scanning electron microscopical and histological studies. I. Maternal vasculature. *Anat. Embryol.* 167, 85-93.

Mossman, H.W. (1926) The rabbit placenta and the problem of placental transmission. *Am. J. Anat.* 37, 433-497.

Nakamura, T., and Ninomiya, H. (1978) A scanning electron microscopic study on the endometrium of the rabbit during early pregnancy. *Proc. Japan Acad. Ser* B 54, 106-110.

Nakamura, T., and Ninomiya, H. (1979) Vascular architecture at the implantation site of the rabbit. *Proc. Japan Acad. Ser.* B 55, 441-444.

Rogers, P.A.W., and Gannon, B.J. (1981) The vascular and microvascular anatomy of the rat uterus during the estrous cycle. *AJEBAK* 59, 667-679.

Steven, D.H. (1983) Interspecies differences in the structure and function of trophoblast. In: *Biology of Trophoblast*, (ed.) Loke, Y.W., and Whyte, A., Amsterdam, New York, Oxford: Elsevier, pp. 111-136.

Tsutsumi, Y. (1962) The vascular pattern of the placenta in farm animals. *J. Facul. Agr. Hokkaido Univ. Sapporo* 52, 372-482.

Wynn, R.M., and Davies, J. (1965) Comparative electron microscopy of the hemochorial placenta. *Am. J. Obstet. Gynecol.* 91, 533-549.

# FETAL CIRCULATION

# THREE-DIMENSIONAL REPRESENTATION OF THE FETAL VESSEL SYSTEM IN THE HUMAN PLACENTA[*]

## - A Review -

Peter Kaufmann[1], Michael Luckhardt[2], and Rudolf Leiser[3]

[1]Abt. Anatomie, RWTH Aachen
Melatener Strasse 211
D 5100 Aachen, West Germany

[2]Universitäts-Frauenklinik  Hamburg
Martinistrasse 52
D 2000 Hamburg 20, West Germany

[3]Institut für Tieranatomie, Universität Bern
Laengassstrasse 120
Ch 3001 Bern, Switzerland

## INTRODUCTION

As compared to the maternal vascularization of the human placenta, the fetal vessels have been of minor interest throughout the past two decades. This is evident, too, from the monograph by Ramsey and Donner (1980) dealing with placental vascularization and circulation. About 5% of the volume is devoted to the fetal aspects. Among the 14 "areas of ignorance" recommended for future work, the fetal vessels of the placenta are not mentioned. This is no criticism of this outstanding monograph, but rather a strong argument that the classical studies by Boe (1953) and Arts (1961) have been fundamental, clear and sufficiently detailed to meet the requirements for the interceding 20 to 30 years.

However, following review of recent physiological and clinical publications, several gaps in our knowledge concerning the fetal vessels became evident. A subdivision of the fetal placental vessels into different segments, comparable to the vessel classification of Rhodin (1967, 1968, 1974) was largely missing. Detailed information regarding position and functional importance of the "sinusoids" was not available. Recent studies of placental vessel architecture have demonstrated the usefulness of scanning electron microscopy on vessel casts (Thiriot and Panigel, 1978; O'Neill, 1983; Habashi et al., 1983; Lee and Yeh, 1983). Methodological advances in this field (cf. Leiser and Kohler, 1983, 1984; Leiser, 1985) and the combination of scanning electron microscopy of vessel casts with three-dimensional reconstruction of serial semithin sections seemed to be a good basis for a de novo study of the fetal vascularization of the human placental villi. The above combination of methods proved to be necessary since scanning electron

[*] Dedicated to Professor Fritz Strauss, Bern, on the occasion of his 80th birthday

microscopy of vessel casts as the single method has two major disadvantages. The exact type of vessels cannot be identified by their casts alone, and different vessel types cannot be associated with the surrounding villous structures. This, however, seems to be mandatory for a useful description of the vessel arrangement, since the peripheral villous tree can be subdivided into 4 distinct villous types (Kaufmann et al., 1979), which primarily differ from each other with respect to the vascularization.

To resolve the above problems, we have studied the fetal vascularization in term placentae by means of scanning electron microscopy and serial semithin histology with subsequent three-dimensional reconstruction (Leiser et al., 1985; Kaufmann et al., 1985). In the present survey, the respective results shall be reviewed in comparison to the classical studies of Boe (1953) and Arts (1961). New findings concerning the clinical-pathological relevance of this subject will be emphasized.

## MATERIALS AND METHODS

Even though most of our results presented in this review are already published together with a detailed description of the methods (Leiser et al., 1985; Kaufmann et al., 1985), essential parts of the technical procedures are summarized since differences in the methods used when compared with other publications, may partially explain differences in the results.

From 46 normal term human placentae obtained during cesarean section, placental villi were obtained via needle puncture from of the in situ and still maternally perfused placenta. The biopsy was aspirated directly into 2.2% glutaraldehyde in phosphate buffer (pH 7.3, 340 mosm) and embedded in Epon. Semithin cross sections of the villi, about 1 μm thick, were stained with toluidine blue. The villous cross sections were classified according to stromal structure following the classification of Kaufmann et al. (1979). The vessel types were identified as far as possible in semithin sections, following the classification of Rhodin (1967, 1968, 1974). Four specimens were cut serially on a length of about 3,000 μm in order to follow the course of villous ramifications and to analyze the three-dimensional vessel arrangement. A complete terminal part of one villous tree, consisting of a stem villus (350 μm in diameter) with its ramifications was chosen for reconstruction based upon a length of 3,000 μm (Figure 1B). The sections were photographed. The vessel arrangement was reconstructed by transferring the type and the position of the vessel cross sections as seen in the serial microphotographs into a two-dimensional drawing (Figure 1C). The results of this reconstructed specimen were analyzed in comparison with those of single random sections from all other placentae.

The vessel casts obtained from four other human term placentae following uncomplicated pregnancies were prepared according to Leiser and Kohler (1983) and Leiser (1985). One large fetal artery of the chorionic plate supplying several fetal cotyledons was cannulated and gently perfused under manual pressure with warm saline containing 5,000 I.U./l Heparin and 0.5% Procaine-HCl. To obtain optimal distention of the capillary system and to remove residual blood, the corresponding vein was also cannulated and the perfusion was continued alternating between artery and vein until the outflow of both vessels was free of blood. Batson No 17 corrosion compound (Polysciences, Inc., Warrington, PA, USA) was freshly prepared and cooled in ice water to retard its polymerization for about 10 minutes. This time was sufficient to instill the plastic with a flow rate of about 5 ml/min into the perfused artery. While maintaining the manual pressure, both the artery and the vein were clamped for preventing efflux of plastic. Then the injected sector was placed in a water bath at 20°C for half an hour, followed by 80°C for 4 hours to allow the plastic to harden. Corrosion of injected placental tissue was accomplished by alternating immersion in 40% KOH and distilled water at 60°C for a few days. To cut well injected cotyledons (cf. Figure 3A) in suitable pieces the material was embedded in warm 20% gelatin solution which was hardened by cooling to about -5°C and thus could be easily cut with a knife into smaller pieces. The corroded casts were repeatedly washed at room temperature in distilled water and 5% neutral Extran (Merck, Darmstadt, FRG). From the cut, air-dried casts suitable specimens were selected and mounted on stubs (Figure 3B), sputter-coated with gold (30 nm) and examined with a Philips 500 and a Zeiss Novascan scanning electron microscope.

The morphometrical comparison of vessel calibers of terminal villi in semithin sections as compared to scanning electron micrographs of vessel casts was thought to be a useful method to estimate the kind and the extent of artificial lumen deformation. Caliber estimation was performed on scanning electron micrographs (magnification X680) by measuring the thickness of the individual capillary casts vertical to their longitudinal axis about every 10 µm. The caliber measurements in photographs of semithin sections (magnification X1,000) were performed in a similar way. For each section of a vessel lumen the longitudinal axis was defined. The diameter was then measured every 5 µm vertical to the longitudinal axis. The resulting data were calculated and classified with a VIDEOPLAN-System (Kontron).

## RESULTS AND DISCUSSION

### Villous Types

The human placental villi can be classified into 4 different types, which have been described in detail by Kaufmann et al., 1979, Sen et al., 1979, and Kaufmann, 1982. The stem villi form the central part of the villous tree. They start with a truncus chorii originating from the chorionic plate (Figure 1A); the truncus ramifies four times into four generations of larger branches, so-called rami chorii of the first to fourth order; the latter branch up to ten times giving rise to the ramuli chorii of the first to about tenth order. Histologically these three types of stem villi are defined on the basis of a stroma rich in connective tissue fibers and of blood vessels containing a media identifiable by light microscopy (Figure 3C). The diameter ranges from approximately 3,000 µm (largest trunci) down to 50 µm (small ramuli of tenth order).

The stem villi branch into bundles of slender, slightly curved, mature intermediate villi or into thicker, bulbous, immature intermediate villi (Figure 1B). Both connect nearly all of the peripherally positioned terminal villi to the stem villi. In the immature placenta the thicker type, the so-called immature intermediate villi (diameter 60 to 500 µm) prevail. However, small numbers of this

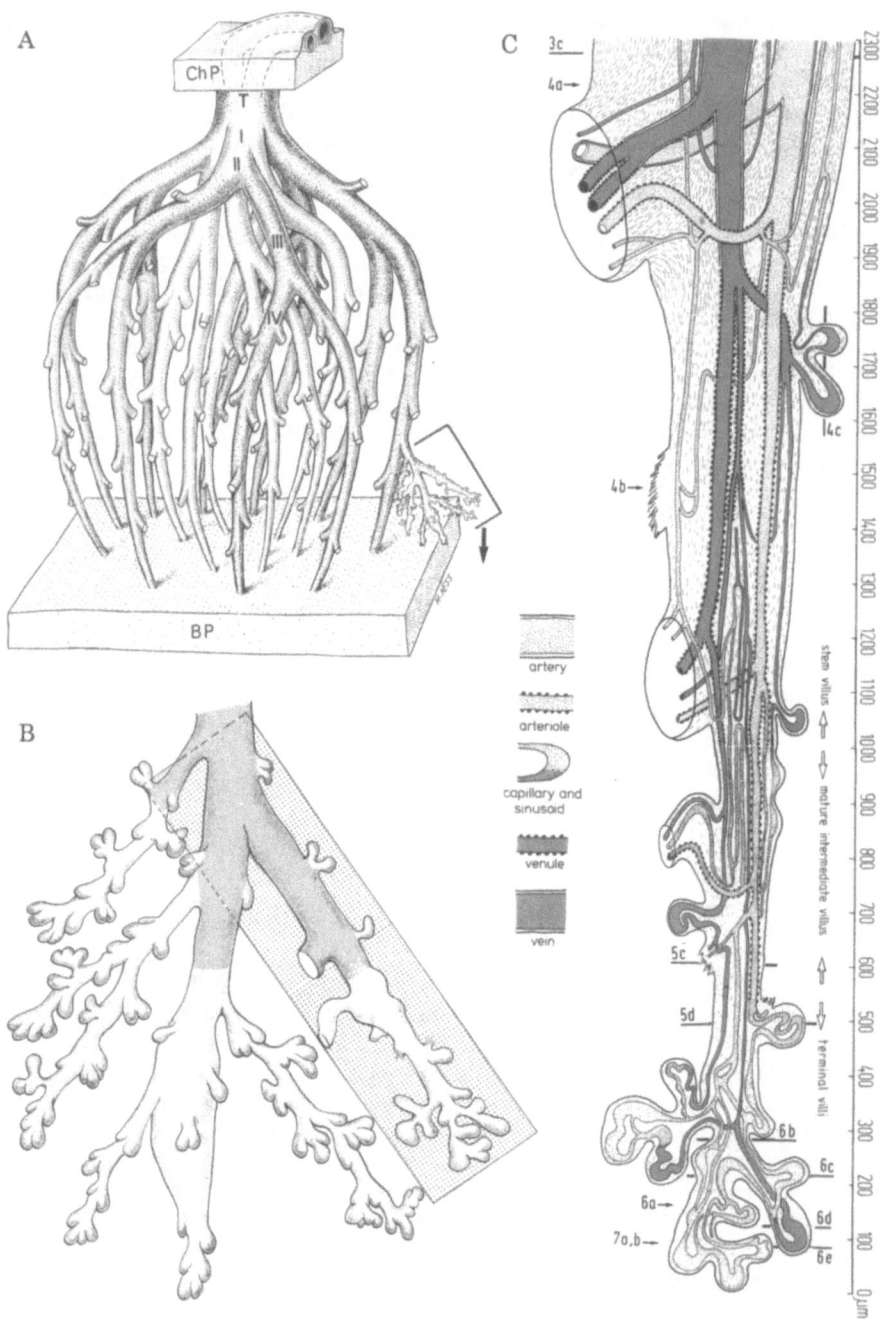

Figure 1A. Schematic drawing of the larger stem villi of the villous tree. ChP = chorionic plate; BP = basal plate; T = truncus; I, II, III, IV: rami chorii of the 1st to the 4th order (dense point shading); the remainder of the peripheral branches depicted in this drawing are ramuli chorii of the 1st to about the 10th order. The marked peripheral ramulus with its branches refers to Figure 1B.  1B). Higher type are present in the centers of the villous trees even in the mature placenta (cf. Schuhmann, 1981). Histologically they are characterized by a reticular stromal pattern poor in connective tissue fibers, as well as by a poorly developed fetal vascularization, mainly consisting of some smaller arterioles and venules accompanied by scarce capillary networks.

In the mature placenta the slender, slightly curved, mature intermediate villi (diameter 40 to 80 μm) dominate. They bear about 95% of all terminal villi. A very loose, unoriented connective tissue occupies more than half of the villous volume (Figure 5C). Most of the fetal vessels are narrow capillaries, in addition a few very small arterioles and venules can be seen.

The terminal villi are the final branches of the villous tree. The diameter ranges from 30 to 80 μm (Figure 6) and thus largely overlaps with that of all foregoing villi. Thus the diameter is not a useful parameter for the definition of this villous type. The terminal villi are supplied by narrow as well as by dilated fetal capillaries occupying more than half of the villous stroma (Figure 6C). Arterioles and venules are absent.

### Umbilical Vessels and Vessels of the Chorionic Plate

The vessels of the umbilical cord normally consist of 2 umbilical arteries with a luminal diameter of about 3 mm as well as of one umbilical vein with a luminal diameter of 5.5 to 6 mm. In approximately 1% of the cases, there is only one umbilical artery (Boyd and Hamilton, 1970). This abnormality is not necessarily combined with other fetal malformations. In the neighborhood of the chorionic plate in most cases, both arteries are connected to each other by a short transverse connecting branch, the so-called Hyrtl anastomose (Hyrtl, 1870), rather than by local fusion of both arteries. Normally arteries and vein follow a spiral course, the vein surrounding the more centrally positioned twisted arteries. Counter-

magnified branches of the villous tree. A peripheral stem (grey shaded) branches into several mature intermediate villi (slender) and one immature intermediate villus (thicker). Whereas the immature intermediate villus displays only a few terminal villi, the mature ones are more densely packed with terminal villi. The rectangular area corresponds to the reconstructed branches depicted in Figure 1C. 1C). Two-dimensional simplified drawing of a peripheral stem villus, continuing into a mature intermediate villus, extending into several terminal villi, reconstructed from serial semithin sections. The marked cross-sectional levels (black lines) refer to corresponding or identical semithin sections depicted in this publication. The arrows refer to comparable figures of scanning electron micrographs of vessel casts. Length and caliber of the villi are drawn on the same scale, whereas the diameter of the vessels is reduced to two thirds. This was necessary because of the two-dimensional representation of a three-dimensional system. Some occasional spots of fibrinoid necrosis on the villous surface are marked by line hatching (Figures 1B and 1C: modified from Leiser et al., 1985).

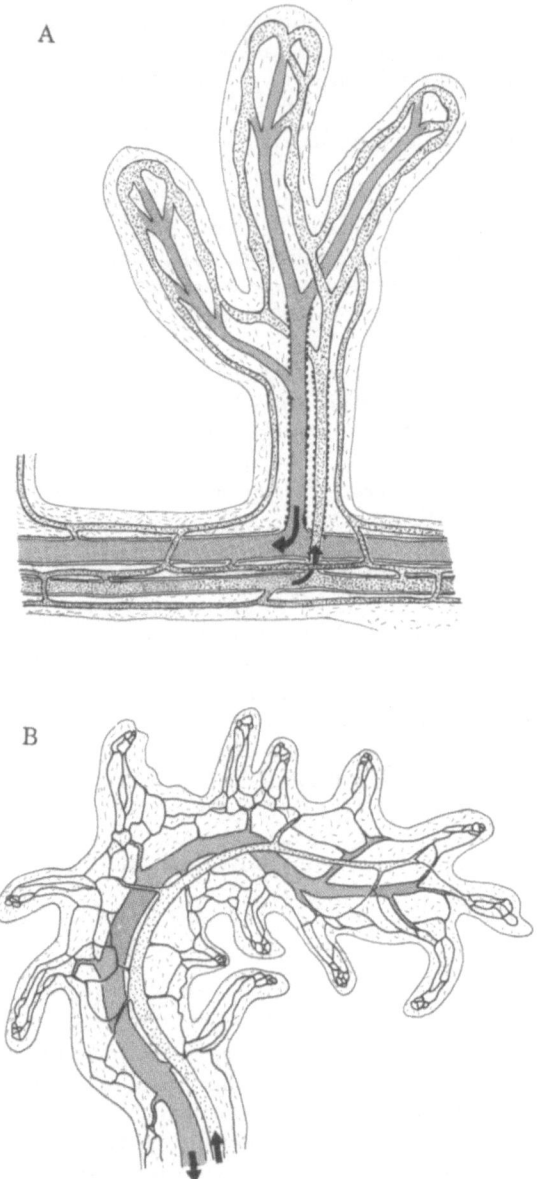

Figure 2.  Classical schematic representations of villous vascularization (Figure 2A: adapted from Arts, 1961; Figure 2B: adapted from Boe, 1969). Figure 2A. The diagram of Arts comes very near to the current observations. The major difference is that following Arts, each single terminal villus has its own supplying arterial branch.  Thus, the terminal villi are capillarized in parallel whereas the current study described mainly serially capillarized terminal branches.  Figure 2B. Following Boe's results the terminal capillaries originate from the paravascular net of the stem villi.  This situation was observed in only immature intermediate villi.

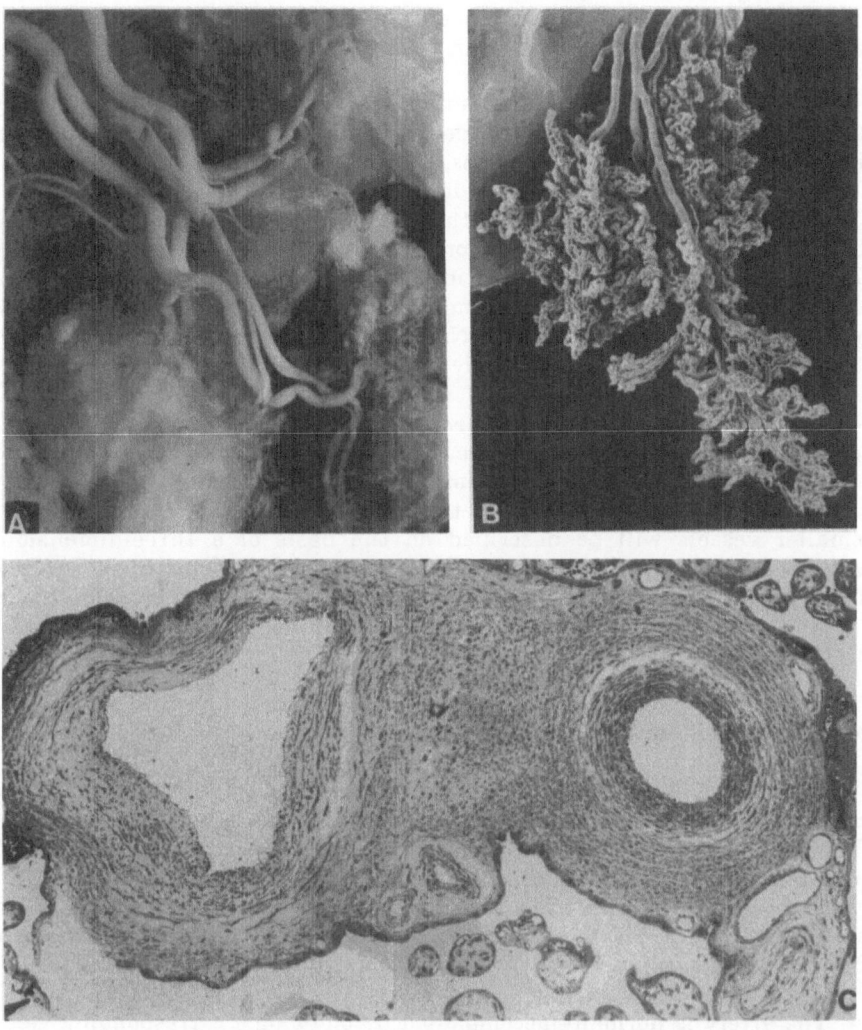

Figure 3A. Fetal vascular cast as seen from the fetal surface of the placenta. Several arteries and accompanying veins are seen, which continue into the roundish and oval cotyledons (fetal villous trees), 5 of which are depicted here. X1. 3B). A vessel cast of an isolated peripheral portion of one of the cotyledons, corresponding to that villous portion schematized in Figure 1B. X35. 3C). Semithin cross-section of a ramulus chorii. Note that the adventitia of the artery (right) and of the vein (left) directly continues into the surrounding dense fibrous stroma of the villus. Superficially numerous smaller vessels of the paravascular net are seen. X110. (Figures 3B and 3C from Leiser et al., 1985 with permission).

clockwise turns are more often to be seen than clockwise ones. From 0 to 380 spiral turns have been reported (Boyd and Hamilton, 1970). It should be noted that except for the first centimeter of the cord near the umbilicus, the following placental vessels are free of nerves (Lachenmayer, 1971, Nikolov and Schiebler, 1973).

Entering the chorionic plate the umbilical arteries branch dichotomously up to four times giving rise to 16 to 24 larger chorionic arteries (Figure 3A). Since the umbilical vein branches up to 5 times, which is different from the cord in the chorionic plate, the numerical relation for arteries and veins is approximately 1:1. A total of 60 to 70 vertical branches of the above arteries and veins enters the same number of stem villi (Boyd and Hamilton, 1970). Each stem villus is supplied by a single artery measuring up to 1.5 mm in diameter and by a single vein measuring up to 2.0 mm in diameter (Schiebler and Kaufmann, 1981). Much larger calibers of these truncal vessels as reported by O'Neill (1983) for vessel casts obviously do not represent in vivo conditions but probably are due to the high infusion pressure.

The truncal vessels start branching dichotomously parallel to the branching patterns of the villous tree (Figure 1A), and only a few millimeters below the chorionic plate. The arrangement and branching patterns of those larger stem vessels have been reported in detail by O'Neill (1983). The arrangement of the smaller vessels will be described on the basis of a three-dimensionally reconstructed specimen of a mature villous tree, which is depicted in Figures 1B and 1C. This is a specimen with a length of 2,300 µm, consisting of a small bulbous stem villus, a mature intermediate villus, continuing in several terminal villi (Figure 1C).

## Larger Vessels of Stem Villi

The stem villus normally contains one single small artery in a nearly central position. Since the degree of arterial constriction is largely varying, the in vivo luminal width cannot be estimated. It roughly may amount to one third of the villous caliber. The endothelial cells are surrounded by a media composed of 3 to 5 layers of smooth muscle cells. The adventitia, which is two to three times as thick as the media in most cases, is continuous with the surrounding villous stroma without a sharp demarcation line (Figure 3C).

The artery is normally accompanied by one single corresponding vein the luminal width of which in our preparations does not usually exceed that one of the artery (Figures 4A and 4B). This relationship is in agreement with the description of most other authors (Boyd and Hamilton, 1970). However, it must be admitted that this might be different under in vivo conditions. In addition to these two main vessels varying numbers of smaller arterioles and venules do exist.

Smaller stem villi of approximately 80 to 150 µm in diameter (ramuli from the 7th to 10th order) represent the last generation of stem villi, which directly branch or continue into mature intermediate villi (Figures 1B and 1C). Arteries and veins of the larger stem villi are transformed into arterioles and venules surrounded by 1 to 2 layers of muscle cells. The tiny venules have only one more or less complete layer of muscle cells (Figure 4C). Some of the venules are surrounded only by pericytes and thus apparently correspond to the collecting venule of Rhodin (1968) despite the differences in diameter. Very often arterioles and venules of these villous segments are so similar to each other regarding structure, luminal width and thickness of the vessel wall, that they cannot be identified upon cross-sectioning but can be only when following their course in the three-dimensional reconstruction of serial sections.

## Paravascular Net of Stem Villi

Superficially, facing the trophoblast, numerous cross-sections of normal capillaries appear (Figure 3C). These capillaries belong to the so-called paravascular net (Boe, 1953) (Figure 2B). Following this author, the paravascular capillaries constitute a system of arterio-arterial shunts or even arterio-venous shunts between afferent arterioles and efferent venules of the terminal branches. Following the results of Arts (1961) (Figure 2A) and previous studies (Leiser et al., 1985) (Figure 1C). This interpretation is not valid at least for the typical terminal branches of the mature placenta. The immature placenta has not been studied. For terminal villi derived from immature intermediate villi, one cannot exclude the situation depicted by Boe (Figure 2B). Terminal villi arising directly from stem villi (upper half of Figure 1C and Figure 4C) may receive their capillary loops directly from the paravascular net. However, the overwhelming number of terminal villi in the mature placenta, i.e., about 95%, are terminal ramifications of the mature intermediate villi (lower end of Figure 1C). The capillary loops of the latter, however, derive from their own arterioles and venules and show only occasional connection to the paravascular net (cf. Figure 2A).

Following recent results in this laboratory and in agreement with the famous drawing of Arts (1961) (Figure 2B), the results of Thiriot and Panigel (1978) as well as Habashi et al. (1983), these paravascular capillaries follow a rather straight course, mostly parallel to the longitudinal villous axis (Figures 4A and 4B). Net-like cross connections are uncommon. They are connected to the arteries and veins by rather short arteriolar and venular segments measuring 40 to 100 μm in length. In many cases these capillaries form hairpin-like loops, their connection to the arterioles and venules being close together (Figure 4B).

Most authors describe ample communication of the paravascular net of the stem villi with the capillary loops of the terminal villi, whereas our results point to two largely different and separate capillary systems (Figure 1C). The erroneous impression of more communications among both capillary systems may be explained by two findings. Firstly, superficially positioned capillaries of the paravascular net are sometimes locally coiled and sinusoidally dilated, bulging against the trophoblastic surface of the stem villus, and forming small isolated terminal villi (cf. upper right of Figure 1C and Figure 4C). These terminal villi are serially intercalated into the paravascular net. Secondly, long venous capillary limbs of the terminal villus capillary system may reach the stem villi and only then enter venules and veins. These venous capillaries limbs are as straight as the paravascular capillaries (Figure 1C). They are usually intermingled with the latter but normally not connected to them, their existence may cause confusion.

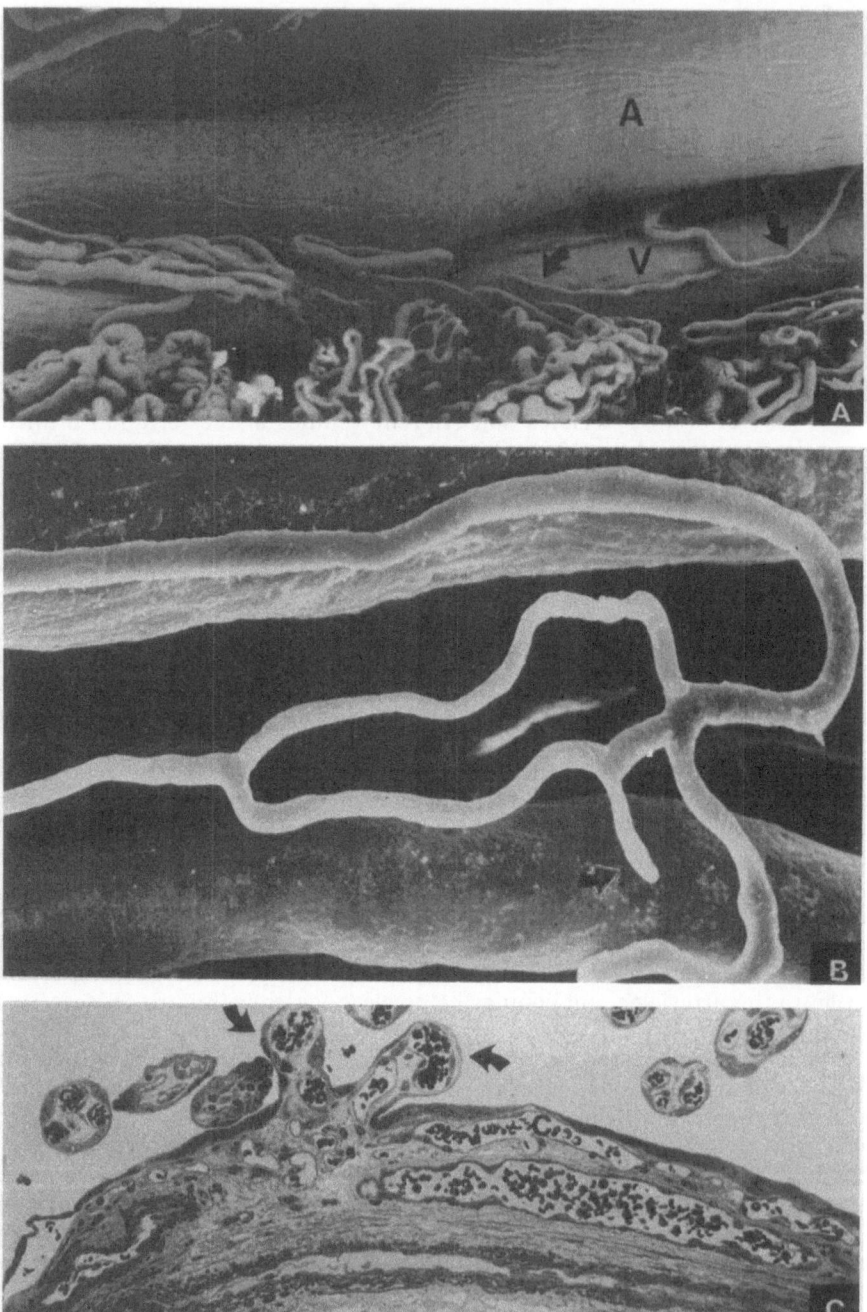

Figure 4.  Stem villi. 4A). Vessel casts of a larger stem villus surrounded by
numerous terminal villi. The paravascular net (arrows) accompanying the stem
artery (A) and the stem vein (V) was partly removed during the preparation of the
specimen. X120.   4B).  Higher magnification of a similar cast demonstrates the

Following the individual capillaries of the paravascular net from the arteriolar beginning to the venular end, results in an average length of 1,000 to 2,000 μm. Arterio-venous shortcuts as described by Boe (1953, 1969) nor arterio-arterial connections in this system could be detected.

The functional relevance of the paravascular network is still a matter for discussion. Thiriot and Panigel (1978) suggested that it was a site for effective feto-maternal exchange. This assumption is not refuted; however, the fact that the capillary loops are often arranged in a hairpin-like manner (Figure 4B) allowing retro-diffusion, as well as the long materno-fetal diffusion length, make this interpretation rather implausible. The assumption of Arts (1961) that the paravascular net may be of nutritional importance for the stem villi is unlikely also according to the considerations of Zeek and Assali (1950). The latter authors point to the fact that the stroma of the stem villi persists even after fetal death, which indicates that this villus receives its nutrition directly from the intervillous space. Boyd and Hamilton (1970) described the paravascular net to be simply a residual indication of better vascularization in earlier stages of development. Keeping in mind that the developmental forerunners of stem villi were immature intermediate villi with a similar vessel arrangement (Kaufmann, 1982), the paravascular net represents the remainder of the immature placenta where terminal villi with their effective exchange system were largely missing and the paravascular network had to sustain materno-fetal exchange. The development of better vascularized terminal villi will render it largely unfunctional.

### Vessels of the Immature Intermediate Villi

Immature intermediate villi are infrequent structures in the full term placenta. In earlier stages of pregnancy they are thought to be the site for the branching of the villous tree (Kaufmann, 1982). Later on they undergo progressive stromal fibrosis and thus are transformed into stem villi. Accordingly their vessel arrangement is comparable to that of the stem villi. A few larger arterioles and venules with a more central position are surrounded by a loosely arranged net of paravascular capillaries, which are directly continuous with the foregoing generation of stem villi. As compared with the paravascular net of the stem villi, the capillaries of the immature intermediate villi are more contorted and

---

arrangement of the paravascular capillaries, predominantly arranged in loops parallel to the longitudinal villous axis. Following our serial semithin sections blind-ending capillaries (arrow) are actual blind-ending outgrowths rather than artifactual results of incomplete filling. X540. 4C). Longitudinal semithin section of a stem villus with two terminal side-branches (arrows). As is obvious from the section as well as from the corresponding part of the drawing (Figure 1C), the sinusoidally dilated capillary loops of the 2 terminal villi originate from the paravascular capillaries (C). (Figures 4A, 4B, and 4C from Leiser et al., 1985, with permission).

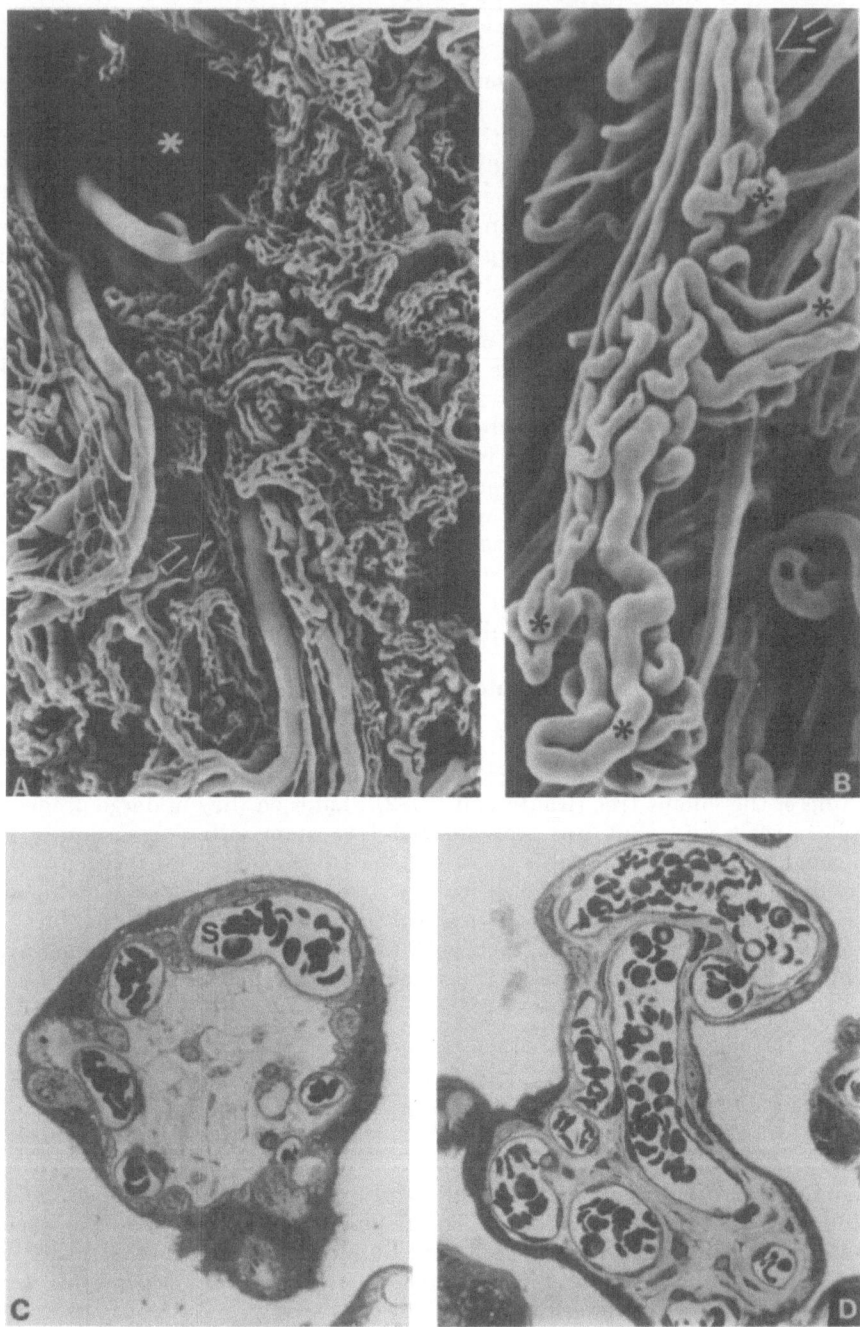

Figure 5. Intermediate villi. 5A). Basal view of the cotyledonary surface demonstrating the central cavity (*) situated beneath the maternal arterial inlet, as well as some surrounding immature intermediate villi (arrows). The latter are

sometimes even arranged in a net-like manner (Figure 5A). Sinusoidal dilations are normally missing.

## Vessel Arrangement in the Mature Intermediate Villi

The mature intermediate villi serve as junctional segments between the smallest stem villi and about 95% of the terminal villi. Their vessels are the direct continuations of the last generation of stem villi. One to two small arterioles with luminal diameters ranging from 20 to 40 μm appear as bare endothelial tubes, accompanied by occasional smooth muscle cells. Precapillary sphincters or comparable narrow segments with complete circular muscular sheets have not been observed. Rather those terminal arterioles continue directly into one or two capillaries by gradual reduction of their luminal diameters and loss of the smooth muscle cells (Figure 1C). In contrast to the more centrally located arterioles, one or two corresponding venules occupy a more superficial position. Also their number normally does not exceed that of the arterioles, their diameter appears to be considerably smaller in most preparations, usually 15 to 20 μm. Following the classification of Rhodin (1968), the term postcapillary venule is deemed to be most appropriate because of the absence of muscle cells and the existence of a more or less complete layer of pericytes. Arterioles and venules are accompanied by the most peripheral loops of the paravascular capillary net of the stem villi, extending about to the middle of the mature intermediate villi (Figure 1C). In the more peripheral parts of the mature intermediate villi, paravascular capillary loops are absent. Instead of those, the first segments of the terminal capillary system appear, originating via gradual transformation of arterioles and venules as described above. The abrupt end of the paravascular net and the step-by-step appearance of the terminal capillaries cause a sharp demarcation line between the more proximal and capillary dense region and the more peripheral and capillary less dense region of the mature intermediate villi (Figures 5B, 5C, and Figure 1C).

Different from the paravascular capillaries the terminal capillary loops form curves and sometimes even coilings. Locally highly dilated segments may

---

characterized by irregularly arranged web-like capillary networks being similar to those depicted by Boe (1969), cf. Figure 2B. X90. 5B). A vessel cast of the most peripheral part of a mature intermediate villus (arrow), branching into a group of terminal villi (*). Note the straight vessel arrangement of the mature intermediate villi as opposed to the capillary coiling in the terminal branches. X250. 5C). Semithin section of the peripheral half of a mature intermediate villus. Note the reduced number of capillaries, the partly sinusoidal dilatations (S), the superficial position of the vessels, and the extremely loose connective tissue as typical features of this particular villous segment. X770. 5D). Zone of transition (lower half) of a mature intermediate villus into terminal villi, together with a typical terminal branch (upper half). Note the increasing diameter of the sinusoidally dilated capillaries as opposed to Figure 5C. X770. (Figures 5C and 5D from Kaufmann et al., 1985; with permission).

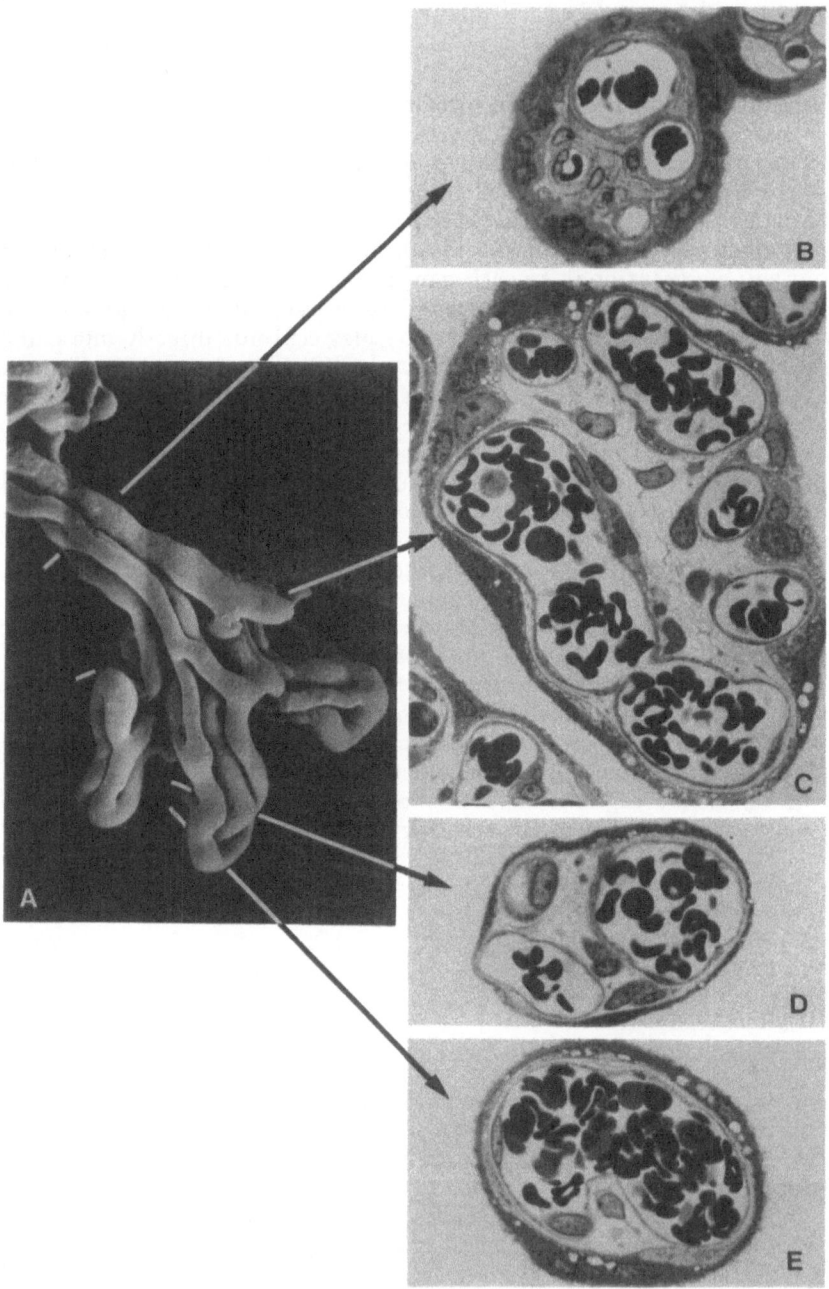

Figure 6. Terminal villi. 6A). Vessel cast of a neck region (upper half) branching
into 3 terminal villi. Comparable to mature intermediate villi, the capillaries of
the neck region are straight and parallel, however, the diameter of the villus is
much smaller. X600. 6B-6E). Corresponding semithin sections of the neck region
(B), the basis of the branching terminal villi (C), a single terminal villus near its

bulge against the trophoblast and thus cause the formation of typical epithelial plates, knob-like small terminal villi or even typical terminal branches (Figure 5D). Coming nearer to the peripheral end of the mature intermediate villi, the number and extent of coilings increases and thus the number of terminal side branches covering the surface of the mature intermediate villi (Figure 1C). The most peripheral end is regularly covered by a big cluster of terminal villi whereas the lateral surface is covered by more single terminal branches (Figure 5B). Each single one causes a slight curve of the mature intermediate axis in the opposite direction.

### Capillary Loops of the Terminal Villi

The terminal villi develop from the mature intermediate villi by continuous transformation of arterioles and venules into almost bare endothelial loops, by enlargement of the capillary diameter, and by reduction of connective tissue (Figure 5D). Since this is a continuous process, a sharp demarcation between both villous types is practically missing. The term "terminal villus" is used for a villous segment that 1. contains no vessels other than capillaries and dilated sinusoids and 2. has the vessel lumina comprising at least half of the stromal volume (Figures 6B-6E).

The capillary loops of the peripheral clusters of terminal villi spread out directly from the terminal arterioles. Only sometimes they show cross connections to the peripheral extensions of the paravascular capillary net as depicted by Arts (1961) (cf. Figure 2A). It should be noted that the capillary loops of neighboring terminal villi are serially connected to each other (Figure 6A). Thus, the blood leaving the terminal arterioles will normally pass through the capillaries of 3 to 5 terminal villi in series before entering either a postcapillary venule or a straight venous capillary passing through the mature intermediate villus (Figure 1C).

The mean capillary length of the terminal capillaries is estimated to range from 3,000 to 5,000 µm. On the other hand, as reported above, the corresponding paravascular capillary loops are only 1,000 to 2,000 µm in length. Since shortcuts at the base of the capillary loops are uncommon, shorter passages for the blood are the exception (Figures 7A and B).

The three-dimensional reconstruction reveals only occasional branching capillaries rather than highly branched capillary networks which are different

---

tip (D), and a flat section of the terminal villous tip (E). The fetal capillaries and the highly dilated sinusoids mostly amount to more than 50% of the stromal volume. X730 (Figures 6A-6E: adapted from Kaufmann et al., 1985; with permission).

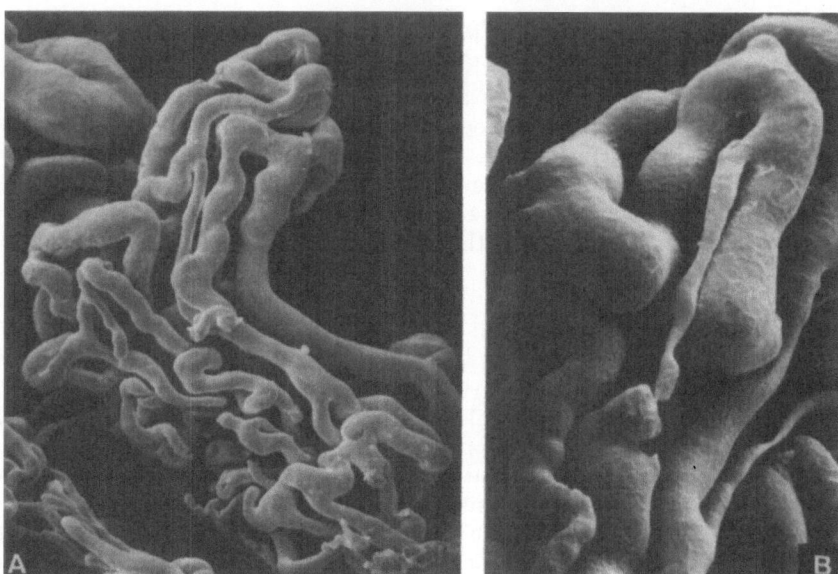

Figure 7. Two vessel casts of terminal villi exhibiting a moderate range of caliber variation (7A) and a maximum range from 2 μm to more than 30 μm (7B). Because of the highly complex arrangement of the terminal capillary convolutes, it is difficult to analyze their true nature. Based upon the reconstruction in Figure 1C, net-like branching is less expressed than highly complex coiling. Figure 7A: X500; 7B: X600 (from Kaufmann et al., 1985; with permission).

from the scanning electron micrographs of vessel casts as well as from most preceding results in the literature (Boe, 1953, 1968; Arts, 1961; Boyd and Hamilton, 1970; Thiriot and Panigel, 1978; Habashi et al., 1983). The few existing branchings mostly form parallel loops which continue into two different terminal villi. On the other hand capillary loops seemingly arranged in parallel to each other very often prove to be continuous, the wrong impression caused by multiple coilings only. These results are contradictory to those of Boe (1968), too, where each single villus is described as one circulatory unit with the paravascular net as the only vascular communication to the single terminal villi. One may argue that the above mentioned number of thorough investigations of large amounts of villi cannot be refuted by a single study dealing with the three-dimensional reconstruction of a few terminal villi, only. However, even looking at optimally preserved vessel casts one probably will not be able to trace a single capillary from the arterial to the venous end (Figure 7A). This is only possible in a reconstruction of serial sections. Only when tracing capillaries in full length will one realize what is capillary mesh-work and what is coiling.

## Classification and Structure of Terminal Capillaries

Those peripheral villous branches which by definition should be called terminal villi (Kaufmann et al., 1979) are characterized by the presence of capillaries, only. Whether a subdivision into arterial and venous capillaries or pre- and post-capillaries with different structure (Rhodin, 1967, 1968, 1974; Nikolov and Schiebler, 1973, 1981) is possible, cannot be decided from the histological material or from vessel casts. Rhodin has developed his capillary classification by studying the monolayer of microcirculatory vessels of the rabbit muscle fascia. These vessels are different from those of the placental villi in several aspects, regarding luminal diameters, thickness, and layers of the vessel wall. Nikolov and Schiebler (1973, 1981) tried to transfer Rhodin's data to the fetal villous vessels using transmission electron microscopy on villous cross sections without exact location and orientation within the villous microvascular bed. Thus an exact definition of the single capillary segment was impossible. This subject requires further investigation.

The same problems do exist for the description of the structure and the continuity of the endothelial wall. Rhodin and Terzakis (1962), Nguyen Anh and Panigel (1964), Becker and Seifert (1965), Tedde (1973), Nikolov and Schiebler (1973, 1981), Heinrich et al. (1976) describe structural details of the capillary wall but do not deal with structural differences along the full length of the capillary loops. As indicated by Becker and Seifert (1965), Heinrich et al. (1976), as well as Heinrich et al. (1987), the fetal capillaries of the human placenta seem to have a continuous endothelium which is different from the situation described for several other hemochorial placentae. Whether this is valid for all segments from the arterial beginning to the venous end of the long capillary loops, of both the paravascular as well as the terminal capillary bed, is still unresolved.

### Diameters of the Capillaries

Typical features of the terminal villi in mature placentae are the so-called sinusoids, enlarged capillary segments attaining diameters up to 50 μm (Figures 6C, 6D, 6E, and 7B). As opposed to sinusoids in liver, spleen, and bone-marrow, they possess a continuous endothelium and a complete basal lamina. In semithin sections, the sinusoids are normally positioned near the villous tips. Vessel casts, however, reveal that they are not dilatations of defined segments of the capillary loops but rather randomly scattered local enlargements. They may narrow and dilate serially several times (Figure 1C). Such dilatations occur more frequently in proximity to the villous tip and along the venous limbs of the loops, as well as at points of branching and fusion. With an increasing rate of dilatation the sinusoids become more tortuous. Measurement of the capillary diameter in the terminal villi from semithin sections and vessel casts produced largely consistent values. The mean diameters varied from 12.2 μm ± 0.58 (SEM) to 14.4 ± 1.94 μm (semithin sections). The maximum values were 39 μm (SEM) and 45 μm (semithin sections). Depending upon the method used, 60 to 80% of the vessel lumina exhibited diameters larger than 10 μm. These data are consistent with those reported by Becker (1962), Becker and Seifert (1965), Boyd and Hamilton (1970). Smaller diameters have been reported by Habashi et al. (1983), describing a maximum of only 20 μm, as well as by O'Neill (1983) giving a range of 4 to 7 μm. Looking at the vessel casts by the latter two authors, it is supposed that their lower figures have been caused by incomplete filling and incomplete distention of the fetal vessel system. A physiological study of Penfold et al. (1981) using perfusion of microspheres of varying diameters, resulted in different data also. The authors stated that as many as 25% of the capillaries may be less than 4 μm in diameter, and that there are virtually none exceeding 11 µm in diameter. These results have already been refuted by Habashi et al. (1983), since based on the erroneous assumption that narrow and dilated capillary loops are arranged in parallel. In fact, they narrow and dilate serially. Thus, while using microsphere perfusion the diameter of the narrowest segment can only be estimated. However, even the estimation that 25% of the capillary loops should have the narrowest segment of less than 4 µm appears to be unacceptable.

### Functional Relevance of Sinusoids

It is evident from the current results that the sinusoidal dilatation cannot be regarded as dilated venous limbs of the capillary loop which allow for a retarded venous back flow as has been suggested by Nikolov and Schiebler (1973). The localization of the sinusoids near to the villous tips may support the conclusion of Arts (1961) that the sinusoids locally decelerate the blood flow, thus providing ample opportunity for feto-maternal exchange. This possibility would be in accordance with the fact that the sinusoids are regularly situated contiguous to the epithelial plates (Boyd and Hamilton, 1970; Nikolov and Schiebler, 1973, 1981). Whether the reduced blood flow velocity can facilitate the materno-fetal exchange in excess of the negative influence of increased materno-fetal diffusion distance from the center of the sinusoids to the villous surface is still uncertain. It cannot be excluded that the negative effect of the increased materno-fetal diffusion distance may compensate or even exceed the positive effect of retarded blood flow. Another explanation for the existence of sinusoids could be that they serve as functionally specialized capillary segments devoted to specific transport processes. Nikolov and Schiebler (1981) have described two different types of endothelial cells. However, both seem to be evenly distributed in both, narrow capillaries as well as dilated sinusoids, not serving as arguments for a functional specialization of the two vessel segments.

Another explanation for the existence of sinusoids is that sinusoids are built up at the end of pregnancy (Becker, 1981) as soon as peripheral ramifications of the villous tree achieve the highest degree of branching and twisting and as soon as the terminal capillary loops reach the maximum length. On the other hand, sinusoids are absent in immature placentae exhibiting shorter capillary loops. These sinusoids are also largely absent within the shorter paravascular capillaries. They are not found in labyrinthine placentae like that of the guinea pig (Kaufmann and Davidoff, 1977) and of the tupaia (Luckhardt et al., 1985). Both placental types display an average fetal capillary length of 250 to 1,000 µm. Only animal placentae like that of the goat having comparable long capillary loops as does the human placenta (Dantzer et al., 1987; Leiser, 1987) seem to form sinusoids. According to the law of Hagen-Poiseuille, the blood flow resistance is reduced by the fourth power of the vessel radius. It, therefore, can be concluded that even limited sinusoidal dilatation of the terminal capillary convolutes may decrease blood flow resistance to such an extent that it does not exceed that of the much shorter paravascular capillaries (Figure 8A and 8B). An even blood flow distribution can be guaranteed for all capillaries independent of their length, only, as soon as the longer ones exhibit focal sinusoidal dilations. In addition for the fetal circulatory system, the perfusion of the huge extracorporal organ becomes much easier.

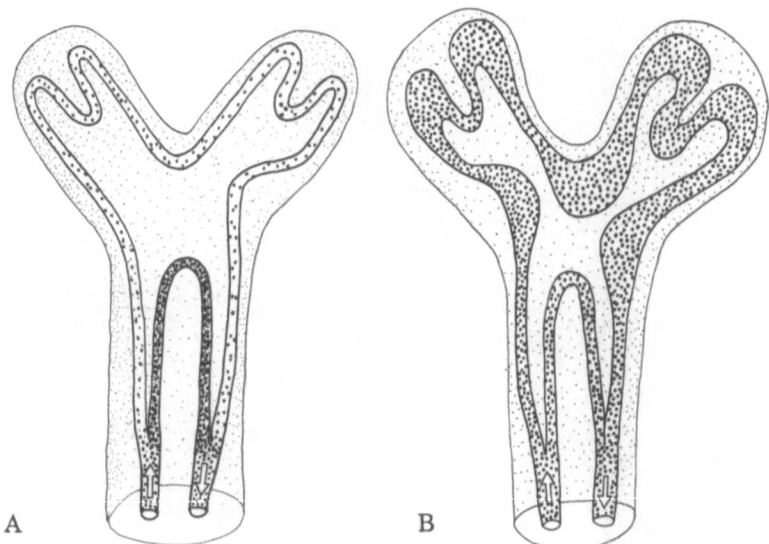

Figure 8. Functional relevance of sinusoids. 8A). Because of the different mean length of the terminal capillary loops (3,000 to 5,000 μm, light stippling) and of the paravascular capillary loops 1,000 to 2,000 μm, densely dotted), in the case of similar diameters of both capillary loops, the latter ones will become predominantly perfused. 8B). Focal sinusoidal dilation of the terminal capillary loops (mean: 14 μm, max.: 45 μm) as compared to the mostly narrow paravascular capillaries (mean: about 7 μm) will decrease blood flow resistance in the larger terminal capillaries to such an extent that an even distribution of flows can be guaranteed.

## Development of Terminal Villi as Induced by Capillary Growth

The above results and interpretations lead to a diagnostically interesting hypothesis for pathology, which is in agreement with a thorough investigation of the capillary arrangement in abnormally matured terminal villous ramifications (Kaufmann, unpublished observation). Most terminal villi arise from the surfaces of mature intermediate villi by bulging of coiled capillaries. So-called "hypermature villi" (Salvatore, 1968; Kaufmann, 1982) show an increased number of terminal villi, together with larger and more coiled capillary loops. Cases of "terminal villi deficiency" (Schweikhart and Kaufmann, 1982) exhibit just the opposite, nearly naked mature intermediate villi, almost devoid of terminal villi, presenting long, usually uncoiled capillaries with a few sinusoidal dilatations, only. It is concluded from these observations that the development of terminal villi is influenced by the balance of the longitudinal growth of mature intermediate villi with their capillary loops (Figure 9). The more longitudinal capillary growth exceeds the longitudinal growth of mature intermediate villi, the more the capillaries become coiled and the more terminal villi are produced.

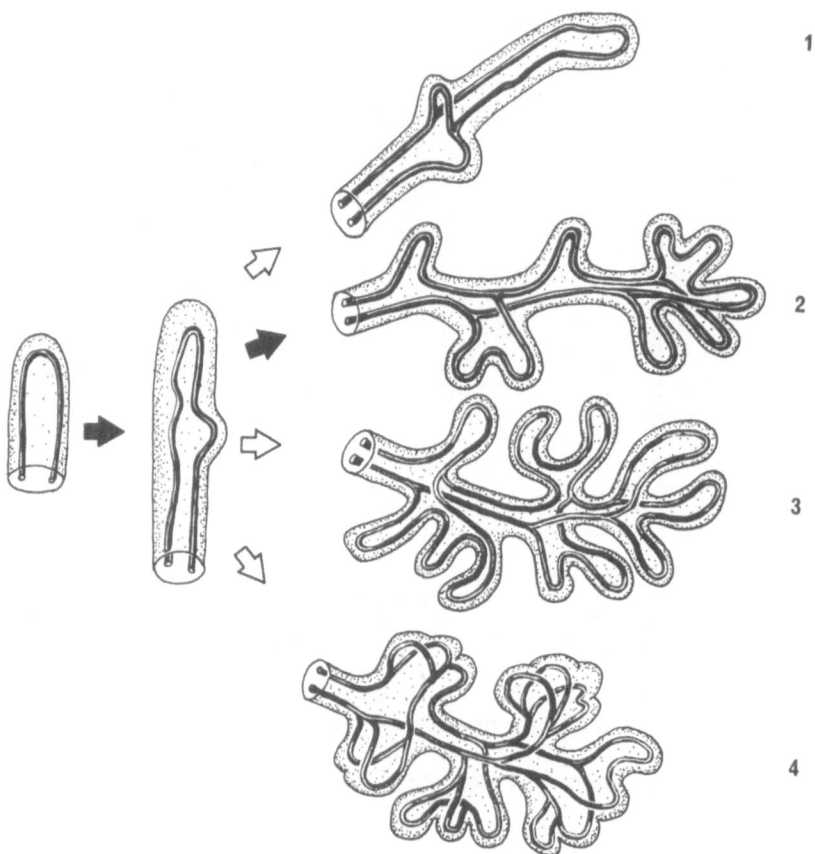

Figure 9.  Highly simplified diagram of terminal villus development in relation to capillary growth.  As long as capillary growth corresponds to the longitudinal growth of the mature intermediate villus (left side) the latter remains straight and does not form side branches.  As soon as the longitudinal capillary growth exceeds the longitudinal villous growth, capillary loops are formed bulging against the surface and hence causing the development of terminal villi.  Varying degrees of imbalance between villous and capillary growth result in different  types of terminal villous development, such as terminal villi deficiency (1), normal mature placenta (2), hypermaturity (3), and hypoxic hypervascularization (4) (Modified and extended from Kaufmann et al., 1985).

It is a well known fact that capillary growth is regulated by  oxygen supply. We have recently demonstrated that this is also valid for the placenta(Bacon et al., 1984).  Long term hypoxia in the pregnant guinea pig resulted in stimulated fetal capillary growth and in a reduced capillary diameter at the same time.  It is very unlikely that longitudinal capillary growth without capillary branching as a response to hypoxia would be accompanied by a reduction of the mean capillary diameter since this would increase blood flow resistance to an incompatible degree. It is concluded that hypoxic capillary growth is mainly a result of capillary branching and formation of parallel loops, thus decreasing blood flow resistance.

If capillary proliferation reflects the terminal villous branching patterns, hypoxic capillary growth, which leads to the formation of parallel loops, will have to induce a development of multiply bulged, short, knob-like terminal villi, originating from a rather short mature intermediate villous axis (Figure 9). Indeed, very often this kind of villous maldevelopment has been observed following pre-eclampsia which is regularly combined with intrauterine malperfusion. These "hypercapillarized" placentae following hypoxic conditions normally are characterized by narrow capillary cross-sections, similar to the findings in the hypoxic guinea pig placenta (Bacon et al., 1984). This pathohistological finding is in agreement with the observations of Tominaga and Page (1966) as well as Chabes et al. (1967), concerning the human placenta.

In contrast terminal villi deficiency (Schweikhart and Kaufmann, 1982) (Figure 9) should be discussed as a result of increased placental oxygen supply. Understimulated capillary growth which does not exceed the longitudinal growth of the mature intermediate villus will not cause capillary coiling and branching. Thus bulging of the villous surface with formation of terminal villi would be a rare event. Accordingly, histological preparations of placentae with terminal villi deficiency are characterized by straight, naked, mature intermediate villi which are poorly vascularized by narrow short capillary loops. There is no information available to date defining the underlying hyperoxic conditions. This type of villous malformation several times has been noted in this laboratory in combination with hyperthyreosis.

If the current hypothesis proves to be correct then overstimulated longitudinal capillary growth without branching-off of newly formed capillary side branches is not caused by hypoxia but rather as a result of capillary growth. This capillary growth may be taking place too early in short mature intermediate villi or also lasting over a too long period of time. In this respect, maturitas praecox placentae (Becker, 1981), placental hypermaturity under normoxic conditions (Salvatore, 1968) or even post term pregnancy could serve as the clinical correlate. Indeed, in most cases of premature maturation of the placenta and in some cases of post term pregnancy, villous trees with increased numbers of terminal villi which were long, slender, and winding were observed. The increased mean capillary length in these cases usually  was indicated by enormous sinusoidal dilatation.

It is still a matter of discussion whether the above four types of villous malformations are results of abnormal conditions long before term, or whether they can be induced even during the last few weeks of pregnancy. Many authors have stated that there is no further growth of the placental villous trees during the last month. Some morphological results in the term placenta give evidence that villous development is still in progress. Vessel casts sometimes show stub-like or longer, blind-ending outgrowths of the capillaries (Figure 4B). Comparable structures have been described by Thiriot and Panigel (1978). Considering only the vessel casts, these outgrowths may be interpreted as a result of incomplete filling. However, reconstruction studies of semithin sections in this laboratory reveal the same features; some of which continue into massive endothelial strings. The endothelial cells, the surrounding connective tissue cells, as well as the accumulations of cytotrophoblast in these regions are signs of intense villous proliferation, which indicates that even at term the development of the vascular system as well as of the villous trees is still in progress.

## SUMMARY

The fetal vessels of the term human placenta are described mainly on the basis of three-dimensional reconstruction of semithin serial sections and of scanning electron microscopy of vessel casts. According to stromal structure and fetal vascularization, the placental villi can be classified into four different types, namely stem villi, immature intermediate villi, mature intermediate villi, and terminal villi. These peculiarities in terms of vascularization are discussed: stem villi are characterized by the presence of arteries and veins, and/or arterioles and venules, as well as capillaries of the so-called paravascular net. Smaller arterioles and venules plus paravascular capillaries continue into both types of intermediate villi. The terminal villi are vascularized by terminal capillary loops originating directly from the most peripheral ends of arterioles and venules and exhibit only poorly developed connections to the paravascular net. Sinusoidal dilatations of the terminal capillaries with diameters up to 45 $\mu$m are interpreted as mechanisms to reduce blood flow resistance in the 3,000 to 5,000 $\mu$m long capillary loops. The paravascular capillaries with an average length of only 1,000 to 2,000 $\mu$m accordingly do not produce such dilated segments. The terminal capillary arrangement is discussed in the relationship to villous development. Several types of villous maldevelopment have to be interpreted as results of under- or overstimulated capillary growth.

## REFERENCES

Arts, N.F.T. (1961) Investigations on the vascular system of the placenta. Part 1. *Am. J. Obstet. Gynecol.* 82, 147-158.

Bacon, B.J., Gilbert, R.D., Kaufmann, P., Smith, A.D., Trevino, F.T., and Longo, L.D. (1984) Placental anatomy and diffusing capacity in guinea pigs following long-term maternal hypoxia. *Placenta* 5, 475-488.

Becker, V. (1962) Mechanismus der Reifung fetaler Organe. *Verh. Dtsch. Pathol. Ges.* 46, 309-314.

Becker, V. (1981) Pathologie der Ausreifung der Plazenta. In: *Die Plazenta des Menschen* (ed.) V. Becker, T.H. Schiebler, and F. Kubli, Stuttgart: Georg Thieme, pp. 266-281.

Becker, V. and Seifert, K. (1965) Die Ultrastruktur der Kapillarwand in der menschlichen Placenta zur Zeit der Schwangerschaftsmitte. *Z. Zellforsch.* 65, 380-396.

Boe, F. (1953) Studies on the vascularization of the human placenta. *Acta Obstet. Gynecol. Scand.* 32, Suppl. 5, 1-92.

Boe, F. (1968) Studies on the human placenta. II. Gross morphology of the foetal structures in the young placenta. *Acta Obstet. Gynecol. Scand.* 47, 420-435.

Boe, F. (1969) Studies on the human placenta. III. Vascularization of the young fetal placenta. A. Vascularization of the chorionic villus. *Acta Obstet. Gynecol. Scand.* 48, 159-166.

Boyd, J.D. and Hamilton, W.J. (1970) *The Human Placenta*, Cambridge: Heffer.

Chabes, A., Peroda, J., and Perez, J. (1967) Morphometry of human placenta at high altitude. Abstract. *Am. J. Pathol.* 50, 14a-15a.

Dantzer, V., Leiser, R., Kaufmann, P., and Luckhardt, M. (1987) Comparative morphological aspects of placental vascularization. *Trophoblast Research* 3, 235-260.

Habashi, S., Burton, G.J., and Steven, D.H. (1983) Morphological study of the fetal vasculature of the human placenta: scanning electron microscopy of corrosion casts. *Placenta* 4, 41-56.

Heinrich, D., Metz, J., Raviola, E., and Forssmann W.G. (1976) Ultrastructure of perfusion-fixed fetal capillaries in the human placenta. *Cell Tissue Res.* 172, 157-169.

Heinrich, D., Aoki, A., and Metz, J. (1987) Overview on fetal capillary organization in different types of placenta. *Trophoblast Research* 3, 149-162.

Hyrtl, J. (1870) *Die Blutgefaesse der menschlichen Nachgeburt in normalen und abnormen Verhlaeltnissen.* Wien: Braumueller.

Kaufmann, P. (1982) Development and differentiation of the human placental villous tree. *Bibltheca. Anat.* 22, 29-39.

Kaufmann, P. and Davidoff, M. (1977) The guinea-pig placenta. *Adv. Anat. Embryol. Cell Biol.* 53, 1-90.

Kaufmann, P., Sen, D.K., and Schweikhart, G. (1979) Classification of human placental villi. I. Histology. *Cell Tissue Res.* 200, 409-423.

Kaufmann, P., Bruns, U., Leiser, R., Luckhardt, M., and Winterhager, E. (1985) The fetal vascularization of term human placental villi. II. Intermediate and terminal villi. *Anat. Embryol.* 173, 203-214.

Lachenmayer, L. (1971) Adrenergic innervation of the umbilical vessels. Light and fluorescence microscopic studies. *Z. Zellforsch.* 120, 120-136.

Lee, M.M.L. and Yeh, M.N. (1983) Fetal circulation of the placenta: a comparative study of human and baboon placenta by scanning electron microscopy of vascular casts. *Placenta* 4, 515-526.

Leiser, R. (1985) Fetal vasculature of the human placenta: scanning electron microscopy of microvascular casts. *Contr. Gynecol. Obstet.* 13, 27-31.

Leiser, R. (1987) Mikrovaskularisation der Ziegenplazenta dargestellt mit rasterelektronisch untersuchten Gefaessausguessen. *Schweiz. Arch. Tierheilk.* 129, 59-74.

Leiser, R. and Kohler, T. (1983) The blood vessels of the cat girdle placenta. Observations on corrosion casts, scanning electron microscopical and histological studies. I. Maternal vasculature. *Anat. Embryol.* 167, 85-93.

Leiser, R. and Kohler, T. (1984) The blood vessels of the cat girdle placenta. Observations on corrosion casts, scanning electron microscopical and histological studies. II. Fetal vasculature. *Anat. Embryol.* 170, 209-216.

Leiser, R., Luckhardt, M., Kaufmann, P., Winterhager, E., and Bruns U. (1985). The fetal vascularisation of term human placental villi. I. Peripheral stem villi. *Anat. Embryol.* 173, 71-80.

Luckhardt, M., Kaufmann, P., and Elger, W. (1985) The structure of the tupaia placenta I. Histology and vascularisation. *Anat. Embryol.* 171, 201-210.

Nguyen H. Anh, J., and Panigel, M.M. (1964) Observations sur l'ultrastructure des capillaires foetaux dans les villosites du placenta humain. *CR. Acad. Sc. Paris* 258, 1056-1058.

Nikolov, S.D. and Schiebler, T.H. (1973) Ueber das fetale Gefaessystem der reifen menschlichen Plazenta. *Z. Zellforsch.* 139, 333-350.

Nikolov, S.D. and Schiebler, T.H. (1981) Ueber Endothelzellen in Zottengefaessen der reifen menschlichen Plazenta. *Acta Anat.* 110, 338-344.

O'Neill, J.E.G. (1983) Vascularizacao da placenta humana. *Dissertacao Universidade Nova de Lisboa*, Portugal.

Penfold, P., Wootton, R., and Hytten, P.E. (1981) Studies of a single placental cotyledon in vitro: III. The dimensions of the villous capillaries. *Placenta* 2, 161-168.

Ramsey, E.M. and Donner, M.W. (1980) *Placental Vasculature and Circulation*. Stuttgart: Georg Thieme.

Rhodin, J.A.G. (1967) The ultrastructure of mammalian arterioles and precapillary sphincters. *J. Ultrastruct. Res.* 18, 181-223.

Rhodin, J.A.G. (1968) Ultrastructure of mammalian venous capillaries, venules, and small collecting veins. *J. Ultrastruct. Res.* 25, 452-500.

Rhodin, J.A.G. (1974) *Histology. A Text and Atlas*. London, Toronto: New York-Oxford University Press.

Rhodin, J.A.G. and Terzakis, J. (1962) The ultrastructure of the human full-term placenta. *J. Ultrastruct. Res.* 6, 88-106.

Salvatore, C.A. (1968) The placenta in acute toxaemia. *Am. J. Obstet. Gynecol.* 102, 347-352.

Schiebler, T.H. and Kaufmann, P. (1981) Reife Plazenta In: *Die Plazenta des Menschen*, (ed.), V. Becker, T.H. Schiebler, and F. Kubli, Stuttgart: Georg Thieme, pp. 51-100.

Schuhmann, R. (1981) Plazenton: Begriff, Entstehung, funktionelle Anatomie. In: *Die Plazenta des Menschen*, (ed.), V. Becker, T.H. Schiebler, and F. Kubli, Stuttgart: Georg Thieme, pp. 199-207.

Schweikhart, G. and Kaufmann, P. (1982) Histologie und Morphometrie der Placenta bei intrauteriner Mangelentwicklung des Feten. 44. *Tagung Deutsche Ges. Gynaek.* Geburtsh., München.

Sen, D.K., Kaufmann, P., and Schweikhart, G. (1979) Classification of human placental villi. II. Morphometry. *Cell Tissue Res.* 200, 425-434.

Tedde, G. (1973) Caratteristiche morfologiche dei periciti dei capillari del villo coriale umano e loro ruolo nei fenomeni immunologici materno-fetali. *Arch.Ital. Anat. Embriol.* 78, 203-216.

Thiriot, M. and Panigel, M. (1978) Microcirculation. La microvascularisation des villosites placentaires humaines. *CR. Acad. Sci. Paris Ser. D.* 287, 709-712.

Tominaga, T. and Page, E.W. (1966) Accomodation of the human placenta to hypoxia. *Am. J. Obstet. Gynecol.* 94, 679-691.

Zeek, P.M. and Assali, N.S. (1950) Vascular changes in the decidua associated with eclamptogenic toxemia of pregnancy. *Am. J. Clin. Pathol.* 20, 1099-1109.

Trophoblast Research 3:139-148, 1988

# MONOCLONAL ANTIBODIES TO PLACENTAL VASCULAR STRUCTURES

Bae-Li Hsi and Chang-Jing G. Yeh

INSERM U210
Faculté de Médecine
Avenue de Vallombrose
06034 Nice-Cedex, France

## INTRODUCTION

In the human placenta, the maternal blood flows from the uterine arteries to fill the intervillous space where it is in direct contact with the syncytiotrophoblast of the chorionic villi. On the other hand, the fetal placental vascular structures form a complex network inside the villous stroma. The placental barrier which consists of trophoblast, chorionic stroma, and endothelium of the fetal blood vessels controls the major traffic of the interchange of materials between maternal and fetal blood (Boyd and Hamilton, 1970). The maturation and differentiation of the chorionic villi are related to the development of fetal blood vessels in the stroma (Fox, 1968; Kaufmann et al., 1985; Leiser et al., 1985). Abnormalities of the fetal blood vessels often lead to pathological changes in the chorionic villi (Fox, 1978). Since the placenta contains a very rich source of fetal vascular structures, it is not surprising that several monoclonal antibodies derived from a mouse which was immunized with cell membrane preparations from a full term placenta demonstrated specific reactivities to vascular structures. Although these antibodies are not specific only to placental vascular structures, they offer useful markers for the endothelium and differentiate several different vascular structures in the placenta. The reactivity of four monoclonal antibodies, GB37, GB40, GB41, and GB42 on the term human placenta is reported.

## MATERIALS AND METHODS

### Tissues

Term human placental tissues were collected from normal pregnancies by vaginal delivery at the Clinique St. George, Nice, France. Specimens of reflected amniochorions were sandwiched between two thin slices of rabbit liver. Placental tissues were collected from the maternal surface (basal plate) and fetal surface (chorionic plate) of each placenta. A segment of umbilical cord from each placenta was also collected. These tissues were wrapped with aluminum foil and snap-frozen in liquid nitrogen cooled iso-pentane (Hsi and Yeh, 1986a). The frozen tissues were kept at -80° C until use.

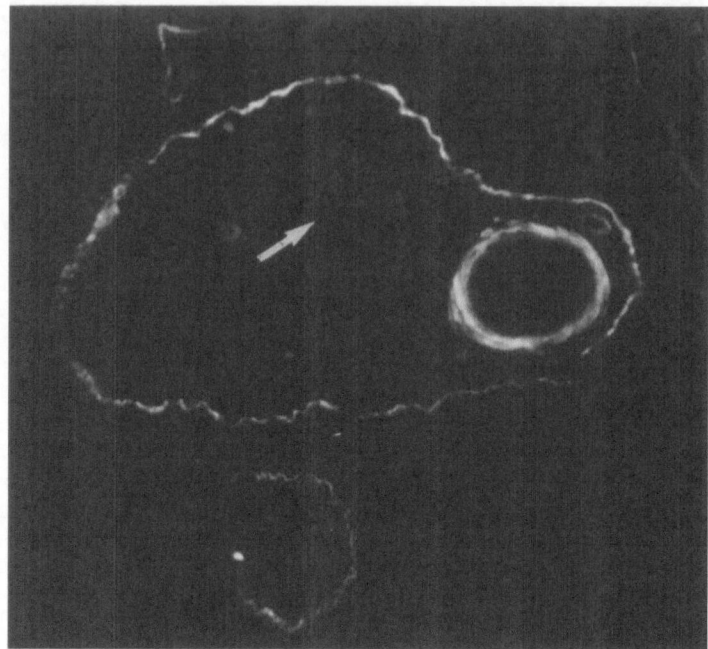

Figure 1.  The reactivity of GB37 on the placenta studied by immunofluorescence. The reactivities are located under the syncytiotrophoblast and around one chorionic stem vessel.  Notice that the other stem vessel is negative (arrow) X300.

## Monoclonal Antibodies

        GB37, GB40, GB41, and GB42 were mouse monoclonal antibodies secreted by hybridoma cell lines established from a fusion of P3-NS1/1-Ag4-1 (NS-1) cells and the spleen cells of a mouse immunized with placental microvilli prepared by differential ultracentrifugation (Smith et al., 1974).  The production procedures were as described by Hsi and Yeh (1986b).  GB37 and GB41 were IgG1, GB40 was IgM, and GB42 was IgG3 as determined by Ouchterlony immunodiffusion using a mouse monoclonal antibody typing kit (Serotec Ltd., Bicester, Oxon, England). Culture supernatants of the hybridoma cell lines were used for the study.

## Immunohistological Procedures

        Frozen sections (4.5 µm) were prepared using a cryostat and air-dried.  For double labeling immunofluorescence, the sections were first incubated with 40 µl of 1:100 dilution of tetramethyl rhodamine isothiocyanate conjugated anti-factor VIII (Atlantic Antibodies, Scarborough, Maine, USA) for 20 minutes, washed in 0.15 M phosphate buffered saline (PBS), pH 7.2 for 10 minutes, then incubated with 40 µl of undiluted monoclonal antibodies for one hour.  After being briefly washed in PBS, the sections were then incubated with 40 µl of 1:40 dilution of fluorescein isothiocyanate conjugated rabbit anti-mouse Ig (Dakopatts, Copenhagen, Denmark) for 20 minutes, washed in PBS then mounted in 50% AF1 mounting medium (Citifluor Ltd., London, England). For immunoperoxidase experiments, the sections were fixed in acetone for 10 minutes, then incubated with monoclonal antibodies for one hour. After being briefly washed in 0.05 M Tris-buffered saline (TBS), pH 7.6, the sections were further incubated with 40 µl of 1:400 dilution of biotinylated rabbit anti-mouse Ig (Dakopatts) for 30 minutes, washed in TBS and incubated with avidin-biotinylated horseradish peroxidase complex (ABC) (Dakopatts) for 30 minutes. After the final wash in TBS, the chromogenic reactions were developed in 40 µl of diaminobenzidine tetrahydrochloride (0.6 mg/ml) and 0.03% $H_2O_2$, counterstained with hematoxylin and mounted with the mounting medium (Technicon Chemical Co., Orcq-Tournai, Belgium). The sections were examined with a Zeiss Universal microscope and photographed as previously described (Hsi and Yeh, 1986a).

## Hemagglutination

Normal human blood (200 µl) was collected in 1 ml of 0.15 M PBS, pH 7.2, and washed with 3 ml of PBS. The cell suspension (5 µl) was added to 10 µl of each monoclonal antibody on a 4-well microscopic slide and gently mixed for 3 minutes.

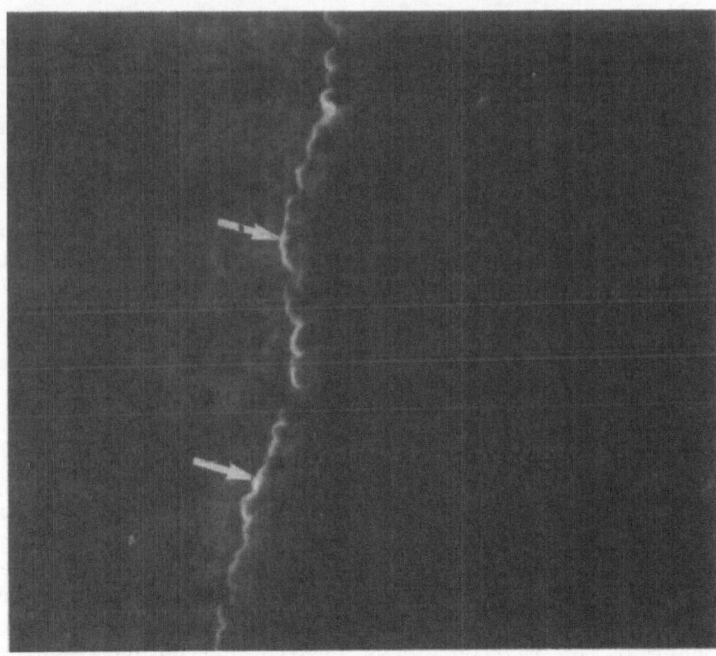

Figure 2. The reactivity of GB37 on the reflected amnion studied by immunofluorescence. The reactivity is localized on the surface of amniotic epithelium (arrows) X300.

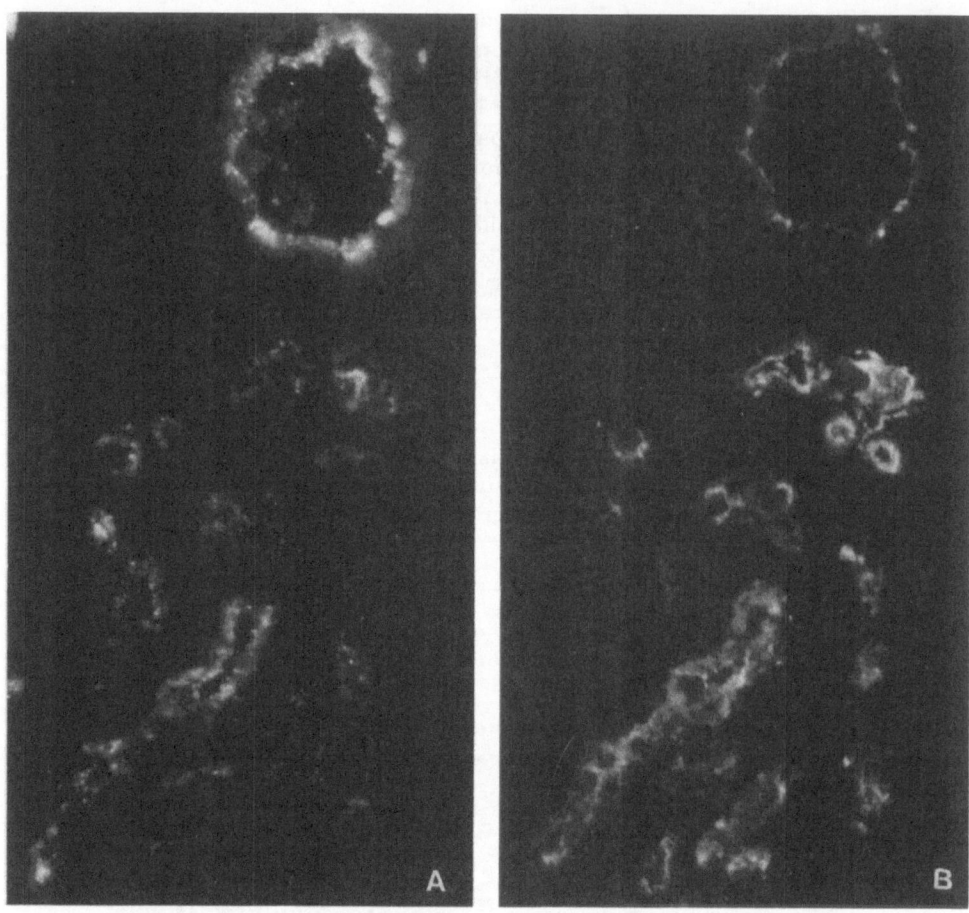

Figure 3. The reactivities of anti-factor VIII and GB40 on the placenta studied by double labeling immunofluorescence X300. A) The granular reactivity of anti-factor VIII is located on the fetal blood vessels. B) The endothelium of the same blood vessels reacts with GB40.

## RESULTS

### GB37

Three types of reactivity for GB37 could be identified in the placenta: (1) a thin, continuous layer between the chorionic stroma and syncytiotrophoblast (Figure 1); (2) around some fetal blood vessels (Figure 1); and, (3) on the surface of amniotic epithelium (Figure 2). The reactivity of GB37 between the stroma and syncytiotrophoblast could be seen in most chorionic villi (Figures 1 and 7A). However, whether the reactivity was located on the basal surface of the syncytiotrophoblast or was situated in the trophoblastic basement membrane could not be resolved by using immunohistology at light microscopic level. The reactivity of GB37 on the fetal blood vessels formed several thick layers around the endothelial basement membrane. Many nuclei could be seen in these layers. The endothelial cells were negative (Figures 1 and 7A). The fetal blood vessels which were positive for GB37 could be seen in both stem villi and terminal villi, and the sizes of the positive vessels varied greatly. Although the reactivity could also be identified on the muscular walls of the chorionic vessels and of the umbilical vessels, the reactivity on the vessels in the chorionic plate and the umbilical cord was much more diffuse and weaker than that of the vessels in the chorionic villi. The epithelial cells of both reflected and placental amnion reacted with GB37. The reactivity was mostly limited to the surface of the epithelial cells (Figure 2).

## GB40

GB40 reacted with the endothelium of all the blood vessels in the placenta as shown by the double labeling immunofluorescence experiments using anti-factor VIII and GB40 (Figure 3). The reactivity of GB40 gave a very clear outline of the endothelium. In addition, weaker reactivites could also be found in the intervillous spaces and to less extent, in the fetal blood vessels (Figure 4). These results suggested that GB40 might also react with erythrocytes. The hemagglutination experiments showed that indeed, GB40 recognized an antigen expressed on the cell membrane of erythrocytes. Of all the four monoclonal antibodies to the placental vascular structures, only GB40 agglutinated human erythrocytes.

## GB41

As GB40, GB41 also reacted with the endothelium of the blood vessels in the placenta. However, its reactivity pattern was very different from that of GB40 and was much weaker. GB41 gave a filament-like reactivity on the endothelium of all the fetal blood vessels in chorionic villi (Figure 5). Under higher magnification, this reactivity was found to be fine, granular, and located between the endothelial cells (Figure 6). The endothelium of all the blood vessels including capillaries, stem vessels, chorionic vessels, and umbilical vessels reacted with this antibody.

## GB42

GB42 reacted with the muscular walls of fetal stem vessels. Unlike GB37, the reactivity pattern of GB42 was much more diffuse and extended deeper into the chorionic stroma. However, there is no relationship between the GB37-positive and GB42-positive blood vessels (Figure 7). As described previously (Hsi and Yeh, 1986c), almost all of the chorionic villi which had GB42-positive vessels showed fibrinoid necrosis of the syncytiotrophoblast on their surface.

### DISCUSSION

The results of this study demonstrated the reactivity of four monoclonal antibodies GB37, GB40, GB41, and GB42 on the vascular structures in term human placentae. All four antibodies were derived from a mouse which was immunized with syncytiotrophoblastic microvilli prepared according to Smith et al. (1974). Totally, 34 different hybridoma cell lines were established from the spleen of this mouse. Eleven of them produced monoclonal antibodies which reacted with the antigens on the placental syncytiotrophoblast (WHO Workshop for Contraceptive

Vaccine, 1986, Toronto, Canada; Hsi and Yeh, 1986b; Hsi and Yeh, 1987). The identification of clones which produced antibodies with specificities to chorionic stromal structures and fibrinoid (Hsi and Yeh, 1987) indicates that the microvilli vesicles prepared by differential ultracentrifugation were probably contaminated by chorionic stromal tissues.

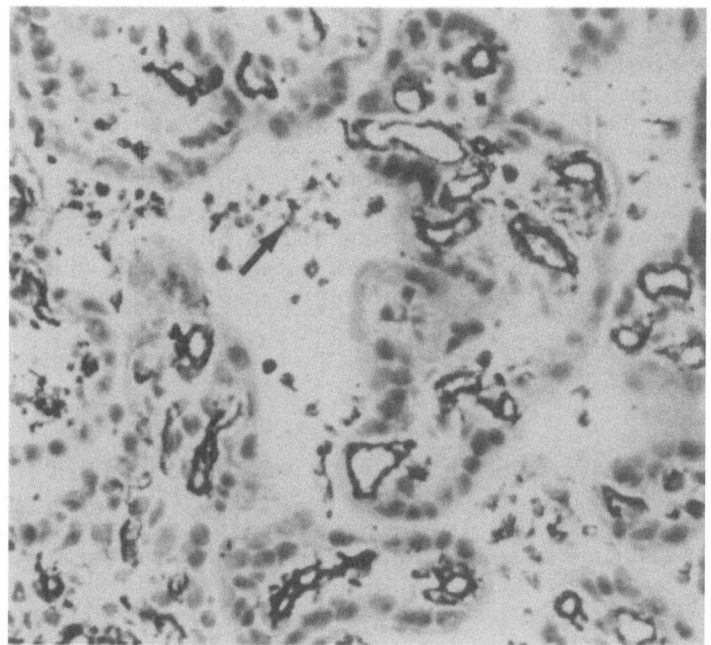

Figure 4. The reactivity of GB40 on the placenta studied by immunoperoxidase. GB40 reacted with the fetal blood vessels. Notice that some reactivity can also be identified in the intervillous space (arrow) X300.

---

Figure 5. The reactivity of GB41 on the placenta studied by immunofluorescence. The filament-like reactivity can be identified on the fetal blood vessels X300.

Figure 6. The reactivity of GB41 on the placenta studied by immunoperoxidase. The reactivities of GB41 on the fetal stem vessels are located between the endothelial cells (arrows) X400.

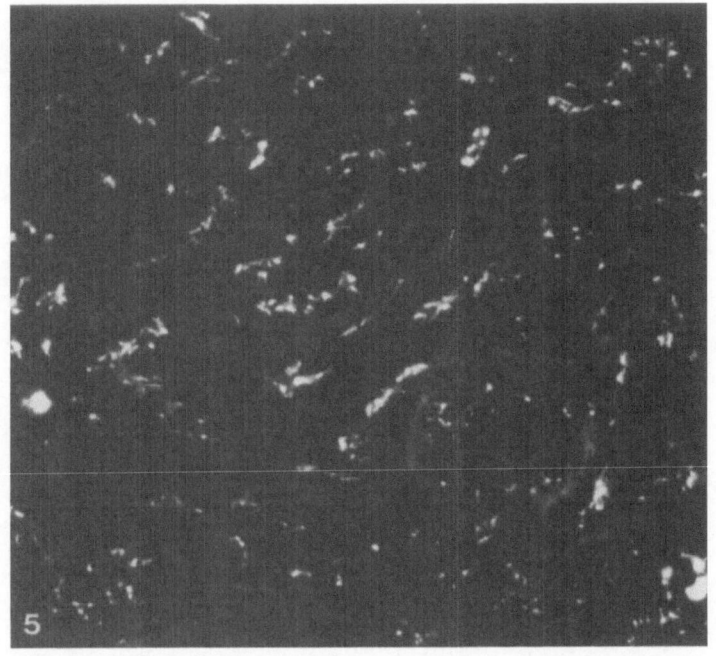

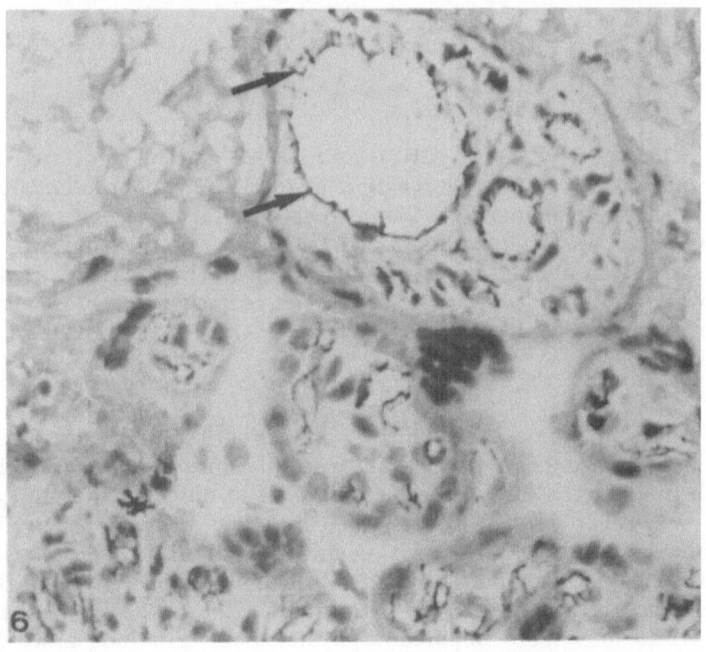

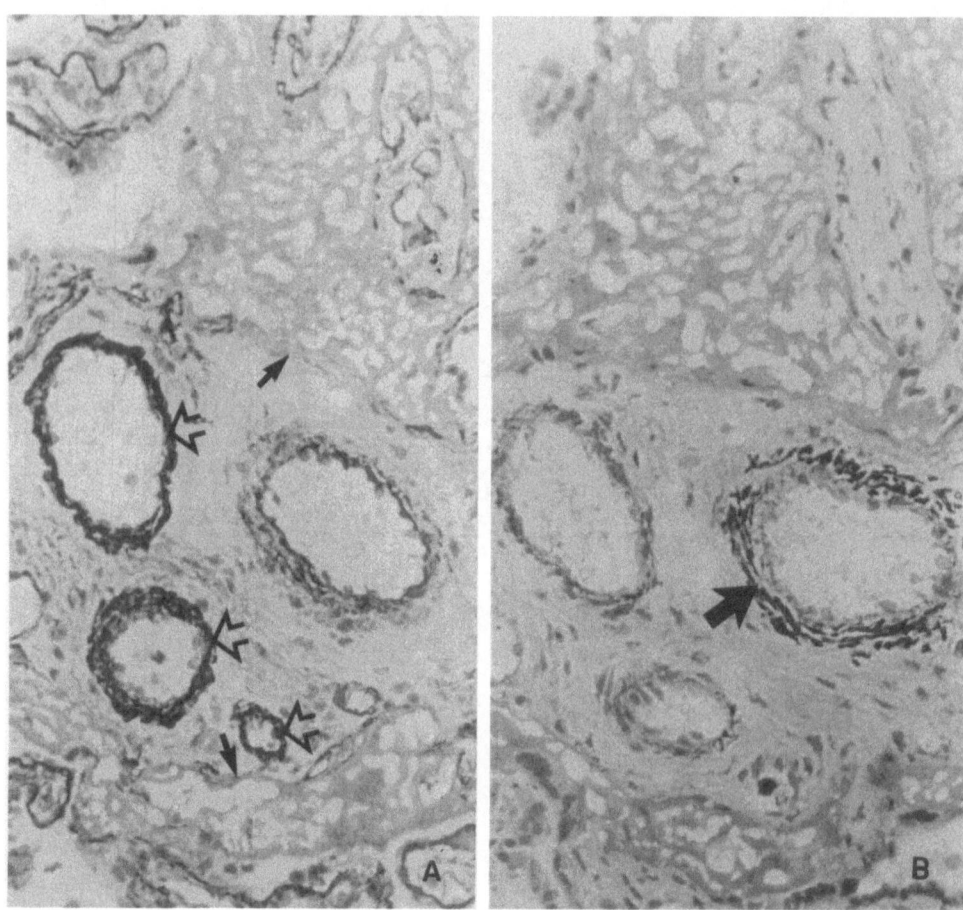

Figure 7. The reactivities of GB37 and GB42 on the placenta studied by immunoperoxidase X200. A) The reactivities of GB37 can be identified on three fetal blood vessels (open arrows). Some reactivities can also be seen under the syncytiotrophoblast in the terminal villi. However, on the chorionic stem villi, where the syncytiotrophoblast is replaced by the fibrinoid, GB37 is not reactive (small arrows). B) Parallel section of Figure 7A reacted with GB42. Positive cells are found around one fetal stem vessel which is only weakly reactive with GB37 (big arrow).

Although all four monoclonal antibodies reacted with the vascular structures in the placenta, none of them were placenta-specific. GB40 and GB41 reacted with the endothelium of the blood vessels in different human tissues (data not shown). However, both of them tended to show stronger reactivity with the placental blood vessels. GB40 was especially valuable as a marker for the endothelium, since it gave a better outline of the endothelial cells than the granular reactivity pattern of anti-factor VIII (Beranek et al., 1985). Furthermore, the antigen of GB40 may have important physiological functions since it was also identified on the erythrocyte membrane. GB42 reacted with the cells which formed many circles around the chorionic stem vessels, whereas the vessels in the terminal villi were completely negative. Even around the chorionic vessels and umbilical vessels, the reactivity of GB42 was much more dispersed. Also, the GB42-positive blood vessels were often associated with C1q and fibrinoid deposits in the chorionic villi (Hsi and Yeh, 1986c). On the other hand, the epidermal growth factor receptors had similar distribution on the placental vascular structures as did GB42 (Magid et al., 1985). These results suggest that the elevated density of GB42-positive cells around the placental stem vessels may represent a physiological response of these cells to the immune complexes as a result of the reaction of maternal anti-allotype antibodies to fetal antigens around these vessels. The most puzzling reactivity in this study was that of GB37. By morphological examination, it is difficult to differentiate the GB37-positive and GB37-negative blood vessels. Although more detailed examination using immuno-electron microscopy is still needed, the reactivity on the surface of amniotic epithelial cells suggests that GB37 probably recognized a cell surface antigen, rather than an extracellular antigen.

In conclusion, this report demonstrated the preliminary results of 4 monoclonal antibodies GB37, GB40, GB41, and GB42 on the vascular structures of placenta. Many more experiments are still required to tackle the biochemical nature of the antigens recognized by these antibodies and their physiological functions. In the meantime, these four monoclonal antibodies offer valuable probes for various placental vascular structures in the morphological studies.

## SUMMARY

Four monoclonal antibodies with specificities to placental vascular structures were identified during the screening of monoclonal antibodies raised against the term human placenta. GB37 recognized the interface between syncytiotrophoblast and villous stroma, some fetal blood vessels, and amniotic epithelium. GB40 reacted strongly with the endothelium of fetal blood vessels in the placenta, as well as the erythrocytes. GB41 gave a filament-like reactivity pattern on the endothelium of all the fetal blood vessels in the chorionic villi. GB42 reacted only with the cells in the muscular walls of some chorionic stem vessels. These data indicated that several different types of blood vessels exist in the chorionic villi. The availability of these four monoclonal antibodies should facilitate further investigations of the various fetal vascular structures in the human placenta.

## REFERENCES

Beranek, J., Hsi, B.-L., and Ortonne, J.P. (1985) Occurance of factor VIII-related antigen positive cells in perivascular infiltrates of venous stasis dermatitis. *Br. J. Dermatol.* 113, 651-659.

Boyd, J.D. and Hamilton, W.J. (1970) *The Human Placenta.* London:Heffer.

Fox, H. (1968) Villous immaturity in the term placenta. *Obstet. Gynecol.* 31, 9-12.

Fox, H (1978) *Pathology of the Placenta.* London:W.B. Saunders Co.

Hsi, B.-L. and Yeh, C.-J.G. (1986a) Monoclonal antibodies to human amnion. *J. Reprod. Immunol.* 9, 11-21.

Hsi, B.-L. and Yeh, C.-J.G. (1986b) Monoclonal antibody GB25 recognizes human villous trophoblasts. *Am. J. Reprod. Immunol. Microbiol.* 12, 1-3.

Hsi, B.-L. and Yeh, C.-J.G. (1986c) Studies of C1q deposits in the human placenta using monoclonal antibodies to human extra-embryonic tissues. *Trophoblast Research,* 2, 223-231.

Hsi, B.-L. and Yeh, C.-J.G. (1987) Monoclonal antibody GB36 raised against human trophoblast recognizes a novel epithelial antigen. *Placenta* 8, 209-217.

Kaufmann, P., Bruns, U., Leiser, R., Luckhardt, M., and Winterhager, E. (1985) The fetal vascularization of term human placental villi. II. Intermediate and terminal villi. *Anat. Embryol.* 173, 71-80.

Leiser, R., Luckhardt, M., Kaufmann, P., Winterhager, E., and Bruns, U. (1985) The fetal vascularization of term human placental villi. II. Peripheral stem villi. *Anat. Embryol.* 173, 203-214.

Magid, M., Nanney, L.B., Stoscheck, C.M., and King, L.E., Jr. (1985) Epidermal growth factor binding and receptor distribution in term human placenta. *Placenta* 6, 519-526.

Smith, N.C., Brush, M., and Luckett, L. (1974) Preparation of human placental villous surface membranes. *Nature* 252, 302-303.

Trophoblast Research 3:149-162, 1988

# FETAL CAPILLARY ORGANIZATION IN DIFFERENT TYPES OF PLACENTA

## - A Review -

Dirk Heinrich[1], Augustin Aoki[2], and Jürgen Metz[3,4]

[1]Universitäts-Frauenklinik  Heidelberg
Vosstr. 9, D-6900 Heidelberg, West-Germany

[2]Centro de Microscopia Electronica
Universidad Nacional de Cordoba, Casilla Postal 362
5000 Cordoba, Argentina

[3]Anatomisches Institut der Universität Heidelberg
Im Neuenheimer Feld 307, D-6900 Heidelberg, West-Germany

## INTRODUCTION

The chorioallantoic placenta is the principal organ of exchange processes between mother and fetus in most higher mammals.  Three fetal components, namely trophoblast, connective tissue, and capillary wall, build the histological barrier in hemochorial placentae.  Species specific variations of the trophoblast are well known, examples of which are hemomonochorial (man, guinea pig), hemodichorial (rabbit), and hemotrichorial (rat, mouse) organizations.  The hemochorial condition is subdivided into labyrinthine pattern in rat, guinea pig, rabbit, and mouse, and a villous arrangement in man.

Studies available dealing with ultrastructural diversities in the organization of the fetal capillaries within the various placentae are limited (Heinrich et al., 1977).  In some publications species specific arrangement and fine structure of the capillary  wall are described e.g., in man (Heinrich et al., 1976; Nikolov and Schiebler, 1981), in the guinea pig (Sibley et al., 1982; Orgnero de Gaisan et al., 1985), and and in the rat (Metz et al., 1976).  Distinct permeability properties of the fetal capillaries have been reported in the guinea pig (Sibley et al., 1981 and 1983; Orgnero de Gaisan et al., 1985), and in the rat (Aoki et al., 1978).

The aim of this contribution is to provide an overview of the fetal capillary organization in different species.  Ultrastructurally placental capillaries are comparable to those from other organs.  Since variables like concentration of a substance in fetal and maternal bloods, the amount of substance metabolized by the placenta during passage and the rate of maternal blood flow are important, ultrastructure consequently reflects only a few of the variables in transfer.

[4]To Whom Correspondence Should Be Addressed

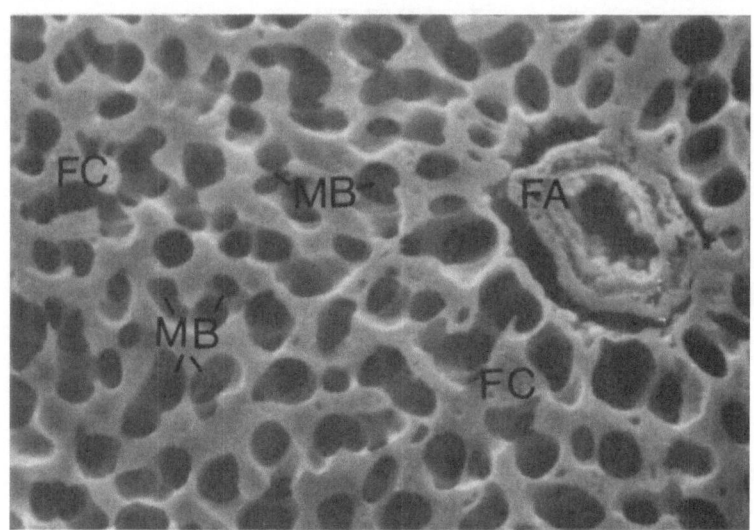

Figure 1.  Rat placenta:  Scanning electron microscopic (SEM) picture of the placental labyrinth after perfusion fixation from maternal side.  The maternal blood spaces (MB) are empty.  The fetal blood capillaries (FC) within the primary labyrinthine lamellae contain erythrocytes and are surrounded by the trophoblastic layers.  Fetal artery (FA).  X200

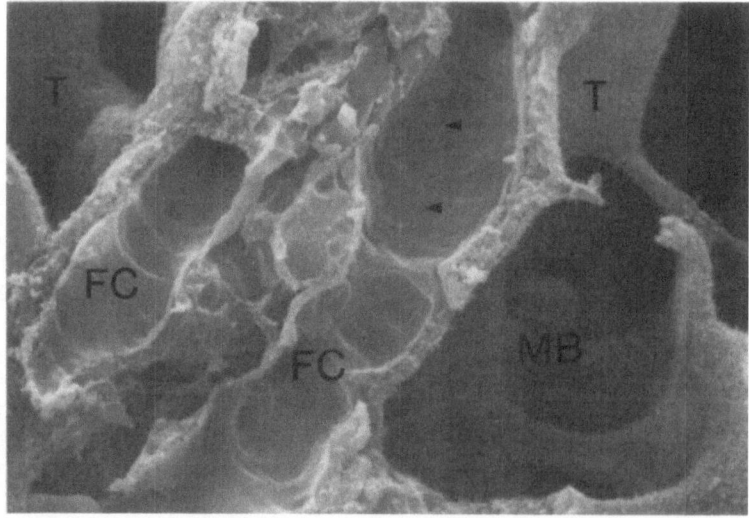

Figure 2.  Rat placenta:  SEM of the placental labyrinth after perfusion fixation from fetal and maternal sides.  Within the fetal capillaries (FC), endothelial cells with intercellular clefts (arrows) are seen.  Connective tissue stroma (S).  Surface of the trophoblast (T) facing the maternal blood space (MB).  X4000

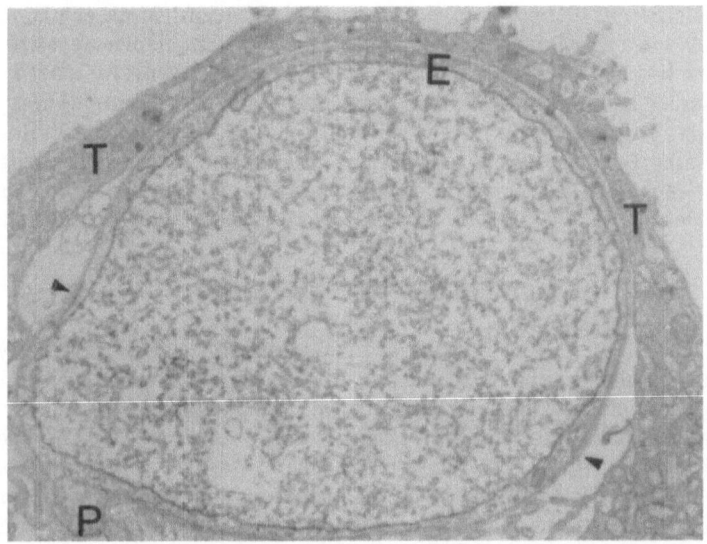

Figure 3.  Guinea pig placenta:  The placenta barrier consists of the trophoblast (T), the basal lamina (arrow), and the fetal capillary endothelium (E).  Pericyte (P). X12000

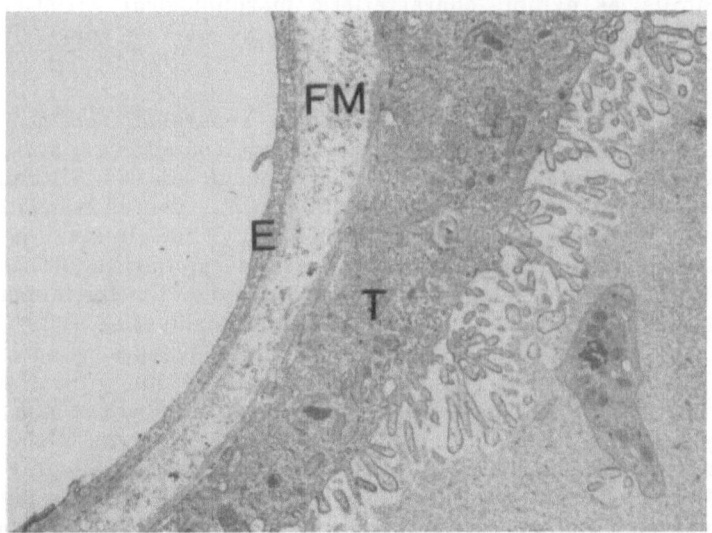

Figure 4.  Human placenta:  Endothelial cell (E) of the capillary is surrounded by a basal lamina  and some fibrous material (FM).  Trophoblast (T).  X12000

## MATERIALS AND METHODS

Placentae of rat, mouse, rabbit, and guinea pig were investigated after perfusion fixation from either maternal or fetal circulation (Metz et al., 1976; Aoki et al., 1978; Orgnero de Gaisan and Aoki, 1985). Human placentae were obtained after normal deliveries or caesarean sections and fixed by perfusion through the umbilical vessels or by immersion of small pieces into 4% phosphate-buffered glutaraldehyde solution (Heinrich et al., 1976; Metz and Weihe, 1980). Transmission electron microscopy of sections and freeze fracture replicas, as well as scanning electron microscopy were performed as reported in earlier publications (Metz et al., 1976; Aoki et al., 1978; Orgnero de Gaisan et al., 1985).

## RESULTS AND DISCUSSION

Fetal capillary organization is investigated within the labyrinthine placenta of rat, mouse, rabbit, and guinea pig, and in the villous placenta of the human. The microvasculature in all placentae is especially developed at the level where the nature and magnitude of the metabolic activities of the trophoblast require an extensive and rapid transfer. In scanning electron microscopy of the rat placental labyrinth the macrovessels such as arteries, veins, or arterioles are viewed as autonomous structures, while the compact primary lamellae suggest that their capillary segments act as functional units together with the surrounding interstitium and the trophoblast (Figures 1 and 2). An extensive study of the capillary organization reveals the existence of discrete segments of the capillary bed within different kinds of villi, which is reflected by a varying morphological arrangement, especially in the human placenta (Kaufmann et al., 1988). The placental capillaries exhibit characteristic morphological variations, which suggest the influence of the microenvironment as well as adaptations of the endothelium.

The fetal blood spaces are found to be separated from the maternal compartments by the vascular wall, interstitial connective tissue, and the trophoblast (Figures 3 and 4). The wall of the exchange vessels is virtually reduced to the endothelium and its basal lamina (Figure 3). The endothelial cells are arranged in a monolayer and are connected by intercellular junctions. A continous endothelium is typically found in fetal capillaries in the placental labyrinth of guinea pig and rabbit, and in the terminal villi in the human placenta (Figures 3, 4, and 5) (Heinrich et al., 1976, 1977; Kaufmann et al., 1982; Orgnero de Gaisan et al., 1985). In the human placenta two different types of endothelial cells have been described within the microvasculature of the villi (Nikolov and Schiebler, 1983). Both cell types contain moderate numbers of plasmalemmal vesicles. Type I cells additionally exhibit contractile filaments (Heinrich et al., 1976; Nikolov and Schiebler, 1981), while type II cells possess a highly developed rough endoplasmic reticulum and secretory granules. In the guinea pig placenta, the continuous endothelium seems to consist of a homogenous cell population. However, quantitative segmental differences in the plasmalemmal expression of the capillary wall are found. There are capillary segments exhibiting only a few vesicles, while in others numerous plasmalemmal vesicles are seen (Figures 5 and 6). Quantitative differences in the formation and turnover of plasmalemmal vesicles between segments in capillary loops in the same organ have also been described by Simionescu and Simionescu (1984). The endothelial cells are interpreted as dynamic features, which are specialized to mediate the bidirectional exchange of substances. Interpretation of interspecies variations by generalization of the formation and turnover of plasmalemmal vesicles within the endothelium is limited. The variations detected have to be referred to the physiological conditions which are reflected in varying morphological substrates (Figures 5 and 6). The ultrastructure of the endothelial surface differentiations demonstrates a frozen state or condition, which may also be influenced by the kind and technique of fixation (Simionescu and Simionescu, 1984).

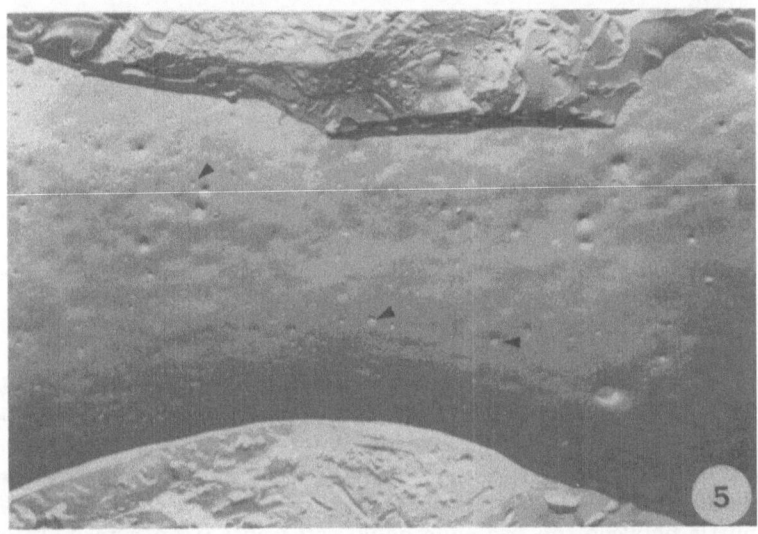

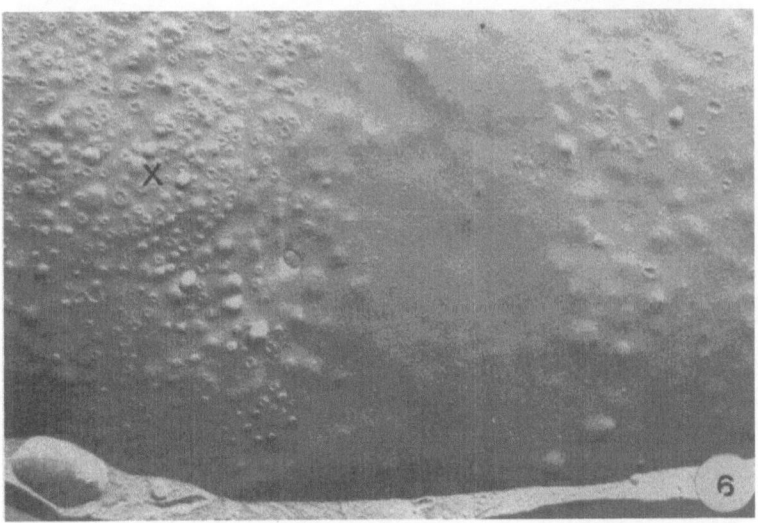

Figures 5 and 6. Guinea pig placenta: Two segments of a capillary loop are seen: one exhibits only a few plasmalemmal vesicles (arrows) (Figure 5), the other shows numerous openings of vesicles (x) (Figure 6). Figure 5 - X5000; Figure 6 - X15000

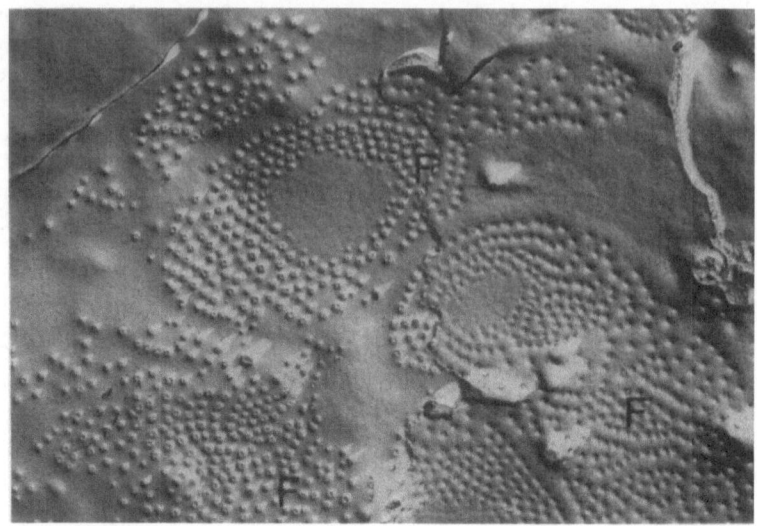

Figure 7. Rat placenta: The fenestrations (F) are often seen to be arranged in "sieve areas". X10000

        The role of the plasmalemmal vesicles in the permeability of the endothelial wall is still a matter of controversy. The endothelial vesicles are suggested to be responsible for the transfer of of larger solutes (Clough and Michel, 1981). In continuous capillaries, probe molecules >1.7 nm in diameter were found to cross the capillary wall primarily via plasmalemmal vesicles, which appear to build a shuttle between the two endothelial cell fronts (transcytosis) (Simionescu, 1983).

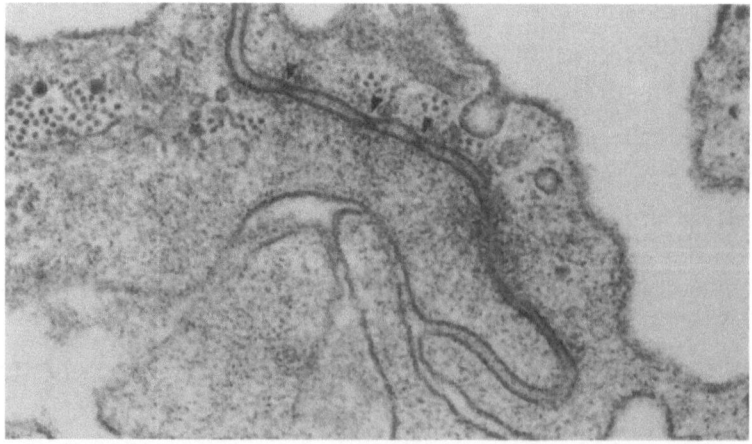

Figure 8. Human placenta: Intercellular cleft between endothelial cells which exhibits numerous membrane appositions (arrows) in the region of the zonula occludens. X60000

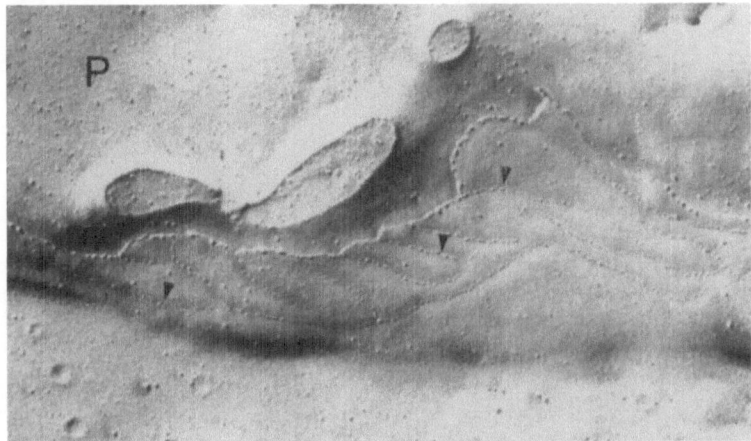

Figure 9. Rabbit placenta: Freeze fracture image of a interendothelial zonula occludens. Three to five strands (arrows) are seen on the P-face (P) of the membrane. X40000

Some investigators believe, however, that plasmalemmal vesicles represent a stable system of cell membrane invaginations (Kobayashi, 1970); associated with one endothelial front or another they may occasionally fuse and form channels (Bundgaard, 1980).

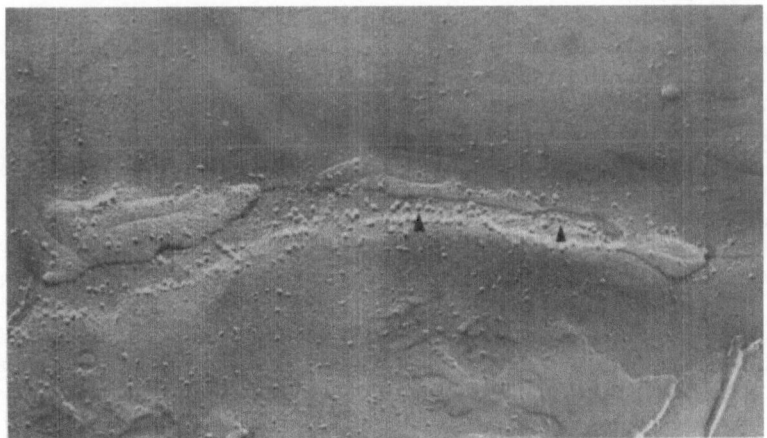

Figure 10. Rat placenta: In the interendothelial cleft, rows of single particles (arrow) and irregular groups of particles are seen. X60000

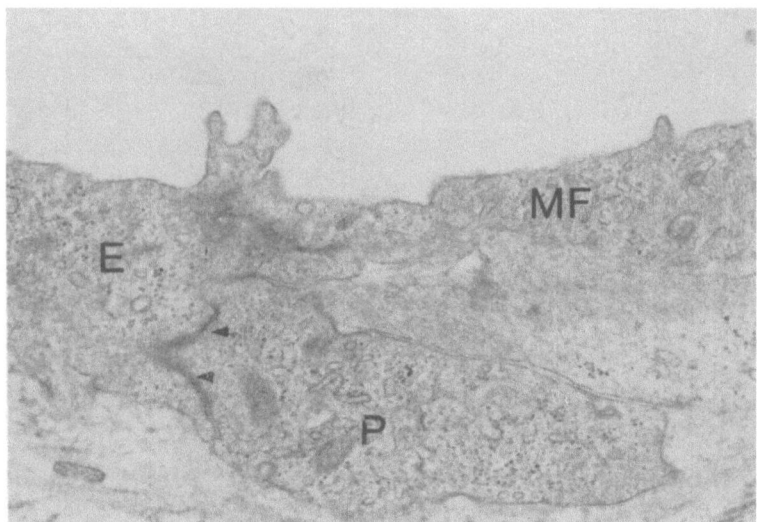

Figure 11. Human placenta: Contact area (arrow) between an endothelial cell (E) and a pericyte (P). The endothelial cell contains considerable amounts of microfilaments (MF). X15000

A fenestrated endothelium is found in the rat and mouse (Metz et al., 1976; Heinrich et al., 1977). Fenestrae are distributed either randomly or in patches (sieve areas) (Figure 7). The diaphragmata within the fenestrations are imposing as melting parts of the endothelial membrane (Rhodin, 1962; Metz et al., 1976). The fenestrae are suggested as labile and dynamic features that can form and disappear under a variety of circumstances. The formation process seems to start from the plasmalemmal vesicles, which appear as highly modulating features (Simionescu and Simionescu, 1984). Single plasmalemmal vesicles or two or more fused vesicles can open concomitantly on both fronts of endothelial cells to form transient, patent transendothelial channels through which plasma and interstitial fluid can communicate directly (Aoki et al., 1978). The ultimate expression of the channels could be considered the fenestrae, a channel reduced to its minimal length. Despite the flexibility of the plasmalemmal vesicle system, genetic factors seem also to be involved in the formation of fenestrations suggesting that endothelial cells with fenestrae belong to a specific type of capillaries.

Large tracers such as ferritin or horseradish peroxidase permeate the fenestrae (Clementi and Palade, 1969; Aoki et al., 1978). Despite this evidence, fenestrated capillaries seem to be less permeable to macromolecules than continuous capillaries, whereas that for glucose is five-fold greater, and the filtration coefficient is 20 times higher (Crone and Christensen, 1978). These physiological data together with the findings that fenestral diaphragms have a high negative charge (Simionescu et al., 1981) suggest that these features may be associated with permeability to water and small solutes, but not to macromolecules (Renkin and Curry, 1978).

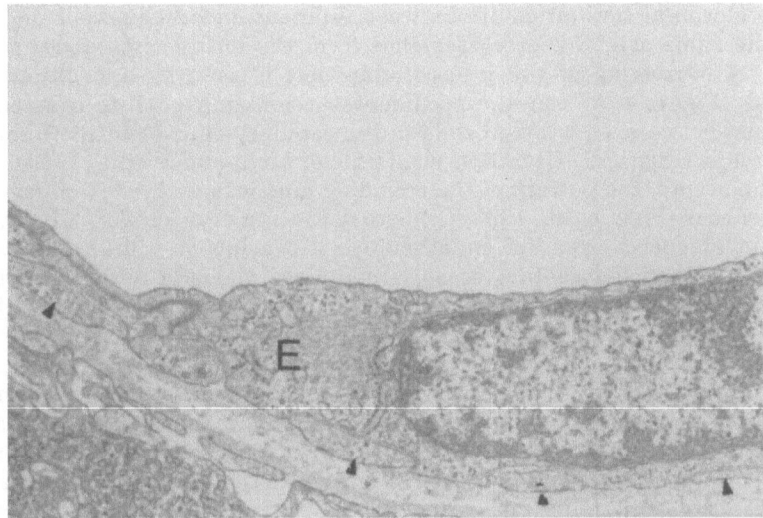

Figure 12.  Human placenta: Pseudopodial extensions (arrows) of other endothelial cells are seen along the capillary endothelium (E).   X20000

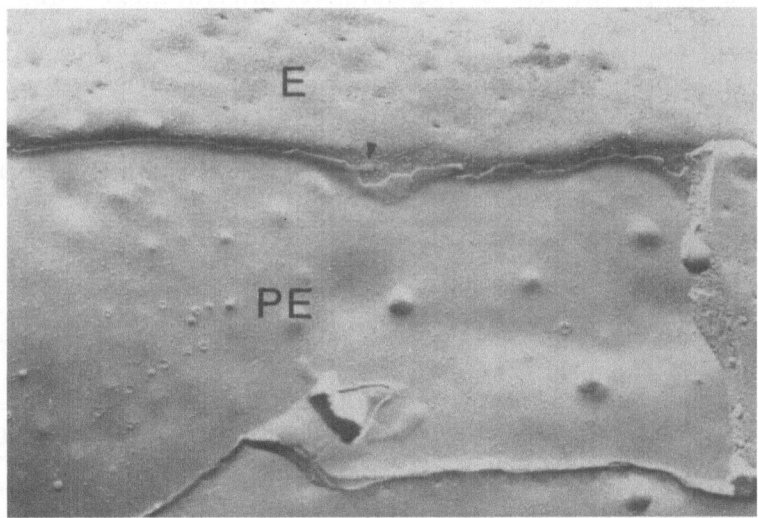

Figure 13. Human placenta: In the contact area between a pseudopodial extension (PE) and an endothelial cell (E) a gap junction (arrow) is seen.  X25000

The different kinds of endothelial connections within the intercellular space are probably derivations of the endothelial membrane. Intercellular spaces within the placental capillaries are between different endothelial cells or between one and the same cell, the processes that form the entire circumference of the capillary. A narrowing of the intercellular cleft is seen by appositions of the membranes (Figure 8). Zonulae occludentes consisting of 3 to 5 strands are mainly found between endothelial cells in the capillary sinuses in the human and rabbit placenta (Figure 9) (Heinrich et al., 1976; Metz and Weihe, 1980). In the guinea pig placenta, the pattern of the occluding junctions within a capillary loop is not homogeneous (Firth et al., 1983; Orgnero de Gaisan et al., 1985). The occluding junctions in extensive areas of endothelial cell overlap may differ in structure from those in restricted contact areas. In the rat placenta very often no tight occluding junctional structures, but only rows of particles are found within the intercellular cleft (Figure 10) (Metz et al., 1976). The ultrastructure of the intercellular junctions suggests a minor paracellular transfer in human and rabbit capillaries. The zonulae occludentes in rat and mouse placental capillaries primarily are more leaky allowing the passage of small as well as large molecular substances (Aoki et al., 1978). However, vasoactive mediators, such as histamine, bradykinin, and serotonin, may influence the permeabilty properties of the intercellular junctions, e.g., allowing extensive extravasation of plasma (Mayno and Palade, 1961; Hultström and Svensjö, 1977).

In conclusion, microvascular endothelial cells within the placenta are envisaged as an active metabolic tissue, which responds to changes in the fetal blood as well as in the interstitium facing the trophoblast. Metabolic factors, which are related to the needs of the fetus and to the supply of the trophoblast are probably reflected in the structural pecularities of the vascular segments involved in the blood tissue transfers. Interspecies variations in ultrastructure of the endothelium appear both as quantitative and qualitative differentiations. Quantitative differentiations are primarily represented by cell constituents such as the plasmalemmal vesicles. Qualitative differences exist in the thickness of the endothelium, expression of fenestrations, and the intercellular junctional tightness. The plasmalemmal vesicles, transendothelial channels, fenestrations, and intercellular junctions are responsible for the regulation of the permeability of the various types of capillaries (Karnovsky, 1968; Casley-Smith and Clark, 1972; Renkin, 1977; Aoki et al., 1978; Kaufmann et al., 1982; Sibley et al., 1982; Orgnero de Gaisan et al., 1985; Firth et al., 1987).

Species differences in the microvascular organization of placentae are also observed in the arrangement of the neighboring cellular layers around the endothelium. Pericytes adjacent to the endothelial cells are found in all placenta types (Figures 3 and 11). The pericytes, which vary considerably, form an incomplete layer around the capillaries. Within the villous human placenta the presence of smooth muscle cells around the capillaries is characteristic (Figure 12) (Heinrich et al., 1976; Metz and Weihe, 1980). The endothelial cells have close contact with defined areas of the pericytic membrane (Figure 11). These pericytic-endothelial contact zones correspond to myoendothelial contacts, which are observed between endothelium and smooth muscle cells (Figure 12). The pericytic-endothelial and myoendothelial contacts are irregularly distributed and have been analyzed as nexus structures (Figure 13) (Metz and Weihe, 1980). The existence of these mini-junctions indicates a close interaction between endothelial cells, pericytes, and smooth muscle cells like a functional syncytium (Barr et al., 1968). Especially within the human placenta an autonomous diameter regulating contractility seems to be of major importance. It is realized by capillary endothelial cells containing considerable amounts of contractile material (Heinrich et al.,1976), the surrounding pericytes, and smooth muscle cells (Granger et al.,1975; Johnson, 1980). Since no innervation is found in the placental vascularization (Lachenmayer, 1971), metabolic factors may probably influence the regulation of the vascular wall.

Finally, the connective tissue within the interstitial space has to be considered in comparison with the microvascular endothelium. The amount of connective tissue varies considerably within the different placentae (Figures 3, 4, and 12). The lamina basalis lining the vascular wall is continuous with the intercellular matrix. It is produced and secreted by the endothelial cells (Jaffe et al., 1976). The importance of the lamina basalis must be evaluated in comparison with the endothelial cells. Although a barrier function for the lamina basalis is only suggested for larger molecules (Caulfield and Farquhar, 1974), considerable variations might exist for the continuous and the fenestrated endothelia. Besides its function as a physical barrier, the lamina basalis builds a rigid skeleton around the capillary (Fung et al., 1966).

## SUMMARY

Various differentiations of the capillary organization have been demonstrated with respect to species specificity. In the hemomonochorial human placenta, a continuous endothelium has been found exhibiting infrequent plasmalemmal vesicles and tight zonulae occludentes. Smooth muscle cells and pericytes around the capillaries were especially prominent as well as a broader connective tissue layer. In the hemomonochorial labyrinthine placenta of guinea pig, a continous endothelium was also observed. Plasmalemmal vesicular expression as well as extent of occluding junctions, exhibited segmental variations. In the hemotrichorial placental labyrinth of rat and mouse, a fenestrated endothelium and leaky occluding junctions were found.

Although the ultrastructural variations of the cellular differentiations mainly reflect dynamic features and adaptations of the endothelium to the metabolic state of the environment, interspecies differences of the microvascular wall may also be influenced to some extent by the variability of the trophoblast.

## REFERENCES

Aoki, A., Metz, J., and Forssmann, W.G. (1978) Studies on ultrastructure and permeability of the hemotrichorial placenta. II. Fetal capillaries and tracer administration into the fetal blood circulation. *Cell Tissue Res.* 192, 409-422.

Barr, L., Berger, W. and Dewey, M.M. (1968) Electrical transmission at the nexus between smooth muscle cells. *J. Gen. Physiol.* 51, 347-368.

Bundgard, M. (1980) Transport pathways in capillaries - in search of pores. *Ann. Rev. Physiol.* 42, 325-336.

Casley-Smith, J.R., and Clark, H.I. (1972) The dimensions and numbers of small vesicles in blood capillary endothelium in the hind legs of dogs, and their relation to vascular permeability. *J. Microsc.* 96, 263-267.

Caulfield, J.P. and Farquhar, M.G. (1974) The permeability of glomerular capillaries to graded dextrans. Identification of basement membrane as the primary filtration barrier. *J. Cell. Biol.* 63, 883-903.

Clementi, F. and Palade, G.E. (1969) Intestinal capillaries. I. Permeability to peroxidase and ferritin. *J. Cell. Biol.* 41, 33-58.

Clough, G. and Michel, C. (1981) The role of vesicles in the transport of ferritin through frog endothelium. *J. Physiol.* 315, 127-142.

Crone, C. and Christensen, O. (1978) Transcapillary transport of small solutes and water. In: *Cardiovascular Physiology III,* (eds.), A.C. Guyton and D.B. Young, Baltimore, MD: University Park, vol. 18, pp. 149-213.

Firth, J.A., Bauman, K., and Sibley, C. (1983) The intercellular junctions of guinea-pig placental capillaries: a possible structural basis for endothelial solute permeability. *J. Ultrastructure Res.* 85, 45-57.

Fung, Y.C., Zweifach, B.W. and Intaglietta, M. (1966) Elastic environment of the capillary bed. *Circ. Res.* 19, 441-461.

Granger, H., Goodman, A., and Cook, B. (1975) Metabolic models of microcirculatory regulation. *Fed. Proc.* 34, 2025-2030.

Heinrich, D., Metz, J., Raviola, E., and Forssmann, W.G. (1976) Ultrastructure of perfusion-fixed fetal capillaries in the human placenta. *Cell Tissue Res.* 172, 157-169.

Heinrich, D., Weihe, E., Gruner, C., and Metz, J. (1977) Vergleichende Morphologie der Placentakapillaren. *Verh. Anat. Ges. Anat. Anz.* 71, 489-491.

Hultström, D. and Svensjö, E. (1979) Intravital and electron microscopic study of bradykinin-induced vascular permeability changes using FITC-dextran as a tracer. *J. Pathol.* 129, 125-133.

Jaffe, E.A., Minck, C.R., Adelman, B., Becker, C.G., and Nachman, R. (1976) Synthesis of basement membrane collagen by cultured human endothelial cells. *J. Exp. Med.* 144, 209-225.

Johnson, P.C. (1980) The myogenic response. In: *Handbook of Physiology. The Cardiovascular System. Vascular Smooth Muscle.* (eds.), D.F. Bohr, A.P. Somlyo, and H.V. Sparks, Bethesda, MD: Am. Physiol. Society, Sect, 2, Vol.II, pp. 409-442.

Karnovsky, M.J. (1968) The ultrastructural basis of transcapillary exchanges. *J. General Physiol.* 52, 64-95.

Kaufmann, P., Schröder, H. and Leichtweiss, H.P. (1982) Fluid shift across the placenta: II Fetomaternal transfer of horseradish peroxidase in the guinea pig. *Placenta* 3, 339-348.

Kaufmann, P., Luckhardt, M., and Leiser, R. (1988) Three-dimensional representation of the fetal vessel system in the human placenta. *Trophoblast Research* 3, 113-137.

Kobayashi, S. (1970) Ferritin labeling in the fixed muscle capillary. A doubt on the tracer experiments as the basis for the vesicular transport theory. *Arch. Histol. Jpn.* 32, 81-86.

Lachenmayer, L. (1971) Adrenergic innervation of the umbilical vessels. Light and fluorescence microscopic studies. *Z. Zellforsch.* 120, 120-136.

Mayno, G. and Palade, G.E. (1961) Studies on inflammation. I. The effect of histamine and serotonin on vascular permeability: an electron microscopic study. *J. Biophys. Biochem. Cytol.* 11, 571-605.

Metz, J., Heinrich, D., and Forssmann, W.G. (1976) Ultrastructure of the labyrinth in the rat full term placenta. *Anat. Embryol.* 149, 123-148.

Metz, J. and Weihe, E. (1980) Intercellular junctions within the human full term placenta: II. Cytotrophoblast cells, intravillous stroma cells and blood vessels. *Anat. Embryol.* 158, 167-178.

Nikolov, S.D. and Schiebler, T.H. (1981) Uber Endothelzellen in Zottengefaessen der reifen menschlichen Placenta. *Acta Anat.* 110, 338-344.

Orgnero de Gaisan, E. and Aoki, A. (1985) Permeability studies of the labyrinth in the guinea pig placenta: I. Perfusion of fixatives and tracers into the fetal circulation. *Anat. Embryol.* 171, 71-74.

Orgnero de Gaisan, E., Aoki, A., Heinrich, D., and Metz, J. (1985) Permeability studies of the guinea pig placental labyrinth II. Tracer permeation and freeze fracture of fetal endothelium. *Anat. Embryol.* 171, 297-304.

Renkin, E.M. (1977) Multiple pathways of capillary permeability. *Circ. Res.* 41, 735-743.

Renkin, E.M. and Curry, F.E. (1978) Transport of water and solutes across capillary endothelium. In: *Transport Organs,* (eds.), G. Giebisch, D.C. Tosteson, and H.H. Ussing. Berlin: Springer-Verlag, Vol. 4, pt. A and B, pp. 1-45.

Rhodin, J. (1962) The diaphragm of capilary endothelial fenestrations. *J. Ultrastructure Res.* 6, 171-185.

Sibley, C.P., Baumann, K.F., and Firth, J.A. (1981) Ultrastructural study of the permeability of the guinea-pig placenta to horseradish peroxidase. *Cell Tissue Res.* 219, 637-647.

Sibley, C.P., Baumann, K.F., and Firth, J.A. (1982) Permeability of the foetal capillary endothelium of the guinea-pig placenta to haem proteins of various molecular sizes. *Cell Tissue Res.* 223, 165-178.

Sibley, C.P., Baumann, K.F. and Firth, J.A. (1983) Molecular charge as a determinant of macromolecule permeability across the fetal capillary endothelium of the guinea-pig placenta. *Cell Tissue Res.* 229, 365-377.

Simionescu, N. (1983) Cellular aspects of transcapillary exchange. *Physiol. Reviews* 63, 1536-1579.

Simionescu, M., Simionescu, N., and Palade, G.E. (1981) Differentiated microdomains on the luminal surface of capillary endothelium. Preferential distribution of anionic sites. *J. Cell Biol.* 90, 605-613.

Simionescu, M. and Simionescu, N. (1984) Ultrastructure of the microvascular wall: Functional correlations. In: *Handbook of Physiology. The Cardiovascular System, Microcirculation.* Bethesda, MD: Am. Physiol. Society, Vol. IV, Chap. 3

Weihe, E., Heinrich, D., and Metz, J. (1978) Funktionell morphologische Untersuchungen an der feto-maternalen Placentabarriere des Menschen. *Perinatale Medizin VII,* 515-517.

Trophoblast Research 3:163-177, 1988

# PERMEABILITY PATHWAYS IN FETAL PLACENTAL CAPILLARIES

## - A Review -

J. Anthony Firth[1,3], Karol F. Bauman[1] and Colin P. Sibley[2]

[1]Department of Anatomy, St. George's Hospital Medical School,
University of London, Cranmer Terrace, London SW17 ORE, U.K.

[2]Departments of Child Health and Physiology, University of Manchester
St. Mary's Hospital, Hathersage Road, Manchester M13 OJH, U.K.

## INTRODUCTION

The structural and biochemical complexity of trophoblast reflects its diverse roles in placental synthesis, metabolism, and transport. However, not all of the functions of the placenta can be equated with activities of trophoblast. It is now becoming evident that the permeability properties of the interhemal membrane can only partially be understood if the contribution of the non-trophoblastic layers of the membrane is not recognized.

All types of chorioallantoic placentae include at least one layer (in endotheliochorial, and epitheliochorial placentae two layers) of endothelial cells in series with the epithelial elements. In this paper, attention is confined to hemomonochorial placentae in which the only continuous cellular layers separating maternal from fetal blood are a single layer of syncytiotrophoblast and a single layer of endothelial cells (Figure 1). In particular, the labyrinthine placenta of the guinea pig is examined. The guinea pig is a species which has been extensively used for studies of placental permeability and transfer (Hedley and Bradbury, 1980; Leichtweiss and Schröder, 1981; Reynolds and Young, 1971; Yudilevich et al., 1979). This is a relatively leaky placenta in which significant maternofetal transfer of nonpolar hydrophilic solutes occurs up to molecular weights of 10,000 to 20,000 Da. (Hedley and Bradbury, 1980; Thornburg and Faber, 1977). The identity of the putative water-filled transplacental channels responsible for this permeability has been discussed; the fact that the joint meeting of the European Placenta Group and the Rochester Trophoblast Conference in 1986 was preceded by a workshop entitled, "The Existence of Transtrophoblastic Channels" not only testifies to the interest in this topic but also demonstrates how the choice of a title can shift emphasis from the entire placental membrane to a single component of it.

This study uses morphological and ultrastructural probes to assess the nature and the size restrictions of routes for transfer of hydrophilic molecules

---

[3]To Whom Correspondence Should Be Addressed: Department of Anatomy and Cell Biology, St. Mary's Hospital Medical School (University of London), Norfolk Place, London, W2 1PG, U.K.

across the fetal microvascular endothelium of guinea pig placentae near term. The purpose of this study is to test the null hypothesis that the fetal capillary endothelium is so permeable that placental transfer can be regarded as mainly a trophoblastic function and consequently the placenta can legitimately be treated physiologically as an interface consisting of a single cellular layer.

## MATERIALS AND METHODS

All studies used albino guinea pigs between 60 and 65 days gestation. Single (fetal) side perfusions were carried out on animals anesthetized with intramuscular ketamine supplemented by intravenous pentobarbital using techniques which were described previously (Sibley et al., 1981, 1982). Probe molecules used in tracer studies (Sibley et al., 1982, 1983) were administered during a 15 minute period in a fetal perfusate consisting of TC199 medium supplemented with 3.5% dextran and gassed with 95% $O_2$/5% $CO_2$. Dual perfusions of isolated placentae used the method of Leichtweiss and Schroeder (1981). In all experiments, perfusion pressures and maternal carotid arterial pressures were continuously recorded. Experiments were terminated, and tissue was fixed for electron microscopy by perfusion through the maternal circulation with a glutaraldehyde formaldehyde fixative (Sibley et al., 1981). Histochemical incubation methods for heme tracers, methods for lanthanum perfusion and tannic acid staining, electron microscopic preparative methods, and freeze fracture techniques were those described in previous publications (Sibley et al., 1981, 1982, 1983; Firth et al., 1983).

## RESULTS

### General Morphology of Fetal Placental Capillaries

The labyrinthine placenta of the guinea pig has a highly ordered microcirculatory pattern of which the fundamental unit is the lobe (Figure 2). The centripetal fetal capillaries and the centrifugal maternal lacunae form a countercurrent system (Faber, 1977; Kaufmann and Davidoff, 1977).

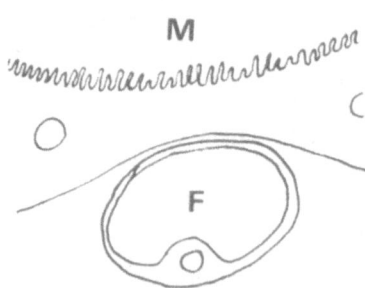

Figure 1. Schema of interhemal membrane of a hemomonochorial placenta. Maternal blood (M) is separated from fetal blood (F) by two continuous cellular layers: syncytiotrophoblast adjoining maternal blood spaces and endothelium bounding fetal capillaries.

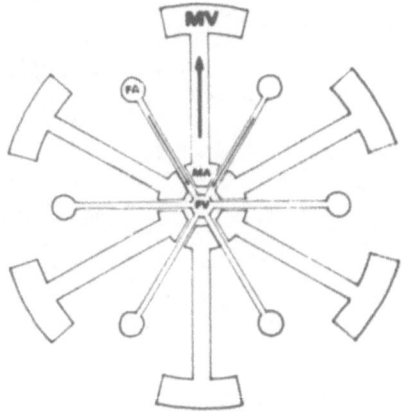

Figure 2. Schema of blood flow within a single lobe of the guinea-pig placenta. Maternal blood flows centrifugally from centrilobar arteries (MA) through syncytium-lined lacunae to peripheral veins (MV): fetal blood flows centripetally from peripheral arteries (FA) to the central vein (FV) through endothelium-lined capillaries.

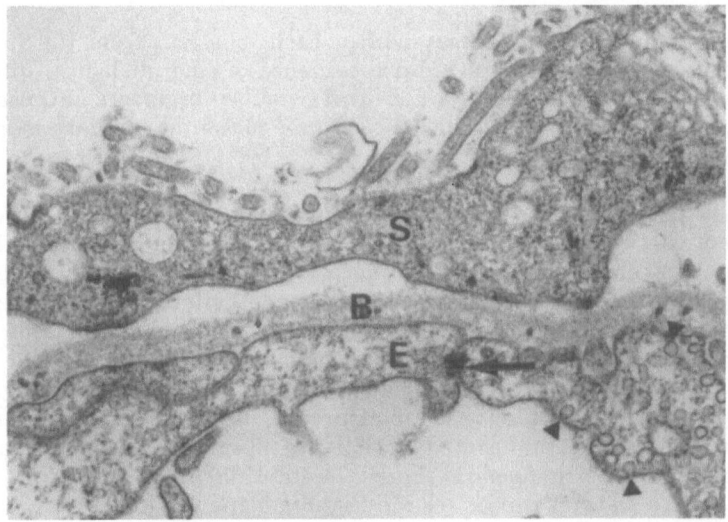

Figure 3. The interhemal membrane of guinea-pig placenta. The syncytiotrophoblast (S) has no evident paracellular or transcellular channels but contains numerous vesicles and other membrane-bounded organelles. The endothelium (E) lacks fenestrae but has paracellular channels (lateral intercellular spaces) which are spanned by junctions (arrow). Endothelium also contains many smooth vesicles and pits (arrowheads). Between syncytium and endothelium is a basal lamina (B). X22,750.

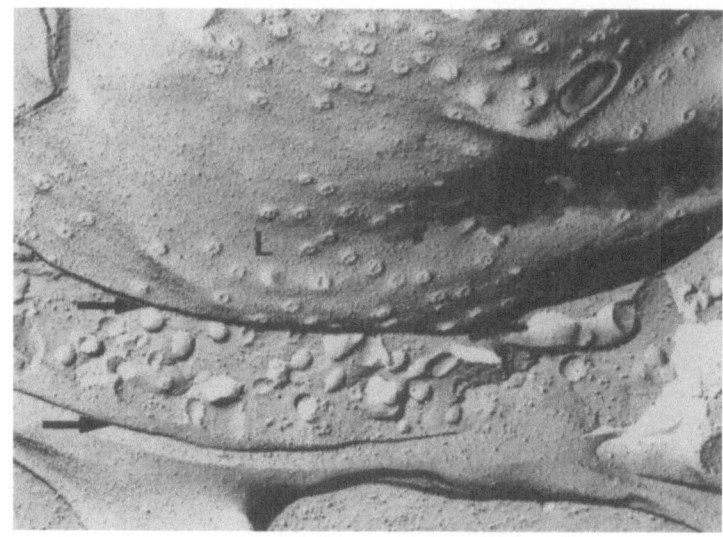

Figure 4. Freeze fracture of endothelium showing luminal plasma membrane (L) with numerous raised crater rims marking sheared necks of epithelial pits. Pits and vesicles are also seen in the cross-fractured endothelial cytoplasm between the arrows. X52,900.

Although the fetal capillaries within each lobe run from the interlobar arteries to the central vein, there is little evidence of morphological differences between the peripheral (arteriolar) and central (venular) segments of these vessels (Firth et al., 1983). A single description of typical placental capillary morphology will therefore suffice.

Guinea pig fetal placental capillaries are in no obvious way different in structure from continuous (non-fenestrated) capillaries from other vascular beds such as that of skeletal muscle (Bundgaard, 1980; Palade et al., 1979). The capillary lumen is bounded by a single layer of endothelial cells which rests on a simple basal lamina which is often fused with that of the trophoblast. One or more lateral intercellular spaces are usually recognizable in any single thin section; along these spaces zonular junctions hold the lateral borders of adjoining cells in close apposition. The endothelial cytoplasm contains a few coated vesicles but much larger numbers of non-coated vesicles of 50-60 nm diameter, and pits (caveolae) of similar size open at both the luminal and abluminal plasma membranes. These features can be seen in Figures 3 and 4.

### Sites of Molecular Sieving in Fetal Capillary Walls

Molecular probes with diameters about 6 nm or less, e.g., microperoxidases, cytochrome C, myoglobin, and horseradish peroxidase, are perfused throughout the fetal vascular bed at physiological pressures. These probes cross the endothelium to appear in the subendothelial space, the basal lamina and sometimes the subtrophoblastic space (Figure 5). Larger molecules such as hemoglobin and ferritin may be seen in capillary lumina adhering to the plasma membrane but fail to cross the endothelium (Figure 6). The permeant tracers label both the lateral intercellular spaces and a large proportion of the pits and vesicles associated with both the luminal and the abluminal plasma membranes, whereas the impermeant probes label only the luminal ends of the lateral intercellular spaces and the luminal population of vesicles and pits. From these results alone it is not possible to deduce the route taken by the permeant probe molecules as these distributions are consistent with at least two alternative mechanisms of probe transfer. The probe could cross endothelial cells by a vesicular transport mechanism; in such a case the apparent filling of the lateral intercellular spaces would be attributable to filling from both ends up to a narrow and unresolved permeability barrier. Alternatively, the probe could pass through permeable lateral intercellular spaces to fill the subendothelial space; it would then have access to both surfaces of the endothelium and could label static or nearly static pits and connected vesicles from each side. It is possible to discriminate between the alternatives by perfusion-fixation of a placenta before perfusion of the fetal circuit with a small, permeant tracer such as lanthanum ions, microperoxidase, or cytochrome C. Such experiments show clearly that labelling of the lateral intercellular spaces, and of its pits and vesicles at both surfaces, takes place even when membrane flow and vesicle traffic have been paralyzed by 15 minutes of perfusion fixation with 2% glutaraldehyde in combination with 2% formaldehyde (Figure 7). It is therefore very likely that most of the transfer of such probes is by a paracellular route through the lateral intercellular spaces of the endothelium.

## Sieve Structures in Endothelial Lateral Intercellular Spaces

Thin section electron micrographs of conventionally fixed and stained lateral intercellular spaces show that each space contains two to five narrow zones at which the intercellular distance is reduced from its normal value of about 20 nm to 8 nm or less. The continuity of such narrow zones in many sections implies that they are zonular structures like epithelial tight juctions rather than punctate attachments like desmosomes or gap junctions. In many cases the membranes at these narrow zones appear to be in contact, but tilting of the specimen with a eucentric goniometer stage reveals that such appearances are nearly all superimposition effects produced by sectioning in a plane not perpendicular to the membrane plane.

Staining techniques which increase membrane contrast, such as the tannic acid-osmium method, reveal dense-staining material within the junctional narrowings of the lateral intercellular space. In sections cut in a plane oblique to the axis of the junction, periodic substructure may sometimes be discerned in this densely-stained intercellular material, and similar periodicity can be revealed in negative contrast by lanthanum perfusion methods. Freeze-fracture replicas of junctional membranes show that periodic structure is also present in junctional elements lying in the membrane plane. Membrane P faces (the membrane leaflet adjacent to protoplasm) show between two and five anastomosing and continuous junctional strands which are formed of linear rows of particles with diameters of $11.5 \pm 1.3$ nm (mean $\pm$ S:D:) and center-to-center spacings of $22.8 \pm 1.8$ nm in peripheral capillaries and $21.6 \pm 3.5$ nm in central ones. The E faces (membrane leaflets adjacent to the intercellular space) carry similarly anastomosing patterns of grooves which lack periodic structure. At sites where the fracture plane has jumped from one membrane to the other it is evident that the P face particle arrays of one cell are complementary to the E face grooves of its neighbor (Figure 8). This provides strong evidence that the particle arrays of the two membranes which participate in the junction are held in register by structures spanning the narrow parts of the lateral intercellular space.

The wide regions of the lateral intercellular space in tannic acid-stained specimens often show bridging structures similar to those seen in desmosomes which are known as linkers (Leeson and Leeson, 1982). These structures appear rather tenuous and do not appear to correspond to any structure visible by freeze fracture in the membrane plane. They are most likely to be condensations of the intercellular matrix or extensions of the glycocalyx. Their periodicity is somewhat striking, but it should be borne in mind that this could be produced by fixation-induced aggregation of a more dispersed meshwork of fibrous macromolecules.

## Sites of Fixed Charge in Endothelial Intercellular Spaces

In all of the tracer perfusion studies, it was noticeable that cationic probes (such as cytochrome C) crossed the endothelium much more readily than similarly sized neutral to anionic molecules (such as myoglobin). The importance of molecular charge for permeation by probes close to the limiting size of the pathway was demonstrated by perfusion of the fetal vessels with media containinig horseradish peroxidase of various cationic (pI = 8.7 - 9.0) and anionic (pI = 4.05 - 5.15) types, both natural and modified.

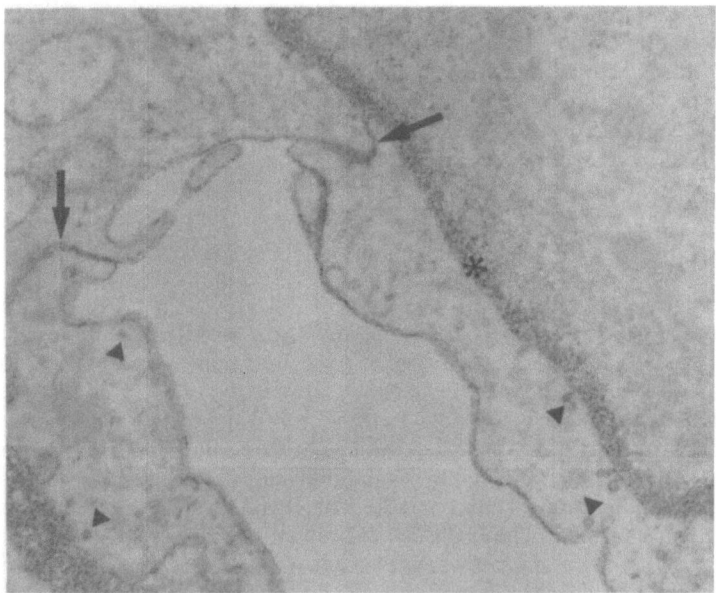

Figure 5. Placenta perfused through fetal circuit with microperoxidase Mp-11. This small probe is found on the endothelial luminal plasma membrane, fills the lateral intercellular spaces (arrows) and binds to the basal lamina (asterisk). Pits and vesicles at both faces of the endothelium are also labeled (arrowheads). X19,500.

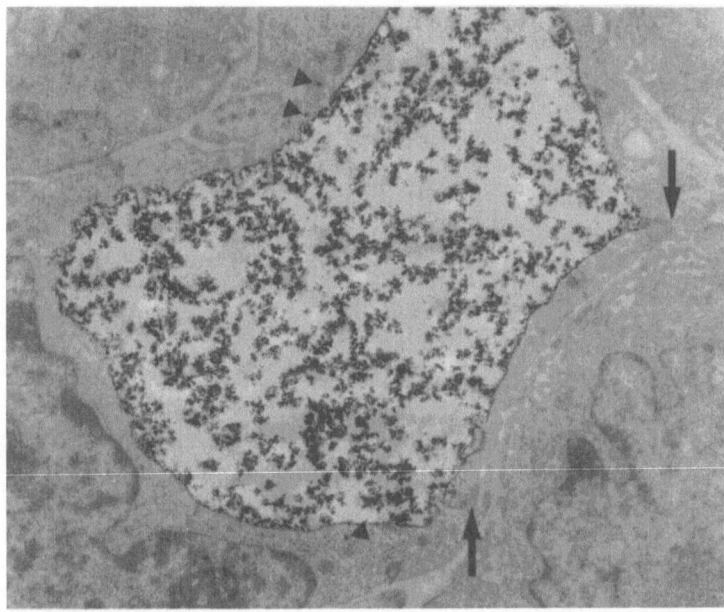

Figure 6. Placenta perfused through fetal circuit with hemoglobin. This larger probe fails to leave the capillaries. Penetration of lateral intercellular spaces is negligible (arrows), and only luminal-side pits and vesicles are labeled (arrowheads). No tracer is seen in the basal lamina. X8,200.

The many items of microscopic information about the structure of the endothelial junctions and their surroundings are summarized in Figure 9. A sample of the micrographs which provide supporting evidence for this model is to be found in Firth et al. (1983). Each zonular junction somewhat resembles a ladder whose rungs hold the two membranes at a constant separation. Each rung probably consists of two half-rungs, one rooted in the hydrophobic zone of each membrane, the extracellular parts of which pair up across the intercellular space. Thus the freeze-fracture P face particles represent the intramembranous parts of the rungs, while the free parts form the junctional bars revealed by tannic acid-osmium staining and by negative staining with perfused lanthanum ions. In a complete lateral intercellular space, two to five such arrays appear to separate luminal and abluminal spaces. The continuity of the freeze-fracture particle arrays and the constant membrane separation at the junctional zones suggest that permeant molecules cross the endothelium by passing through the gaps between the rungs in each array in turn. Permeant molecules must also pass through the intercellular matrix in the wide zones; the spaces in this regions (between linkers seen by tannic acid staining and by negative staining with lanthanum ions) seem relatively large in fixed material.

Horseradish peroxidase is a heme protein with a molecular weight of 40,000 Da. and a diameter approaching 6 nm. In all cases, the lateral intercellular spaces of the capillary endothelium were readily permeable to the cationic probes but impermeable to the anionic forms (Sibley et al., 1983).

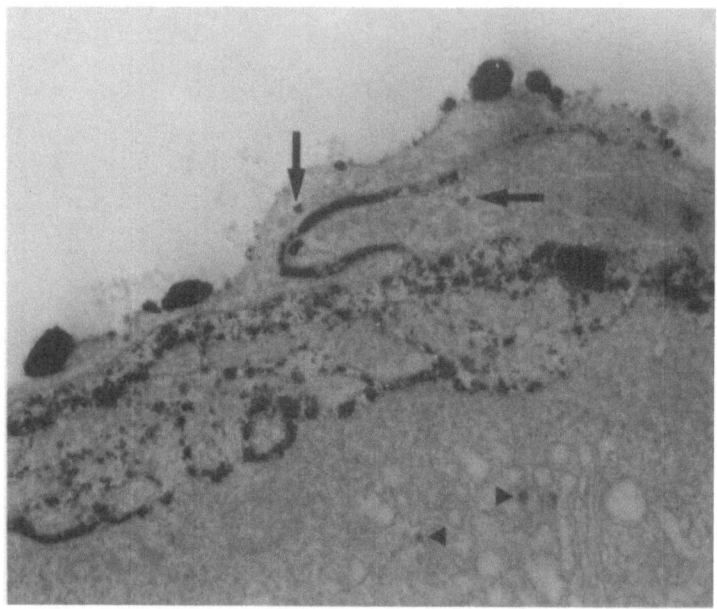

Figure 7. Capillary junctional area from placenta perfused through fetal circuit with lanthanum after fixation. This small probe is seen in the lumen, lateral intercellular spaces, the basal lamina, and at the base of the syncytiotrophoblast. Vesicles still acquire label although vesicle formation has been paralyzed (arrows). Some label has entered small membrane-bounded spaces within the trophoblast (arrowheads). X50,400.

It seems probable that such charge-selective properties of the lateral intercellular space might depend on the distribution of fixed charges on endothelial cell surfaces. Support for this view was provided by experiments in which the perfusate in the fetal circuit contained the large, impermeant probe ferritin (diameter = 11-12 nm) in its cationic form. After perfusion with cationic ferritin, a period of washout with probe-free perfusate was used to elute unbound probe prior to fixation. Firmly bound probe remained in patches on the luminal plasma membrane, and in addition was found at a high density in the lateral intercellular spaces on the luminal side of the first narrow junctional zone (Figure 10). The possibility that there might be more sites of fixed anionic charge deeper in the junctional region could not be tested because of the inaccessibility of these sites to large probes.

## DISCUSSION

### Identification of Limiting Structures for Endothelial Pemeability

These observations concerning the structural features of guinea pig fetal placental capillaries (Firth et al., 1983) are generally confirmed by Orgnero de Gaisan et al. (1985) and are similar to findings on other continuous capillaries such as those of skeletal muscle (Palade et al., 1979), cardiac muscle (Bundgaard,

1984), and mesentery (Simionescu et al., 1975). For more than a decade, the structural identity of the channels or pores predicted on physiological grounds has been a fertile field for the growth of conflicting hypotheses. In particular, the relative merits of the endothelial vesicles and pits and the lateral intercellular spaces have been regularly debated (cf. Crone, 1981; Palade et al., 1979; Simionescu, 1981). In the last few years evidence has steadily accumulated that the "small pore" properties of continuous capillaries can best be understood in terms of the permeability characteristics of the lateral intercellular spaces (Bundgaard, 1984; Bundgaard and Frokjaer-Jensen, 1982; Clough and Michel, 1986; Firth et al., 1983; Wissig, 1979), whereas the endothelial vesicles and pits may have a role in much slower transfer or handling of larger solutes (Clough and Michel, 1981). The hypothesis that endothelial vesicles in continuous capillaries may form transient channels which completely perforate the cell (Palade et al., 1979) is intriguing but has failed to obtain widespread confirmation.

A problem common to all models of the small pore has been the inability of electron microscopy to demonstrate restrictive structures of appropriate sizes to explain the physiological findings. In fact, this very difficulty has helped to advance "fiber matrix" models in which filtration is ascribed to the meshwork of glycoprotein and proteoglycan which fills intercellular spaces and coats plasma membranes (Bundgaard, 1980; Curry and Michel, 1980; Turner et al., 1983) With increasing evidence that endothelial lateral intercellular spaces are the predominant pathway involved in small pore properties, the detailed organization of the endothelial junctions becomes an important problem. These junctions lie at the narrowest regions of the lateral intercellular spaces and so are well placed to act as restricting structures. In the very tight capillaries of the central nervous system the endothelial junctions resemble tight junctions of classical epithelia and are well recognized as important restrictive structures of the blood-brain interface (Brightman and Reese, 1969). However, in the more permeable continuous capillaries found at other sites the junctions are often regarded as discontinuous structures which can be by passed by permeant molecules but which may act as shutters restricting the proportion of the lateral intercellular space which is available for filtration (Bundgaard, 1984).

The guinea pig fetal placental capillaries show some features which are difficult to reconcile with such a model. No evidence was found from either thin-section or freeze-fracture studies that junctions are interrupted in such a way as to offer open routes across the lateral intercellular space. Neither should it be considered that these junctions are in themselves closed to small solutes. Even junctions which show apparent contact between plasma membranes usually reveal a separation of several nm when tilted so as to bring the membranes parallel to the optical axis of the microscope. Therefore, it is suggested that, at least in the particular type of capillary we have investigated, the interstices between the "rung" elements of the zonular junctions may impose major size-based restriction of solute transfer. The size of these pores is difficult to measure with precision. The visible gaps between "rungs" are estimated to be about 6 nm, but we obtain larger spacings (11.5 ± 1.32 nm) for the intramembranous particles seen in freeze-fracture images. The former is likely to be low because of tissue shrinkage during processing and embedding, while the latter figure does not refer to measurement in the intercellular space. Nonetheless, it seems reasonable to conclude that the zonular endothelial junctions form gratings which delineate pores which probably do not have an effective diameter greater than about 10 nm. This is compatible with the range of predictions of capillary small pore sizes based on physiological data (Crone, 1981).

This model is not offered as an alternative to the fiber matrix concept. Rather it is emphasized that the matrix properties of the intercellular spaces are likely to have profound effects both as molecular sieves and as sites of fixed negative charge. We suggest that such a fibrous filter is in series with the (usually multiple) junctional gratings, and that it is possible though not established that the junctions rather than the matrix may set the maximum size limits for permeation of the lateral intercellular space.

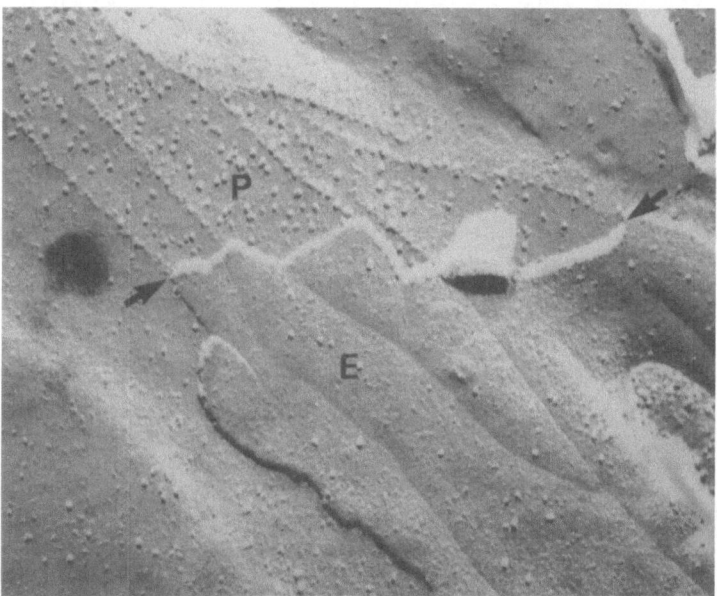

Figure 8. Freeze fracture of endothelial lateral intercellular space showing part of a zonular junction. The zig-zag white band (arrows) is a cross fracture at which the fracture plane has jumped from one membrane to the other across the lateral intercellular space. Two fracture surfaces within plasma membranes are shown: face E is the deep surface of the outer (exoplasmic) leaflet of the nearer cell, and face P is the superficial surface of the inner (protoplasmic) leaflet of the further cell. Junctional grooves on the E face are in register with particle alignments on the P face, implying that intramembrane particles protrude into and interact in the narrow zone of the lateral intercellular space. X80,600.

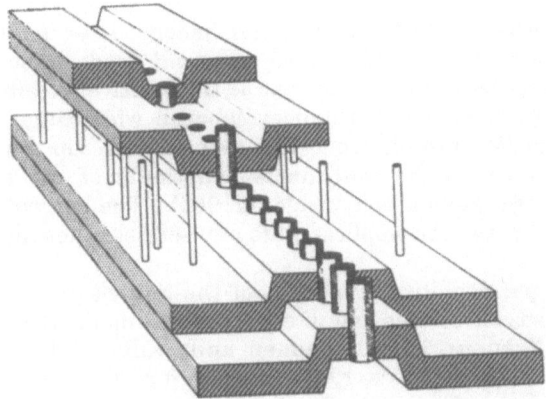

Figure 9. Possible model for part of the endothelial lateral intercellular space based on thin-section and freeze-fracture studies. Narrow zone of space (usually multiple but one shown here) is spanned by a single row of bars rooted in the plasma membrane interiors. Wide regions are spanned by linkers which probably are part of the glycocalyx. Drawing not to scale.

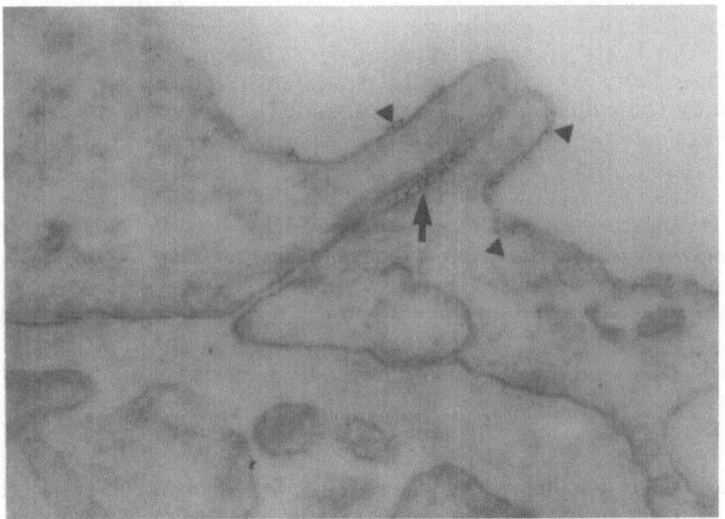

Figure 10. Junctional region of capillary perfused with cationic ferritin then flushed out to remove unbound probe. Clusters of ferritin molecules are bound at anionic sites both on the luminal membrane and its pits (arrowheads) and in the wide part of the lateral intercellular space (arrow). This large probe cannot pass the narrow part of the junction. X64,500.

## Capillary Properties and Placental Permeability

As in most other aspects of placental biology, it is not likely that many useful generalizations can be made which will hold good for both the very tight placentae of the sheep and the horse as well as the relatively leaky placentae of the guinea pig and man. Capillary morphology shows a wide range of variation even within the hemochorial group, from the fenestrated capillaries of the rat's hemotrichorial placenta to the continuous endothelia of the hemomonochorial placentae of people and guinea pigs (Enders, 1965). The current findings are not proposed to have any automatic application to any species other than guinea pigs.

The overall permeability properties of the guinea pig placenta have been studied using a variety of solutes and of experimental methods both in vivo and in vitro (Hedley and Bradbury, 1980; Kelman and Walter, 1977; Leichtweiss and Schröder, 1981; Stulc and Svihovec, 1977; Thornburg and Faber, 1977; Woods et al., Yudilevich et al., 1979). These studies have not shown transplacental transfer through the chorioallantoic placenta of molecules with diameters greater than about 6 nm. Such a restriction is similar to that imposed by continuous capillaries at other sites (Thornburg and Faber, 1977). Thornburg and Faber (1977) also pointed out that attempts to calculate pore radii from restriction and permeability data are only valid if restriction of large molecules occurs at the layer which offers the greatest diffusional resistance to small molecules. This assumption has been proved to be false for the hemodichorial placenta of the rabbit (Thornburg and Faber, 1976) and is thrown into serious doubt for the guinea pig by the demonstration that the fetal capillaries impose important restrictions. Therefore, the size of the limiting pores or transplacental channels of the guinea pig placenta is not known. The current results merely show that the capillaries restrict protein transfer on the basis of size and charge. It seems likely that polarity and molecular specificity in transplacental transfer is imposed by the trophoblast rather than by the endothelium because endothelial selectivity is based on rather simple biophysical criteria rather than receptor-mediated mechanisms.

We have repeatedly emphasised the need to consider the effect of both cellular layers together rather than the trophoblast alone. In so doing, the effects of a third component which is repeatedly seen to bind and trap ultrastructural probe molecules has been ignored. The basal lamina is a continuous fiber matrix in series with the two cellular layers. The contribution of the basal lamina to the permeability properties of the placenta is virtually unknown, but its known importance in the renal glomerulus indicates that serious inquiry is overdue.

## SUMMARY

The placental membrane in hemochorial placentae comprises three main elements in series: trophoblast, basal lamina, and endothelium. In the hemomonochorial placenta of the guinea pig, the continuous fetal endothelium restricts transfer of proteins on the basis both of size and charge. Size selection (sieving) is based on a complex filter composed of the narrow zonular endothelial junctions and probably also of the less structured intercellular matrix. Charge selectivity in favor of cations may depend on fixed negative charges concentrated in the matrix in the wider parts of the lateral intercellular spaces. These systems probably make a significant contribution to the permeability properties of the placental membrane as a whole.

## ACKNOWLEDGEMENTS

We thank the Medical Research Council, the Wellcome Trust, and the North Atlantic Treaty Organization for grant support.

## REFERENCES

Brightman, M.W. and Reese, T.S. (1969) Junctions between intimately apposed cell membranes in the vertebrate brain. *J. Cell Biol.* 40, 648-677.

Bundgaard, M. (1980) Transport pathways in capillaries - in search of pores. *Ann. Rev. Physiol.* 42, 325-336.

Bundgaard, M. (1984) The three-dimensional organization of tight junctions in a capillary endothelium revealed by serial-section electron microscopy. *J. Ultrastruct. Res.* 88, 1-17.

Bundgaard, M. and Frokjaer-Jensen, J. (1982) Functional aspects of the ultrastructure of terminal blood vessels:a quantitative study of consecutive segments of the frog mesenteric microvasculature. *Microvasc. Res.* 23, 1-30.

Clough, G. and Michel, C.C. (1981) The role of vesicles in the transport of ferritin through frog endothelium. *J. Physiol.* 315, 127-142.

Clough, G. and Michel, C.C. (1986) Comparisons between the hydraulic conductance of the walls of single frog capillaries and the ultrastructure of the intercellular clefts. *J. Physiol.* 374, 12P.

Crone, C. (1981) Tight and leaky endothelia. In: *Water Transport Across Epithelia, Alfred Benzon Symposium 15*, (ed.), H.H. Ussing, N. Bindslev, N.A. Lassen, and O. Sten-Knudsen, Copenhagen:Munksgaard, pp. 258-267.

Curry, F.E. and Michel, C.C. (1980) A fibre matrix model of capillary permeability. *Microvasc. Res.* 20, 96-99.

Enders, A.C. (1965) A comparative study of the fine structure of the trophoblast in several hemochorial placentas. *Am. J. Anat.* 116, 29-68.

Faber, J.J. (1977) Steady-state methods for the study of placental exchange. *Fed. Proc.* 36, 2640-2646.

Firth, J.A., Bauman, K.F., and Sibley, C.P. (1983) The intercellular junctions of guinea-pig placental capillaries: a possible structural basis for endothelial solute permeability. *J. Ultrastruct. Res.* 85, 45-57.

Hedley, R. and Bradbury, M.W.B. (1980) Transport of polar non-electrolytes across the intact and perfused guinea-pig placenta. *Placenta* 1, 277-285.

Kaufmann, P. and Davidoff, M. (1977) The guinea-pig placenta. *Adv. Anat. Embryol. Cell Biol.* 53 (2), 1-91.

Kelman, B.J. and Walter, B.K. (1977) Passage of cadmium across the perfused guinea pig placenta. *Proc. Soc. Exp. Biol. Med.* 156, 68-71.

Leeson, T.S. and Leeson, C.R. (1982) The use of lanthanum chloride as a marker for intercellular junctions in rat exocrine pancreas. *Stain Technol.* 57, 245-248.

Leichtweiss, H.-P. and Schröder, H. (1981) Dual perfusion of the isolated guinea-pig placenta. *Placenta (Suppl. 2)*, 119-128.

Orgnero de Gaisan, E., Aoki, A., Heinrich, D., and Metz, J. (1985) Permeability studies of the guinea-pig placental labyrinth. II. Tracer permeation and freeze-fracture of fetal endothelium. *Anat. Embryol.* 171, 297-304.

Palade, G.E., Simionescu, M. and Simionescu, N. (1979) Structural aspects of the permeability of the microvascular endothelium. *Acta Physiol. Scand. (Suppl. 463)*, 11-32.

Reynolds, M.L. and Young, M. (1971) The transfer of free-amino nitrogen across the placental membrane in the guinea pig. *J. Physiol.* 214, 583-597.

Sibley, C.P., Bauman, K.F., and Firth, J.A. (1981) Ultrastructural study of the permeability of the guinea-pig placenta to horseradish peroxidase. *Cell Tissue Res.* 219, 637-647.

Sibley, C.P., Bauman, K.F., and Firth, J.A. (1982) Permeability of the foetal capillary endothelium of the guinea-pig placenta to haem proteins of various molecular sizes. *Cell Tissue Res.* 223, 165-178.

Sibley, C.P., Bauman, K.F., and Firth, J.A. (1983) Molecular charges as a determinant of macromolecule permeability across the fetal capillary endothelium of the guinea-pig placenta. *Cell Tissue Res.* 229, 365-377.

Simionescu, M., Simionescu, N., and Palade, G.E. (1975) Segmental differentiations of cell junctions in the vascular endothelium. The microvasculature. *J. Cell. Biol.* 67, 863-885.

Simionescu, N. (1981) Transcytosis and traffic of membranes in the endothelial cell. In: *International Cell Biology 1980-81*, (ed.), H.G. Schweiger, pp. 657-672. Berlin, Springer-Verlag.

Stulc, J. and Svihovec, J. (1977) Placental transport of sodium in the guinea-pig. *J. Physiol.* 265, 691-703.

Thornburg, K.L. and Faber, J.J. (1976) The steady state concentration gradients of an electron dense marker (ferritin) in the three-layered hemochorial placenta of the rabbit. *J. Clin. Invest.* 58, 912-925.

Thornburg, K.L. and Faber, J.J. (1977) Transfer of hydrophilic molecules by placenta and yolk sac of the guinea pig. *Am. J. Physiol.* 233, C111-C124.

Turner, M.R., Clough, G., and Michel, C.C. (1983) The effects of cationised ferritin and native ferritin upon the filtration coefficient of single frog capillaries. Evidence that the proteins in the endothelial cell coat influence permeability. *Microvasc. Res.* 25, 205-222.

Wissig, S.L. (1979) Identification of the small pore in muscle capillaries. *Acta Physiol. Scand. (Suppl 463),* 33-44.

Woods, L.L., Thornburg, K.L., and Faber, J.J. (1978) Transplacental gradients in the guinea pig. *Am. J. Physiol.* 235, H200-H207.

Yudilevich, D.L., Eaton, B.M., Short, A.H., and Leichtweiss, H.-P. (1979) Glucose carriers at maternal and fetal sides of the trophoblast in guinea pig placenta. *Am. J. Physiol.* 237, C205-C212.

Trophoblast Research 3:179-188, 1988

# REGULATION OF FETAL PLACENTAL BLOOD FLOW

## - A Review -

Debra F. Anderson and J. Job Faber

Department of Physiology, L334
Oregon Health Sciences University
3181 S.W. Sam Jackson Park Road
Portland, Oregon 97201 USA

## INTRODUCTION

The magnitude of blood flow to any organ will be determined by the driving pressure and the vascular resistance. It follows that the regulation of blood flow, that is the maintenance of blood flow within a given set of limit appropriate for the metabolic needs of the tissue, occurs only as a result of changes in driving pressure and/or vascular resistance.

### Local Mechanisms for Regulating Fetal Placental Blood Flow

The mechanisms available for regulation of fetal placental resistance are limited. While the intrafetal umbilical vessels are innervated (Spivack, 1943), it is commonly believed that the extrafetal cord and placenta lack innervation (Spivack, 1943; Bell, 1972; Reilly and Russell, 1977). As a consequence, neural control over placental blood flow is not believed to be of importance. However, there are a number of mechanisms acting locally which are able to alter fetal placental blood flow.

When angiotensin II is exogenously administered to the fetal lamb, an acute increase in umbilical vascular resistance results (Iwamoto and Rudolph, 1981). However, if the angiotensin II blocker [sar$^1$,ile$^8$]-angiotensin II (Rankin and Phernetton, 1978) or [sar$^1$,ala$^8$]-angiotensin II (Iwamoto and Rudolph, 1979) is given to the fetus, no change in umbilical vascular resistance results, suggesting angiotensin II does not exercise a tonic restraint over fetal placental blood flow under resting conditions. Similar results have been noted for catecholamines: exogenous norepinephrine will cause fetal placental vasoconstriction (Rankin and Phernetton, 1976a) while blockade of the alpha receptors will not change fetal placental vascular resistance under normal conditions (Rankin and Phernetton, 1978). Vasopressin has also been given to fetal lambs. Exogenous administration of vasopressin in dosages sufficient to simulate fetal plasma levels during hypoxia causes vasoconstriction of the fetal placental circulation (Iwamoto et al., 1979).

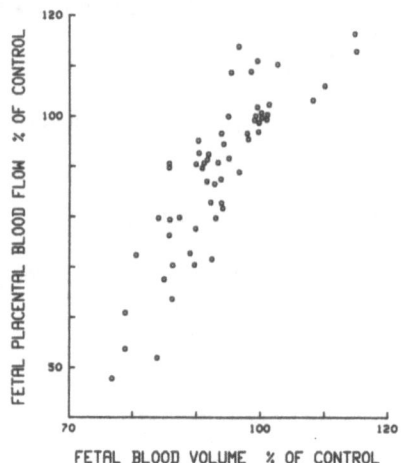

Figure 1. Fetal placental blood flow as a function of fetal blood volume, both expressed as percentages of their control values. (Data adapted from Faber, Gault, Green and Thornburg, 1973.)

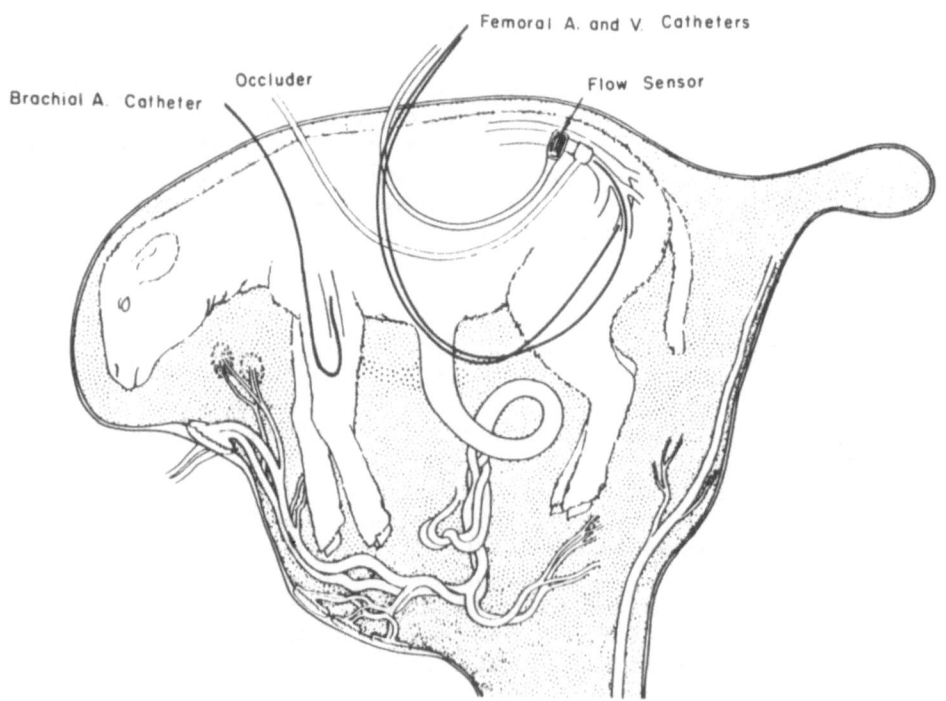

Figure 2. Instrumentation of lamb fetus. Catheters were placed in upper and lower body arteries and veins. An electromagnetic flow sensor was placed around the aorta, below the renal arteries. An inflatable silastic occluder was placed around the aorta, below the flow sensor.

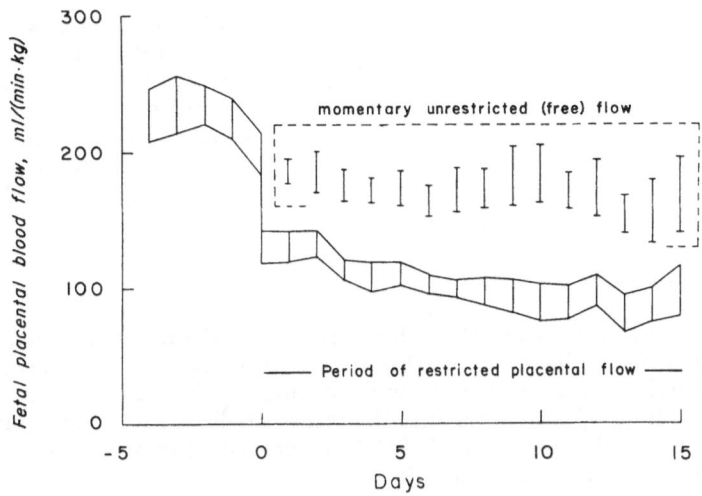

Figure 3. Placental blood flow per kg estimated fetal weight (mean ± sem) before and during restriction of blood flow. Blood flow was reduced at day zero and maintained at this value with only temporary release for estimation of free placental blood flow. (From Anderson and Faber, 1984 with permission of the *American Journal of Physiology*.)

Thus, even though a number of endogenous hormones can elicit vasoconstriction on the fetal side of the ovine placenta, none has been shown to be important for the regulation of fetal placental blood flow under resting conditions. Of course, these hormones may play a more prominent role in the regulation of fetal blood flow under conditions of stress, although it is unclear that vasoconstriction of the umbilical circulation would benefit the fetus. It is noteworthy that no significant umbilical vasodilators have been found.

## Local Matching of Maternal and Fetal Placental Blood Flows

Another aspect of local regulation of fetal placental blood flow is the control of the relative distribution of maternal and fetal blood flows within the placenta. To maximize exchange between mother and fetus, fetal and maternal placental blood flows must be evenly matched. Rankin et al. (1970), using radioactively labeled microspheres, demonstrated that maternal and fetal blood flow distributions were correlated. These results were later confirmed by Power et al. (1981). When maternal placental blood flows were reduced through either ligation of a maternal blood vessel supplying a cotyledon or through embolization using non-radioactive microspheres (Stock et al., 1980), the corresponding umbilical blood flow was significantly reduced after 24 hours. Thus, local reductions of maternal placental blood flow were able to cause local reductions in fetal placental blood flow.

Rankin suggested that, in the sheep, the action of prostaglandin $E_2$ assists the evenness of matching between maternal and fetal placental blood flows.

Prostaglandin $E_2$ acts as a vasoconstrictor on the fetal side of the placenta (Rankin and Phernetton, 1976b). When given to the fetus and allowed to diffuse to the maternal side of the placenta, prostaglandin $E_2$ will cause maternal placental vasodilation (Rankin and Phernetton, 1976c). According to Rankin, if a local reduction of maternal blood flow occurs, the maternal to fetal blood flow ratio would decrease. However, local release of prostaglandin $E_2$ would increase maternal placental blood flow and decrease fetal placental blood flow, bringing the maternal to fetal blood flow ratio closer to one.

## Acquisition of Fluid by the Fetus

Faber and associates (1973) have shown fetal placental blood flow to be dependent upon fetal blood volume (Figure 1). It follows that those factors able to alter fluid acquisition by the fetus will be able to alter blood volume and fetal placental blood flow. Fluid entry into the fetus is believed to occur primarily at the placenta. Faber and Thornburg (1981) have described this movement using the Kedem and Katchalsky (1958) equation:

$$Jv = Lp[\Delta P - \sigma RT \, \Delta C] \tag{1}$$

Jv = ml/sec volume flow per $cm^2$ placenta: cm/sec
Lp = filtration coefficient: $cm^3/ (s \cdot N)$
$\Delta P$ = hydrostatic pressure difference between fetal and maternal placental
         capillaries: $N/cm^2$
$\Delta C$ = concentration difference across the placenta: $mol/cm^3$
R = gas constant
T = absolute temperature
$\sigma$ = reflection coefficient ($\pi$ observed/$\pi$ theoretical)

It can be seen that movement across the placenta occurs as the result of both hydrostatic ($\Delta P$) and osmotic ($\sigma RT \Delta C$) pressure differences between maternal and fetal plasmas. The osmotic pressure is the sum of many osmotic pressures. In the sheep some of these (e.g., those exerted by amino acids and fructose) facilitate water entry into the fetus whereas others (e.g., NaCl) oppose it.

Conrad and Faber (1977) have theoretically shown that, in the sheep placenta, the filtration coefficient, Lp, is without much influence on water acquisition by the fetus because the primary constraint on fluid entry into the fetus is the acquisition of necessary osmotic solutes. This is not surprising in light of the estimated pore diameter of 0.45 nm for the ovine placenta (Boyd et al., 1976). Since small changes in their reflection coefficients can have substantial effects on the entry of solutes into the fetus, water entry is actually facilitated by a reduction in the reflection coefficient for NaCl. The impact of the reflection coefficient in determining fluid movement across the placenta becomes more profound in light of the evidence provided by Faber and Thornburg (1977), by Thornburg et al. (1979), and by Leake and colleagues (1983) that vasopressin may alter the placental reflection coefficient for salt. Therefore, it is possible that, through changes in the placental reflection coefficient, the fetus can alter fluid acquisition and thus regulate its placental blood flow.

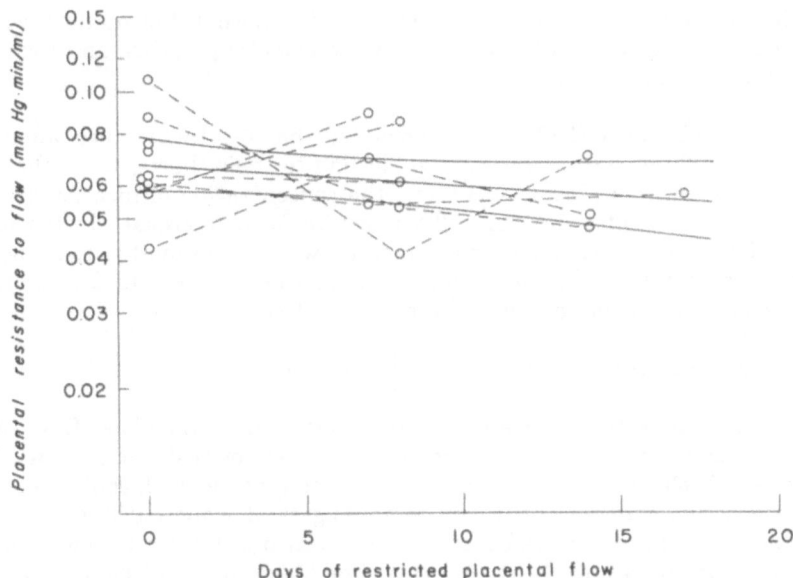

Figure 4.  Placental resistance during control period (before day zero) and during the period of restricted blood flow.  Solid lines, mean placental resistance and its 95% confidence limits.  Dashed lines connect measurements made in the same animal.  Note logarithmic scale.  (From Anderson and Faber, 1984 with permission of the *American Journal of Physiology.*)

        In the hemochorial placenta, there must be at least one class of pores of which the equivalent pore radius is much  greater than in the sheep placenta. Placental permeability is  roughly proportional to the coefficient of free diffusion for hydrophilic solutes up to 5 kilo Da. in size.  The absence of transplacental gradients for crystalloids in the guinea pig (Woods et al., 1978) also suggests that the permeabilities for these ions are large. Anderson and Faber (1982) have demonstrated that fluid moves across the guinea pig placenta in response to changes in the colloid osmotic pressure gradient.  This indicates that the large pore system does not freely admit plasma proteins.  In these placentae, colloid osmotic pressures and hydrostatic pressures may be responsible for fluid movement through a "large" pore system.  Whether there is an additional  small pore system as suggested by Stulc et al. (1969) perhaps similar to that in the sheep is plausible but not yet known.

        In hemochorial placentae, Faber (1972) has proposed the  following mechanism for the regulation of fetal placental blood flow.  In the face of a decreased fetal arterial blood pressure,  there will be a fall in fetal capillary blood pressure.  Fluid  will move from the maternal capillary to the fetal capillary, increasing fetal blood volume.  The increased fetal blood volume will increase venous blood pressure and therefore increase fetal cardiac output, either by Starling's law of the heart or through compensatory ventricular growth.  The increase in cardiac output would restore fetal placental blood flow through an increase in arterial blood pressure. Therefore, fetal placental blood flow would be "self-regulating" due to the interaction of colloid osmotic pressure and hydrostatic pressures acting at the placenta.

Longo and Power (1983) have concluded that fetal water accumulation is closely linked to fetal $CO_2$ production. According to their thesis, when the partial pressure of $CO_2$ in fetal plasma increases, the concentration of bicarbonate ion in the fetal plasma will also increase. This results in an increase in the osmotic pressure of fetal plasma, causing a movement of water from mother to fetus. Once fluid enters the fetal circulation, cardiac output and arterial blood pressure will increase, leading to an increased umbilical blood flow.

## Umbilical Vascular Resistance and Gestational Age

Mechanical factors can also act to change placental blood flow through changes in vascular resistance. During the last third of gestation, the fetal lamb undergoes a 10-fold increase in body weight, yet umbilical placental blood flow remains fairly constant at about 185 ml/min·kg fetal weight (Thornburg et al., 1976; Sheldon et al., 1979). Because fetal arterial blood pressure only increases about 30 mm Hg to 45 mm Hg during this time (Anderson and Faber, 1984), this increase in blood flow must be due to a slow but substantial decrease in umbilical resistance. What governs this decrease is unknown. The following experiments were designed to investigate whether this almost 10-fold decrease in fetal placental resistance was governed by any form of negative feedback control (Anderson and Faber, 1984).

## MATERIALS AND METHODS

Eleven fetal lambs of approximately 116 days gestational age were instrumented with upper and lower body arterial and venous catheters. An electromagnetic flow sensor was placed around the fetal aorta, below the renal arteries. About 75% of the blood flow here is placental flow. A silastic occluder was placed around the aorta, below the flow sensor (Figure 2).

After three days of recovery from surgery, control aortic blood flow measurements were made for approximately 6 days using the electromagnetic flow sensor. Control blood pressure measurements were then made and the distribution of distal aortic flow was determined using radioactive microspheres. The microspheres were injected into the fetal femoral vein while an integrated arterial blood sample was simultaneously withdrawn from the fetal femoral artery. In five fetuses, microspheres of a different label were also injected into the femoral artery; these spheres would be distributed to only the lower body and the placenta. The presence of these spheres in the upper body of the fetus would indicate loss of previously trapped spheres in the time interval between control measurements and necropsy.

Fetal placental vascular resistance was measured by one of two ways. If an umbilical venous catheter was present, fetal placental vascular resistance was calculated as the ratio of the driving pressure (femoral artery minus umbilical vein pressure) and the placental blood flow (flow meter flow corrected for non-placental blood flow).  In fetuses without an umbilical venous catheter when the aortic occluder was partially inflated, femoral artery blood pressure and aortic flow measured.  The slope of the pressure-flow relationship (aortic blood flow corrected for placental flow fraction) was taken as the placental resistance.

Once the control measurements were completed, aortic blood  flow was reduced to 2/3 of control and maintained at that level (Figure 3).  The above measurements were repeated at weekly intervals with the following results.

## RESULTS

Aortic blood flow was reduced for an average of 16 days  (range 7 days to 34 days).  During the control period, fetal arterial pH = $7.37 \pm 0.01$, $PCO_2 = 48 \pm 1$ torr and $PO_2 = 19 \pm 1$  torr (mean ± sem).  After aortic blood flow reduction, pH = $7.32 \pm 0.02$  (P<0.01), $PCO_2 = 52 \pm 1$ torr (P<0.025), and $PO_2 = 16 \pm 1$ torr  (P<0.05).

Mean placental blood flow (flow sensor flow corrected for  non-placental flow fraction) was decreased from $484 \pm 44$ ml/min  during the control period to $303 \pm 23$ ml/min (mean ± sem) during the period of blood flow reduction (P<0.001).

More than 95% of the microspheres injected into the femoral artery catheter remained trapped in the lower body and/or placental tissues.

Upper body arterial blood pressure showed no significant  change (48 mm Hg during the control period (n=7) and 50 mm Hg after restriction (n=6)) while lower body arterial blood pressure decreased from $41 \pm 3$ mm Hg to $27 \pm 2$ mm Hg (P<0.001).  This blood pressure reduction was maintained for the duration of the study.

During the period of aortic blood flow reduction, placental vascular resistance decreased at a rate of 1.2% per day (Figure  4).  This was not different from zero, nor was it different from the normal change in resistance of 2.8% per day.  Therefore, these results did not show any acceleration of the normal decrease in placental vascular resistance after long term aortic blood flow reduction.

## DISCUSSION

From these results, it was concluded that fetal placental  blood flow was not defended by negative feedback control since neither resistance nor driving pressure showed any compensatory changes after a substantial reduction of flow over a long period of time.  Clearly some other form of control, not of a feedback nature, is responsible for the large decrease in fetal placental  resistance and the large increase in placental blood flow seen throughout gestation in the fetal lamb.

All experimental work points to the possibility that the resistance of the fetal vascular bed follows an inflexible, or at least nonregulated, developmental program.  If so, it would be an exception to the rule that vascular resistance adapts to need.  In fact, one would have to hypothesize that the fetus grows within the limits set by its placenta.

## SUMMARY

Changes in blood flow occur through chemically or mechanically mediated changes in pressure and resistance. Application of this principle to the regulation of fetal placental blood flow has not unearthed major physiological principles. The fetal placental circulation appears to be exempt from neural control, insensitive to most chemical mediators known to alter the distribution of blood flow and unaffected by fetal need. While exogenous catecholamines and angiotensin will cause vasoconstriction, blockade of endogenous hormone does not alter vascular resistance. Prostaglandins have not been shown to regulate fetal placental blood flow, though they may help match local fetal placental blood flow to local maternal placental blood flow. If this is true locally, one is almost compelled to believe that it must also be true generally. In that case a generalized maternal underperfusion should result in a generalized fetal placental vasoconstriction. It is curious that such an effect has not yet been described.

Mechanical regulation of umbilical blood flow may act through direct changes in fetal arterial and/or venous blood pressures or through changes in placental vascular resistance. Normally, placental resistance decreases with advancing gestation; what governs this decrease is unknown, except that it is not fetal need. Maintenance of fetal blood pressure ultimately depends upon the ability of the fetus to acquire amounts of water sufficient to maintain its blood volume and cardiac output, suggesting that water acquisition at the placenta may play a role in fetal placental blood flow regulation. Entry of water into the fetus is determined by the balance between the hydrostatic and osmotic forces acting at the placenta, the relative importance of each being dependent upon placental ultrastructure. It has been suggested that vasopressin may act on the placenta to alter transplacental water flux. However, in the sheep, all of these proposed mechanisms failed this laboratory's test that a long term artificial reduction in fetal placental blood flow ought to give rise to a compensatory change in vascular driving pressure or resistance. It is curious that such a simple problem as the governance of fetal placental blood flow should prove so refractory to solution.

## ACKNOWLEDGEMENTS

This work supported in part by NIH grant 5 R01 HL 27194.

## REFERENCES

Anderson, D.F. and Faber, J.J. (1984) Regulation of fetal placental blood flow in the lamb. *Am. J. Physiol.* 247, R567-R574.

Anderson, D.F. and Faber, J.J. (1982) Water flux due to colloid osmotic pressures across the haemochorial placenta of the guinea pig. *J. Physiol.* (London) 332, 521-527.

Bell, C. (1972) Autonomic nervous control of reproduction: Circulatory and other factors. *Pharmacol. Rev.* 24, 657-736.

Boyd, R.D.H., Haworth, C., Stacey, T.E., and Ward, R.H.T. (1976) Permeability of the sheep placenta to unmetabolized polar non-electrolytes. *J. Physiol.* (London) 256, 617-634.

Conrad, E.E. and Faber, J.J. (1977) Water and electrolyte acquisition across the placenta of the sheep. *Am. J. Physiol.* 233, H475-H487.

Faber, J.J. (1972) Regulation of placental blood flow. In: *Respiratory Gas Exchange and Blood Flow in the Placenta,* (eds.), L.D. Longo and H. Bartels, DHEW, Bethesda, MD., pp. 157-177.

Faber, J.J., Gault, C.F., Green, T.J., and Thornburg, K.L. (1973) Fetal blood volume and fetal placental blood flow in lambs. *Proc. Soc. Exp. Biol. Med.* 142, 340-344.

Faber, J.J. and Thornburg, K.L. (1977) Fetal homeostasis in relation to placental water exchange. *Ann. Rech. Vet.* 8, 353-361.

Faber, J.J. and Thornburg, K.L. (1981) The forces that drive inert solutes and water across the epitheliochorial placentae of the sheep and the goat and the haemochorial placentae of the rabbit and the guinea pig. *Placenta* (Suppl. 2), 203-214.

Iwamoto, H.S. and Rudolph, A.M. (1979) Effects of endogenous angiotensin II on the fetal circulation. *J. Develop. Physiol.* 1, 283-293.

Iwamoto, H.S. and Rudolph, A.M. (1981) Effects of angiotensin II on blood flow and its distribution in fetal lambs. *Circ. Res.* 48, 183-189.

Iwamoto, H.S., Rudolph, A.M., Keil, L.C., and Heymann, M.E. (1979) Hemodynamic responses of the sheep fetus to vasopressin infusion. *Circ. Res.* 44, 430-436.

Kedem, O. and Katchalsky, A. (1958) Thermodynamic analysis of the permeability of biological membranes to non-electrolytes. *Biochim. Biophys. Acta* 27, 229-246.

Leake, R.D., Stegner, H., Palmer, S.M., Oakes, G.K., and Fisher, D.A. (1983) Arginine vasopressin and arginine vasotocin inhibit ovine fetal/maternal water transfer. *Ped. Res.* 17, 583-586.

Longo, L.D. and Power G.G. (1983) Long-term regulation of fetal cardiac output. *Gynecol. Invest.* 4, 277-287.

Power, G.G., Dale, P.S., and Nelson, P.S. (1981) Distribution of maternal and fetal blood flow within cotyledons of the sheep placenta. *Am. J. Physiol.* 241, H486-H496.

Rankin, J.H.G. (1976) A role for prostaglandins in the regulation of the placental blood flows. *Prostaglandins* 11, 343-353.

Rankin, J., Meschia, G., Makowski, E.L., and Battaglia, F.C. (1970) Macroscopic distribution of blood flow in the sheep placenta. *Am. J. Physiol.* 219, 9-16.

Rankin, J.H.G. and Phernetton, T.M. (1976a) Effect of norepinephrine on the ovine umbilical circulation. *Proc. Soc. Exp. Biol. Med.* 152, 312-317.

Rankin, J.H.G. and Phernetton, T.M. (1976b) Circulatory response of the near-term sheep fetus to prostaglandin $E_2$. *Am. J. Physiol.* 231, 760-765.

Rankin, J.H.G. and Phernetton, T.M. (1976c) Effect of prostaglandin $E_2$ on ovine maternal placental blood flow. *Am. J. Physiol.* 231, 754-759.

Rankin, J.H.G. and Phernetton, T.M. (1978) Alpha and angiotensin receptor tone in the near-term sheep fetus. *Proc. Soc. Exp. Biol. Med.* 158, 166-169.

Reilly, F.D. and Russell, P.T. (1977) Neurohistochemical evidence supporting an absence of adrenergic and cholinergic innervation in the human placenta and umbilical cord. *Anat. Rec.* 188, 277-286.

Sheldon, R.E., Peeters, L.L.H., Jones, M.D., Makowski, E.L., and Meschia, G. (1979) Redistribution of cardiac output and oxygen delivery in the hypoxemic fetal lamb. *Am. J. Obstet. Gynecol.* 135, 1071-1078.

Spivak, M. (1943) On the presence or absence of nerves in the umbilical blood vessels of man and guinea pig. *Anat. Rec.* 85, 85-109.

Stock, M.K., Anderson, D.F., Phernetton, T.M., McLaughlin, M.K., and Rankin, J.H.G. (1980) Vascular response of the fetal placenta to local occlusion of the maternal placental vasculature. *J. Develop. Physiol.* 2, 339-346.

Stulc, J., Friedrich, R., and Jiricka, Z. (1969) Estimation of the equivalent pore dimensions in the rabbit placenta. *Life Sci.* 8, 167-180.

Thornburg, K.L., Binder, N.D., and Faber, J.J. (1979) Diffusion permeability and ultrafiltration-reflection-coefficients for $Na^+$ and $Cl^-$ in the near-term placenta of the sheep. *J. Develop. Physiol.* 1, 47-60.

Thornburg, K.L., Bissonnette, J.M., and Faber, J.J. (1976) Absence of fetal placental waterfall phenomenon in chronically prepared fetal lambs. *Am. J. Physiol.* 230, 886-892.

Woods, L.L., Thornburg, K.L., and Faber, J.J. (1978) Transplacental gradients in the guinea pig. *Am. J. Physiol.* 235, H200-H207.

# EFFECTS OF ELEVATED UMBILICAL VENOUS PRESSURE ON FLUID AND SOLUTE  TRANSPORT ACROSS THE ISOLATED PERFUSED HUMAN PLACENTAL COTELYDON

Henning Schneider[1,4], Jan Stulc[2],
Claudio Redaelli[3], and Jakob Briner[3]

[1]Division of Perinatal Physiology
Department of Obstetrics and Gynecology
and ·
[3]Department of Pathology
University of Zürich
Frauenklinikstrasse 10
CH-8091 Zürich, Switzerland

[2]Department of Pharmacology, Faculty of Pediatrics
Charles University, Albertov 4,
12800 Prague 2, Czechoslovakia

## INTRODUCTION

Everyone who has perfused the placenta of the guinea pig, rat or rabbit, has observed that the venous outflow rate decreased when the umbilical outflow pressure was elevated.   This observation implies that in the placentae of these species, elevation of the umbilical venous pressure promotes a significant volume flow from the perfused umbilical side of the placenta to the maternal circulation.  The phenomenon has been described in more detail in the placenta of the guinea pig (Dancis et al., 1962), under conditions of in situ perfusion of the umbilical circuit and in the isolated dually perfused preparation (Leichtweiss and Schröder, 1977). Dancis and coworkers observed that water flux from the fetal to the maternal side of the placenta was greatly increased when the umbilical outflow pressure was elevated to about 20 cm $H_2O$, and that labeled albumin and erythrocytes, which had been added to the umbilical perfusion fluid, could readily be detected in the maternal circulation.  In the experiments of Leichtweiss and Schröder, increasing the umbilical venous pressure caused a net fluid movement from the fetal to the maternal side without any observable evidence for sieving off the albumin molecules.   Electron microscopy of the perfused tissue, using horseradish peroxidase as a tracer, demonstrated that wide bag-shaped channels open in the placental trophoblast when the umbilical outflow pressure is increased (Kaufmann et al., 1982). All of the changes described above were reversible. In the course of the vaginal delivery of the human baby, partial or complete compression of the umbilical cord is quite a frequent occurrence which might cause sudden rise of the umbilical venous pressure. It may therefore be of interest for the obstetrician to know whether the events observed in the animal placenta at a high outflow pressure can take place in the human placenta as well.

[4]To Whom Correspondence Should Be Addressed: Department of Obstetrics and Gynecology ,University of Berne, Schanzeneckstrasse 1, CH-3012 Berne, Switzerland

In the following experiments, the effect of elevated umbilical venous pressure on volume flow and solute movement across the human placenta in vitro using the dually perfused cotelydon has been studied. Five substances with different transport characteristics were selected: antipyrine (transferred by simple diffusion predominantly transcellularly), deoxyglucose (transferred transcellularly by the hexose carrier system), L-glucose, dextran 70,000, and horseradish peroxidase (HRP), substances moving across the placenta by simple diffusion through paracellular routes.

## MATERIALS AND METHODS

The placentae were obtained from normal term pregnancies after vaginal delivery or cesarean section. The isolated placental cotyledon was perfused as described previously (Schneider et al., 1972). A chorionic artery and vein supplying a placental cotyledon were cannulated and rinsed with perfusate. For perfusion of the maternal compartment, 4 to 6 fine cannulae with blunt tips were pushed through the decidual plate into the intervillous space. The perfusate returning from the intervillous space through venous openings in the decidual plate was continuously drained by a syphon. The perfusion fluid was composed of Earle's buffered salt solution and NCTC tissue culture medium (1:2) with dextran 40,000 (10 g/l) and human serum albumin (HSA, 2 g/l). The medium was gassed with 95% oxygen and 5% $CO_2$. Roller pumps were used in both circuits which over the perfusion pressures used in this series deliver constant flow volumes with a mean deviation from the preset value of less than 3%. For precise determination of venous outflow rates, the fluid collected over 2 minutes was weighed. Twenty minutes after start of perfusion on the fetal side, the fetal venous outflow was measured. Those preparations were discarded where the difference between arterial inflow as indicated by the pump setting and venous return was greater than 0.5 ml/min. The perfusion rate was about 8 ml/min on the fetal side and 12 ml/min on the maternal side.

The radioactive substances $^3$H-deoxyglucose, $^{14}$C-dextran 70,000, $^3$H-L-glucose, were obtained from New England Nuclear. Horseradish peroxidase (HRP type II) was purchased from Sigma. The experiments for the investigation of the effect of an elevated umbilical venous pressure on volume flow and flux of the four radioactive solutes followed the same general protocol. The placenta was perfused for 20 minutes with the umbilical outflow catheter set at the height of the perfused cotyledon (zero level). Five 2-minute samples of venous effluent were collected from the two sides of the placenta (control period). The venous outflow level was then increased in steps of 10 cm up to 30 cm above the level of the placenta, and then returned to zero level. At each outflow level the placenta was perfused for 12 minutes. Five 2-minute samples of effluent were taken at each level, starting 2 minutes after the outflow level had been changed. Control experiments were run according to the same time schedule with the outflow level remaining zero. At the end of the experiment the decolorized tissue was excised and weighed. The weight was taken to represent the weight of the perfused tissue.

The transfer of $^3$H-deoxyglucose was measured from the maternal to the fetal side (M-F) only. Transfer of antipyrine was measured in the M-F direction in most experiments. Only in 3 experiments the direction was from the fetal to the maternal side (F-M). Transfer of $^{14}C$-dextran and $^3H$-L-glucose was measured in M-F or F-M direction, in the individual experiments the direction was the same for both tracers. With elevation of the umbilical venous pressure, volume flow across the placenta developed, from F-M, as indicated by a negative difference between the pump rate and the measured outflow rate on the fetal side.

The concentration of the radioactive substances was determined by liquid scintillation counting, while antipyrine was measured spectophotometrically (Brodie et al., 1949). The transfer rates of the test substances as calculated from the acceptor side are expressed as clearance which is defined as the rate of transfer across the placenta divided by the inflow concentration on the donor side. Clearance and volume flow are related to the weight of the perfused tissue. The data are represented as means; the limits are S.D., Statistics were applied where appropriate using the paired t-test or the Whitney and Mann U-test.

In order to trace the path of fluid movement and large extracellular markers across the placental barrier, HRP was added to the perfusate on the fetal side at 1.0, 2.0, or 4.0 mg/ml. Perfusion with the enzyme was continued for time periods varying between 5 and 30 minutes. Fetal venous outflow pressures of 10, 15, or 20 cm $H_2O$ were used. For fixation of the tissue, the intervillous space was perfused with cold phosphate-buffered glutaraldehyde (2.5%, pH 7.4) for 10 minutes while perfusion with HRP was continued on the fetal side. After termination of the perfusion pieces of ca. 2 x 2 x 1 mm were cut from the well fixed part of the tissue and immersed in glutaraldehyde at 4° C for further fixation of at least 2 not more than 24 hours. The pieces were cut by hand into thin slices of ca. 0.1 mm using razor blades and washed three times for 15 minutes in 0.2 M tris buffer before incubation at room temperature and complete darkness in 10 ml 0.2 M tris buffer containing 20 mg 3,3 diaminobenzidin-tetra-HCl (Sigma) and 1 ml 0.03% $H_2O_2$. Slices were washed briefly in tris-buffer and post-fixed for 60 minutes in S collidin buffered osmium tetroxide. The material was embedded in epon and semi-thin sections for light microscopy and ultra-thin sections for electron microscopy were prepared using standard procedures.

Table 1

Clearance* of Four Different Compounds Across The Dually
In Vitro Perfused Human Placental Cotyledon

| Antipyrine | $^3H$-Deoxyglucose | $^3H$-L-Glucose | $^{14}C$-Dextran |
|---|---|---|---|
| 104.61 ±41.63 | 64.32 ±24.26 | 32.18 ±13.87 | 1.89 ±1.04 |
| n = 17 | 5 | 12 | 16 |

*μl/min/g
mean ± SD

## RESULTS

The mean weight of the perfused tissue is $28.0 \pm 10$ g (n = 18). The mean clearance values of the four compounds studied normalized for tissue weight as measured under control conditions after 20 minutes are shown in Table 1. The transfer rates of antipyrine, [3]H-L-glucose, and [14]C-dextran are slightly higher in the F-M than M-F direction, but since the difference is not significant, data are pooled. These results are consistent with previous determinations obtained under comparable conditions. Maternal and fetal flow rates, QM and QF, as determined by timed collection of venous outflow were 494 and 318 µl/min/g, respectively and with the fetal venous outflow at the level of the placenta, i.e., under control conditions, there is a slight decrease in fetal outflow rate with time which is significant at 18, 30, 42, and 54 minutes (Figure 1A). Since the pump rate remains constant, this change is suggestive of volume flow in the F-M direction which was between 3 and 5 µl/min/g. There is a decline in maternal flow as well.

However, this was significant only for the value at 54 minutes. When the level of the fetal venous outflow is elevated stepwise above the placenta, the drop in fetal flow is more pronounced and the difference between control experiments and those with elevated outflow levels in the fetal circuit is significant at 20 and 30 cm $H_2O$ (Figure 1B). The volume flow as taken from the difference between pump rate and outflow rate on the fetal side was $12.7 \pm 11.5$ and $25.8 \pm 15.2$ µl/min/g at 20 and 30 cm $H_2O$ umbilical venous pressure, respectively (n=11). The changes in QM are not significant when paired comparison against the zero value is performed. The lack of correlation between changes in QF and QM may be partly explained by the limited precision in timed collection of venous return on the maternal side. The perfusate leaves the intervillous space through multiple openings in the decidual plate and is continuously drained from the surface of the placenta by a syphon. It is quite likely that this collection technique is not sufficiently accurate to detect small changes in flow.

The elevation of outflow pressure has no significant effect on the transfer of deoxyglucose when measured from M-F indicating that the glucose carrier mechanisms are not impaired by the increased pressure. Antipyrine clearance decreased to $83 \pm 5\%$ of the control value at an outflow level of 30 cm. After return to zero, it climbed back to $92 \pm 6\%$ of the control. The spontaneous change in clearance in percent of the baseline value for [3]H-L-glucose and [14]C-dextran is shown in Figures 2 and 3 and in Tables 2 through 5. Both [3]H-L-glucose and [14]C-dextran showed an increase in clearance during perfusion with the rise of transfer from F-M being clearly higher than in the opposite direction (Figures 2A and 2B). Furthermore, the change in clearance with time is most pronounced for dextran when measured from F-M. The effect of fetal venous pressure elevation on clearance is shown in Figures 3A and 3B and Table 4 and 5. The transport from M-F is slightly depressed when compared to the control experiments. The increase in clearance from F-M is similar to the change seen under control conditions. The rise in dextran clearance from F-M with pressure elevation was significant at 30, 42, and 54 minutes. L-glucose and dextran reveal a significant difference. The fetal venous pressure elevation did not lead to a substantial rise in solute flux from F-M.

Table 2

Clearance Changes - Control Experiments
for $^3$H-L-Glucose

| Exp. No. | | 6 min | 18 min | 30 min | 42 min | 54 min |
|---|---|---|---|---|---|---|
| | | M→F | | | | |
| 14 | | -1.4 | + 2.8 | + 2.8 | +10.2 | +14.4 |
| 17 | | +7.2 | +10.8 | +10.8 | +18.0 | +14.4 |
| (n=2) | x̄ | +2.9 | + 6.8 | + 6.8 | +14.1 | +14.4 |
| | | F→M | | | | |
| 18 | | +4.9 | + 7.3 | +13.9 | +18.8 | +18.8 |
| 19 | | - | + 8.2 | +12.5 | +18.1 | +30.6 |
| 20 | | +3.7 | +18.7 | +31.9 | +31.9 | +37.8 |
| (n=3) | x̄ | +2.9 | +11.4 | +19.4 | +22.9 | +29.1 |

Changes are expressed in percent of the baseline value at the beginning of each experiment.

Reviewing the tissue samples from the experiments with HRP revealed considerable heterogeneity in the intensity of the HRP reaction. There was quite a large variability in the degree of staining among experiments and in 4 out of 11, hardly any reaction product could be localized. The heterogeneity was also present within the same villi or among neighboring villi. Apparently this was not related to enzyme concentration, length of exposure or venous pressure in the fetal perfusion circuit.

With electron microscopy which was performed on the specimens with a strong reaction HRP could be localized at the endothelial lining of the fetal capillaries and also within the intercellular junctions (Figure 4). Occasional pinocytotic vesicles with reaction product were found in the cytoplasm of the endothelial cells. In no instance was there any reaction product in the subendothelial basement membrane or within the syncytiotrophoblast. Even with fetal venous pressure elevations up to 20 cm $H_2O$, no signs for the formation of tubules or channels within the trophoblast or any staining of the microvilli could be detected. There was occasional positive reaction in lysosomes or vesicles in the syncytio- or cytotrophoblast.

## DISCUSSION

There was a negative difference between the outflow rate and pump rate on the fetal side under control conditions without a detectable positive difference on the maternal side. The pronounced decrease in the fetal outflow rate, brought about by elevation of the fetal outflow pressure also was not accompanied by a corresponding increase in the outflow rate on the maternal side. The perfusion pumps have been carefully checked for constant pump rate and for independence of pump rate on the perfusion pressure. Nothing to explain the discrepancy was observed. Because the capacity of the fetal vascular bed to store the fluid is limited while the intervillous space is highly distensible some of the fluid not recovered at the fetal outflow may have moved to the maternal side without being promptly detectable as increase in maternal outflow. The volume flow estimated as the difference between the inflow and outflow rate on the fetal side should be taken only as its possible upper limit.

With elevation of the fetal venous pressure to 20 and 30 cm $H_2O$ the fetal outflow rate decreased significantly to roughly 90% of the inflow rate. This, however, is considerably less than what was seen in the isolated guinea pig placenta (Leichtweiss and Schröder, 1977). In this preparation at a pressure of 20 mm Hg, 70-80% of the flow was shifted from the fetal to the maternal side and at 30 mm Hg fetal venous outflow came to a complete stop.

Table 3

Clearance  Changes - Control Experiments
for $^{14}$C-Dextran

| Exp. No. | | 6 min | 18 min | 30 min | 42 min | 54 min |
|---|---|---|---|---|---|---|
| | | M→F | | | | |
| 14 | | - | - | - | + 8.3 | + 8.3 |
| 17 | | +16.7 | +33.3 | +33.3 | + 33.3 | + 33.3 |
| (n=2) | $\overline{x}$ | + 8.4 | +16.7 | +16.7 | + 20.8 | + 20.8 |
| | | F→M | | | | |
| 18 | | +25.6 | +44.2 | +97.7 | +132.6 | +160.5 |
| 19 | | - | + 5.9 | +17.7 | + 29.4 | + 52.9 |
| 20 | | - | +20.9 | +39.6 | + 53.9 | + 64.8 |
| (n=3) | $\overline{x}$ | + 8.5 | +23.7 | +51.7 | + 72.0 | + 92.7 |

Changes are expressed in percent of the baseline value at the beginning of each experiment.

Figures 1A and 1B. Change in maternal (QM) and fetal (QF) flow rate measured as venous outflow against time under control conditions and with elevation of the fetal venous pressure. QM and QF represent venous flow rates. Shown are mean values ± SD. In the control experiments, the drop in QF is significant at 18, 30, 42, and 54 minutes when compared to the 0 value by paired t-test. The change in QM is significant only at 54 minutes. With elevation of fetal venous pressure the drop in QF is significant at 20 and 30 cm $H_2O$ when compared to control experiments (* $p<0.05$, ** $p<0.02$).

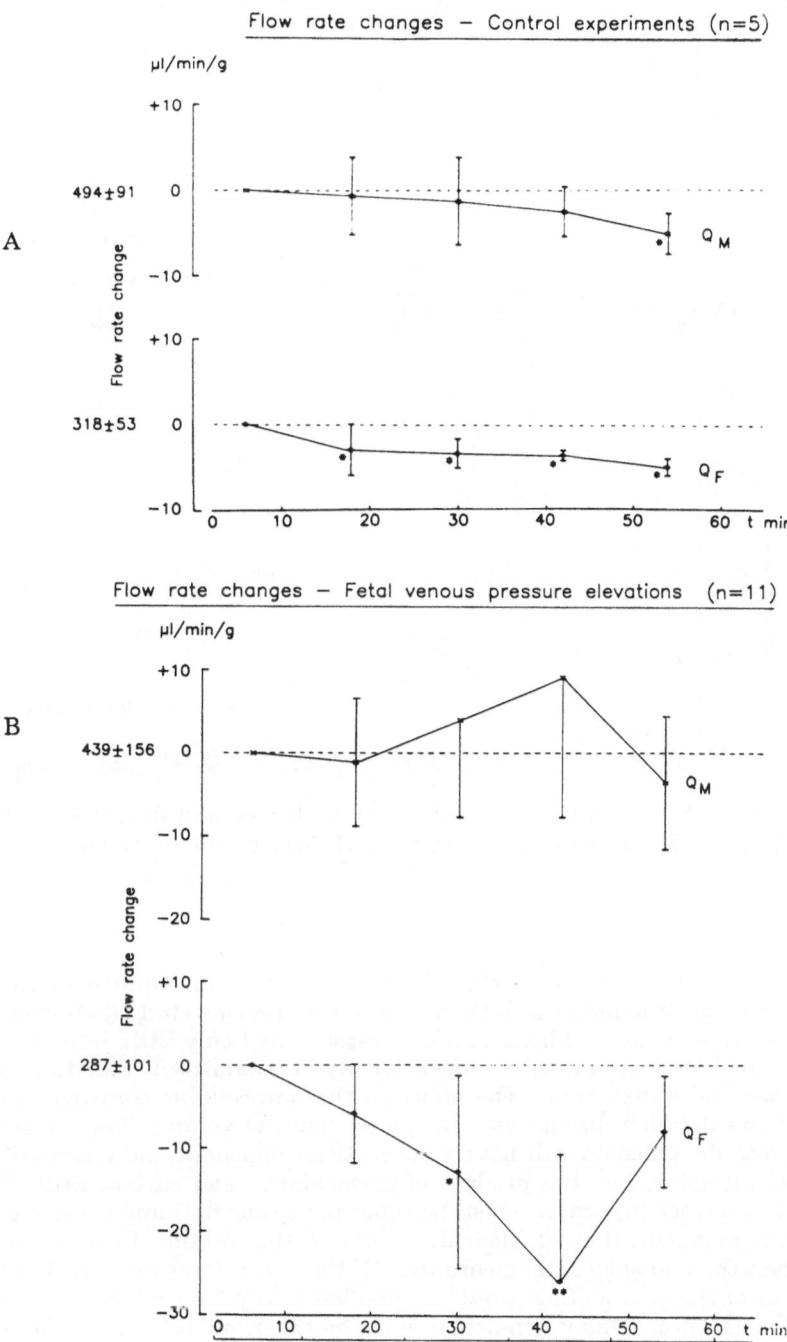

Flow rate changes — Control experiments (n=5)

μl/min/g

A

Flow rate change

494±91

318±53

$Q_M$

$Q_F$

Flow rate changes — Fetal venous pressure elevations (n=11)

μl/min/g

B

Flow rate change

439±156

287±101

$Q_M$

$Q_F$

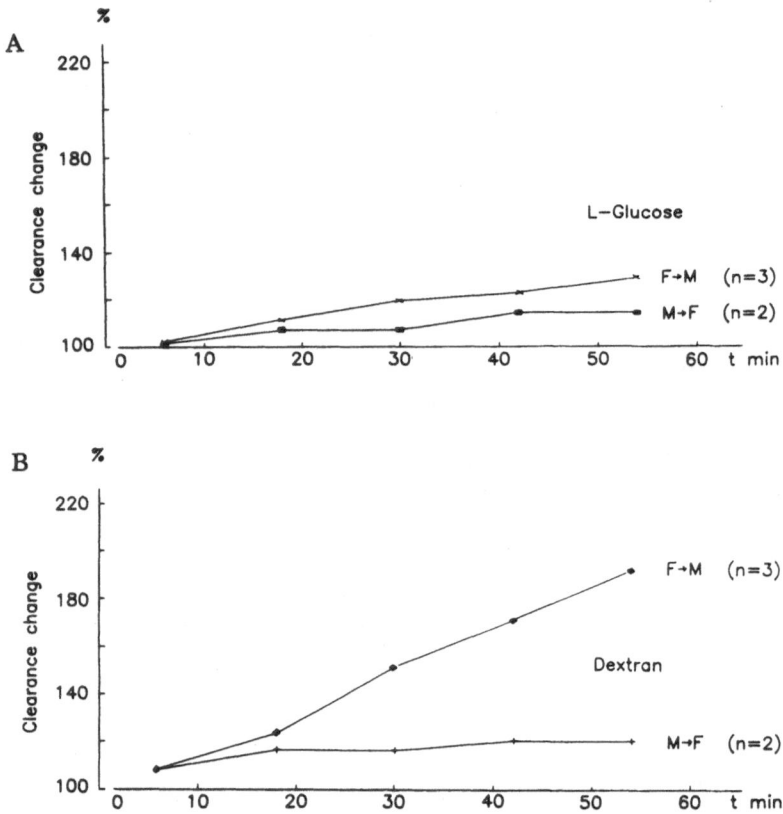

Figures 2A and 2B. Change in clearance of L-glucose and dextran 70,000 from maternal to fetal (M-F) and fetal to maternal (F-M) side under control conditions.

The clearance values determined under control conditions are quite similar to results obtained in this laboratory for a previous study (Schneider et al., 1985). Elevation of the umbilical outflow pressure had only little influence on the transplacental transport of transcellularly transmitted substances ($^3$H-deoxyglucose and antipyrine). The effect on the paracellular transport, however, deserves more detailed discussion. In the presence of volume flow, movement of solutes across the placenta will have a convective component and clearance will be the sum of diffusion, i.e., the product of permeability and surface area (PS) and convection. Convection, can, at most, be equal to volume flow and therefore gives a measurable augmentation of clearance only if the volume flow is not much smaller than the transplacental clearance. Of the test solutes used in this study, a major effect of the volume flow would be predicted only for dextran, since it has a very small clearance. This is consistent with the experimental observation that the increase in clearance was highest for dextran in the direction from F-M, i.e., in the direction of the volume flow.

Table 4

Clearance Changes - Fetal Venous Pressure Elevations
for $^3$H-L-Glucose

| Exp. No. | | 10 cm/18 min | 20 cm/30 min | 30 cm/42 min | 0 cm/54 min |
|---|---|---|---|---|---|
| | | M→F | | | |
| 13 | | + 5.5 | + 6.6 | + 3.3 | +11.1 |
| 15 | | - 3.3 | -11.9 | -10.2 | + 4.9 |
| 16 | | + 5.8 | + 8.7 | + 5.8 | + 8.7 |
| (n=3) | $\bar{x}$ | + 2.7 | + 1.1 | - 0.4 | + 5.0 |
| | | F→M | | | |
| 9 | | - 2.3 | + 7.0 | + 9.2 | + 7.0 |
| 10 | | + 1.5 | +10.9 | +23.1 | +19.6 |
| 11 | | + 8.5 | +25.1 | +54.0 | +49.8 |
| 12 | | +14.9 | +37.4 | +49.0 | +43.5 |
| (n=4) | $\bar{x}$ | + 5.7 | +20.1 | +33.8 | +30.0 |

Changes are expressed in percent of the baseline value with no pressure elevation.

Table 5

Clearance Changes - Fetal Venous Pressure Elevations
for $^{14}$C-Dextran

| Exp. No. | | 10 cm/18 min | 20 cm/30 min | 30 cm/42 min | 0 cm/54 min |
|---|---|---|---|---|---|
| | | M→F | | | |
| 13 | | + 9.0 | +12.1 | + 6.0 | + 15.1 |
| 15 | | - | - 7.7 | - 3.5 | + 6.8 |
| 16 | | + 5.9 | + 8.7 | + 2.7 | + 8.7 |
| (n=3) | $\bar{x}$ | + 5.0 | + 4.4 | - 1.7 | + 10.2 |
| | | F→M | | | |
| 5 | | - | +34.5 | +155.2 | + 55.2 |
| 6 | | +16.7 | +16.7 | + 75.0 | + 75.0 |
| 8 | | - | - | + 27.3 | + 54.6 |
| 9 | | +13.0 | +26.0 | + 78.3 | + 65.2 |
| 10 | | - 7.7 | + 3.8 | + 65.4 | + 57.7 |
| 11 | | + 5.3 | +47.7 | + 78.9 | +100.0 |
| 12 | | +14.3 | +42.8 | +10.71 | + 64.3 |
| (n=7) | $\bar{x}$ | + 5.9 | +24.5 | + 83.9 | + 67.4 |

Changes are expressed in percent of the baseline value with no pressure elevation.

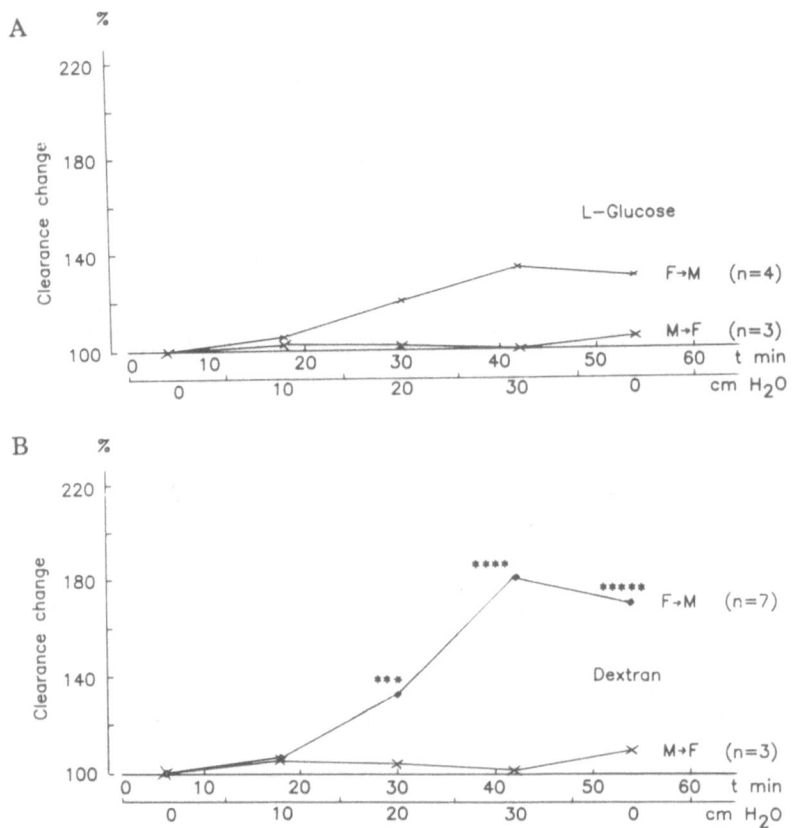

Figures 3A and 3B. Change in clearance of L-glucose and dextran 70,000 from maternal to fetal (M-F) and fetal to maternal (F-M) side with elevation of the fetal venous pressure. Rise in clearance of dextran from F-M was significant at 20 and 30 cm $H_2O$ and also after return to 0 pressure when compared to the initial clearance by paired t-test (*** p<0.01, **** p<0.001, ***** p<0.0005). The rise in clearance of dextran from F-M with elevation of fetal venous pressure to 20 and 30 cm $H_2O$ is significantly greater than for L-glucose when tested by the U-test of Mann and Whitney (p<0.05).


However, the clearance increased spontaneously also when measured in the M-F direction. When clearance is measured in the opposite direction of volume flow, the effect should be negative, and clearance should decrease. The rise in clearance from M-F is best explained by a change in permeability of the placenta for hydrophilic molecules due to in vitro perfusion. Elevation of the fetal outflow pressure had no significant additional effect on clearance of the two solutes. The suppression of the clearance in M-F direction observed only as a trend is consistent with the expected effects of volume flow on transport and is taken as suggestive of additional volume flow across the placenta during the period of elevated venous pressure.

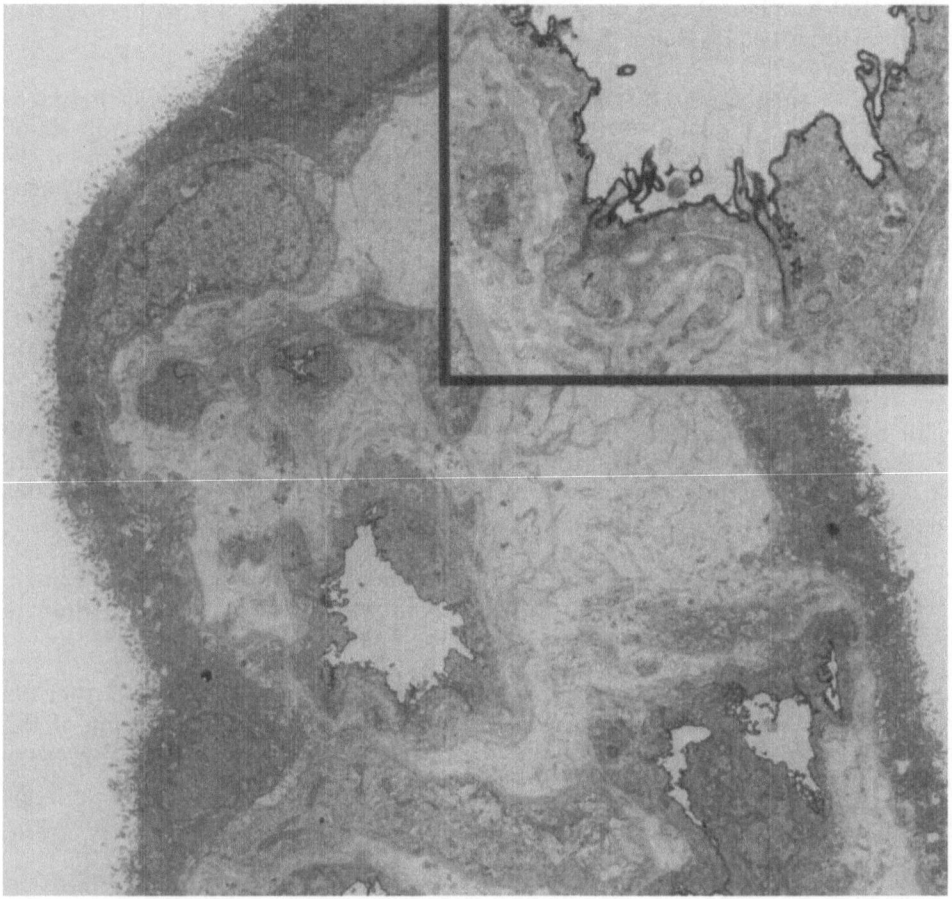

Figure 4. The capillaries of the placental villus show reaction product on the endothelial surface (X3800). Insert shows extension to the outer third along the intercellular junctions of the endothelium (X12,900).

As noticed above for the effect of fetal venous pressure elevation on volume flow, the findings with HRP also differed substantially from what has been described for the isolated dually perfused guinea pig placenta (Kaufmann et al., 1982). In these experiments with regular perfusion, not only the endothelial cells but also the basement membrane of the fetal capillaries were clearly stained by the marker protein which had penetrated through the intercellular junctions. After fetal venous pressure elevation to approximately 20 cm $H_2O$, HRP-positive outlines of bag-like channels suggesting connections between the luminae of fetal capillaries and the maternal lacunae were noticed within the trophoblast. In these studies, even after pressure elevation up to 30 cm $H_2O$ HRP apparently did not penetrate beyond the inner third of the intercellular junctions of the endothelium. This would confirm the species-dependent differences in the tightness of the endothelial portion of the placental barrier within the group of hemochorial placentae described by Heinrich et al. (1976).

With complete occlusion of the umbilical cord as may occur during labor pressure in the umbilical vein may rise to arterial values of approximately 45-50 mm Hg. It cannot be excluded that significant shifts of fluid and solutes from the fetal to the maternal circuit may develop in human labor when umbilical venous pressure rises above the upper limit of 25 mm Hg used in these series.

## SUMMARY

In the in vitro perfused human placenta, there is a spontaneous rise in permeability and volume flow, the latter from fetal to maternal side. This volume flow in the well preserved in vitro perfused human placenta remains, however, small so that its effect on the measured transport rates of most molecules of biological interest is negligible. If, the directions of transport across the placenta are directly compared, volume flow may affect results, in particular for compounds with low placental permeability.

Elevation of fetal venous outflow pressure up to 30 cm $H_2O$ raised the volume flow, but had only limited effect on placental transport. In this respect, the human placental barrier clearly differs from that of the guinea pig.

Even with fetal venous pressure elevations up to 20 cm $H_2O$, no signs for the formation of tubules or channels within the trophoblast or any staining of the microvilli with HRP could be detected. There was occasionally HRP-positive reaction in lysosomes or vesicles in the syncytio- or cytotrophoblast.

## ACKNOWLEDGEMENTS

This research was supported in part by a grant from Schweizerischer Nationalfonds. We are grateful to Mrs. B. Benz and Miss S. Heeb for expert technical assistance.

## REFERENCES

Brodie, B.B, Axelrod, J., Soberman, R., and Levy, B.B. (1949) The estimation of antipyrine in biological materials. *J. Biol. Chem*. 179, 25-29.

Dancis, J., Brenner, M., and Money, W.L. (1962) Some factors affecting the permeability of guinea pig placenta. *Am. J. Obstet. Gynecol*. 84, 570-576.

Heinrich, D., Metz, J., Raviola, E., and Fossman, W.G. (1976) Ultrastructure of perfusion-fixed fetal capillaries in the human placenta. *Cell Tiss. Res*. 172, 157-169.

Kaufmann, P., Schröder, H., and Leichtweiss, H.-P. (1982) Fluid shift across the placenta. II. Fetomaternal transfer of horseradish peroxidase in the guinea pig. *Placenta* 3, 339-348.

Leichtweiss, H.-P. and Schröder, H. (1977) The effect of elevated outflow pressure on flow resistance and the transfer of THO, albumin and glucose in the isolated guinea pig placenta. *Pflügers Arch.* 371, 251-256.

Schneider, H., Panigel, M., and Dancis, J. (1972) Transfer across the perfused human placenta of antipyrine, sodium and leucine. *Am. J. Obstet. Gynecol.* 114, 822-828.

Schneider, H., Sodha, R.J., Proegler, M., and Young, M.P.A. (1985) Permeability of the human placenta for hydrophilic substances studied in the isolated dually in vitro perfused lobe. *Contrib. Gynecol. Obstet.* 13, 98-103.

# EFFECTS OF SOME AUTACOIDS AND HUMORAL AGENTS ON HUMAN FETOPLACENTAL VASCULAR RESISTANCE: CANDIDATES FOR LOCAL REGULATION OF FETOPLACENTAL BLOOD FLOW

- A Review -

M. Helen Maguire, Randy B. Howard,
T. Hosokawa, and Alan M. Poisner

Departments of Pharmacology, Toxicology and Therapeutics,
and Ralph Smith Research Center
University of Kansas Medical Center
39th and Rainbow Blvd.
Kansas City, Kansas 66103

## INTRODUCTION

Mechanisms of local regulation of blood flow through the extensive fetoplacental vascular bed of the mature human placenta are not understood. As the placenta is not innervated, there is no nervous control of vascular resistance. Locally-produced vasoactive autacoids such as prostaglandins and thromboxane could play a role in modulating fetoplacental blood flow, or humoral agents could be involved. Human placenta in the form of in vitro slice preparations has been shown to produce thromboxane $B_2$, the stable metabolite of thromboxane $A_2$, and to convert exogenous arachidonic acid to several prostanoids, including $PGE_2$, $PGD_2$, $PGF_{2\alpha}$ and 6-keto-$PGF_{1\alpha}$ a biologically inactive metabolite of prostacyclin, $PGI_2$ (Mitchell et al., 1982; Makila et al., 1984; Harper et al., 1983). Also, higher levels of iPGE were found in umbilical venous plasma than in plasma from umbilical arteries (Bibby et al., 1979), suggesting that production of PGE by the placenta occurs in vivo. Thromboxane $A_2$, $PGE_2$, and $PGI_2$ are known to have pressor or depressor actions in many vascular beds (Whittle and Moncada, 1984; Kadowitz et al., 1984). We therefore evaluated the effects of $PGE_2$, $PGF_{2\alpha}$, $PGI_2$, $PGE_1$ and the endoperoxide analogue U46619, a thromboxane mimetic (Granström et al., 1983), on the resistance of human fetoplacental vasculature in isolated dual-perfused cotyledons from human term placenta. Furthermore, the formation of a potentially important humoral agent, angiotensin II (AII), within the fetoplacental vascular bed was studied. This pressor peptide, the primary vasoactive component of the renin-angiotensin system, is present in human umbilical blood. In vaginal deliveries, concentrations of cord venous AII were found to be significantly higher than those in cord arterial blood (Lumbers and Reid, 1977; Broughton et al., 1977), suggesting that AII was formed from its inactive precursor AI within the fetoplacental circulation or, as suggested by Symonds (1979), that the complete renin-angiotensin system was functional within the placenta. Using dual-perfused human placental cotyledons it was shown that AII elicited potent dose-related pressor responses in the fetoplacental vascular bed, with a threshold dose of

10 pmoles (Howard et al., 1983). In order to evaluate the possible contribution of in situ generation of AII within the fetoplacental vasculature, the fetoplacental conversion of AI to AII was studied by measuring effects of the peptides on fetal perfusion pressure in dual-perfused cotyledons in the presence of specific antagonists of AII formation and action. The release of renin into fetal and maternal perfusates was also measured to assess involvement of the complete renin-angiotensin system in local control of fetoplacental vascular resistance.

## METHODS

Human placentae from normal full term pregnancies were obtained immediately after spontaneous delivery or delivery by cesarean section. The fetal circulation and intervillous space of a single cotyledon from each placenta were perfused as described elsewhere (Schneider et al., 1972; Howard et al., 1986). Perfusion was performed at constant flow with Earle's salt solution (Earle, 1943) containing dextran, 40 g per l. Maternal perfusate was gassed with 95% oxygen-5% carbon dioxide; the fetal perfusate was gassed similarly or with 94% nitrogen-6% carbon dioxide. Preparation and perfusates were maintained at 37°C. Maternal arterial, fetal arterial, and fetal venous perfusates were sampled with glass syringes from appropriate ports in the perfusion lines. Maternal venous perfusate was sampled by syringe from perfusate outflow adjacent to maternal cannulae. Arterial and venous perfusate gas and pH values were measured with a Radiometer BMS blood gas analyzer and venous values served to indicate adequacy of the maternal perfusion. At the end of each experiment, the fetal circuit was infused with a 1% solution of Coomassie Blue in 0.9% NaCl; the cotyledon so demarcated was dissected and weighed.

Perfusion pressure of the fetal circuit was used as an index of fetal vascular resistance, and was monitored via a Statham P23ID transducer and recorded on a Gilson ICT-2H Duograph (Hosokawa et al., 1985; Howard et al., 1986).

Pressor responses to prostanoids were expressed as mm Hg increase in perfusion pressure over baseline perfusion pressure. For study of vasodilator prostanoids, baseline perfusion pressure was elevated to 50-55 mm Hg by inclusion of 254 nM AII in the fetal perfusate. Depressor responses were expressed as % change in perfusion pressure from the baseline perfusion pressure which was taken as 100%. Within a single cotyledon, responses to each concentration of prostanoid were determined in triplicate.

Increases in perfusion pressure elicited by 1 nmole doses of AI and AII were measured in triplicate. The average increase in perfusion pressure produced by 1 nmole of AII administered before infusion of antagonists was taken as control in each cotyledon; responses to AI, and to AI and AII during and after infusion of antagonists were expressed as a percentage of the average control response to AII. Experimental results are given as means ± SEM. Statistical analysis was performed using Student's t-test or, where groups showed significantly different variances, by the signed Wilcoxon rank test.

Renin (active and inactive) in the perfusates was assayed by a modification of the method of Poisner et al. (1981a). Perfusate samples were centrifuged immediately after collection, decanted from any pelleted debris, and stored at -20°C until assay. Forty μl of perfusate were preincubated for 30 minutes at room temperature in the presence or absence of 2 μg per ml of trypsin, to differentiate between active and inactive reinin, and then incubated for 3-20 hours at 37°C with sheep renin substrate. Angiotensin generated was assayed by radioimmunoassay as described elsewhere (Poisner et al., 1981a; Poisner and Poisner, 1987). Total renin (active plus inactive) was measured and expressed as μU per ml of perfusate. The Human Renin International Standard was used. The detection limit of the assay was 0.1 μU per ml.

$PGF_{2\alpha}$, AII, AI, captopril and saralasin were dissolved in 0.9% NaCl. Stock solutions of $PGE_2$ in 1.9 mM $Na_2CO_3$ and U46619 in ethanol were diluted with 0.9% NaCl. $PGI_2$ was dissolved in 50 mM $Na_2CO_3$-$NaHCO_3$ buffer, pH 10.5, and diluted with ungassed Earle's salt solution pH 8.5. Prostaglandins and peptides were administered via close arterial injection in boli of 50-100 μl. Solutions of captopril and saralasin were infused to give final concentrations of 2.2 μM and 94 nM, respectively; infusions commenced 10 minutes before injections of AI and AII.

Prostaglandins were obtained from the Upjohn Company, AI from Bachem Inc., AII (Hypertensin) from Giba-Geigy Corp., captopril from E.R. Squibb & Sons, Inc. and saralasin acetate from Norwich-Eaton Pharmaceuticals Inc. Human renin standard was provided by the National Institute for Biological Standards, London. $I^{125}$ labeled AI and AI antiserum were obtained from New England Nuclear.

## RESULTS

### Perfusion Parameters

Flow rates, pH and gas values of fetal and maternal perfusates are summarized in Table 1. Twenty-five cotyledons were used in study of the actions of prostanoids on fetal perfusion pressure, and in these experiments fetal perfusate was gassed with 95% oxygen-5% carbon dioxide. Six cotyledons were used in the study of the conversion of AI to AII, and in these preparations the fetal perfusate was gassed with 94% nitrogen-6% carbon dioxide. Under the latter conditions, arteriovenous increase in fetal perfusate oxygen tension indicated that perfusion of the maternal circuit resulted in substantial maternal to fetal oxygen transfer consistent with the arteriovenous fall in maternal perfusate oxygen tension (Table 1). Under the former conditions, in which fetal perfusate was gassed with 95% oxygen-5% carbon dioxide, arteriovenous differences in pH and gas tensions indicated release of $CO_2$ and consumption of oxygen by the cotyledons (Table 1).

### Responses to Prostanoids

$PGE_2$ elicited reversible increases in perfusion pressure, but although the response increased with increasing concentration of the prostanoid, in the range of 14 to 280 nmoles, it was not possible to obtain a precise log concentration-effect relationship because sensitization occurred with repeated dosing. Furthermore, after a strong vasoconstriction to $PGE_2$, e.g. 30-50 mm Hg, desensitization to subsequent doses was often observed. $PGF_{2\alpha}$ also caused reversible increases in perfusion pressure but did not exhibit conspicuous self-sensitization. Dose-related increases in perfusion pressure were seen in the range of 10-31 nmoles of $PGF_{2\alpha}$

(Figure 1). U46619 was a potent vasoconstrictor in the fetoplacental vascular bed, and elicited reversible increases in perfusion pressure which were dose-related over the range of 14-57 pmoles (Figure 1). Responses to this prostanoid were consistent in seven cotyledons studied, particularly when several intermediate-range "conditioning" doses were given before commencing dosing to obtain the log concentration-effect curve. However, both sensitization and desensitization were observed in different cotyledons after doses of U46619 > 86 pmoles which caused > 80 mm Hg increases in perfusion pressure.

$PGI_2$ and $PGE_1$ elicited reversible dose-related decreases in fetoplacental perfusion pressure in perfused cotyledons in which baseline perfusion pressure was elevated to 50-55 mm Hg by infusion of AII (Figure 2). $PGI_2$ was more potent than $PGE_1$; threshold doses were $\leq 10$ pmoles and $\leq 140$ pmoles, respectively. Reversible vasodilatation was also elicited by $PGI_2$ and $PGE_1$ in preparations with

Table 1

Mean Fetal and Maternal Flow Rates, Perfusate Gas Tensions and pH, and Cotyledon Weights of Dual-Perfused Cotyledons.

| | Wt g | Q ml min⁻¹g⁻¹ | pO$_2$ mm Hg | | pCO$_2$ mm Hg | | pH | |
|---|---|---|---|---|---|---|---|---|
| | | F | $F_A$ | $F_V$ | $F_A$ | $F_V$ | $F_A$ | $F_V$ |
| Mean | 16.6* | 0.34 | 502 | 379 | 34.6 | 41.1 | 7.39 | 7.32 |
| SEM | 1.4 | 0.033 | 6 | 12 | 0.3 | 1.1 | 0.002 | 0.01 |
| | | M | $M_A$ | $M_V$ | $M_A$ | $M_V$ | $M_A$ | $M_V$ |
| Mean | | 1.1 | 557 | 416 | 34.1 | 40.3 | 7.38 | 7.34 |
| SEM | | 0.09 | 7 | 13 | 0.3 | 1.0 | 0.002 | 0.07 |
| | | F | $F_A$ | $F_V$ | $F_A$ | $F_V$ | $F_A$ | $F_V$ |
| Mean | 14.3** | 0.49 | 27 | 195 | 43.0 | 43.2 | 7.34 | 7.35 |
| SEM | 2.0 | 0.07 | 2 | 14 | 0.5 | 1.3 | 0.01 | 0.02 |
| | | M | $M_A$ | $M_V$ | $M_A$ | $M_V$ | $M_A$ | $M_V$ |
| Mean | | 1.56 | 547 | 331 | 33.2 | 38.9 | 7.40 | 7.35 |
| SEM | | 0.23 | 6 | 26 | 0.7 | 2.6 | 0.003 | 0.01 |

* n = 25: $Q_F$ and $Q_M$ n = 25; fetal gas values n = 21-23; maternal gas values n = 10-14.
** n = 6

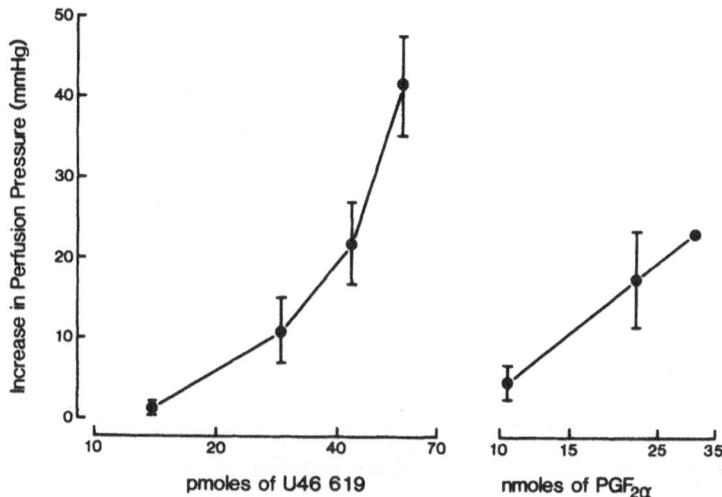

Figure 1. Log dose-response curves for increases in fetoplacental perfusion pressure elicited by U46619 and $PGF_{2\alpha}$. Curves are composites of 6 individual log dose-response curves for U46619 and 4 for $PGF_{2\alpha}$. Points signify a mean of 2 values or, where vertical bars indicate ± S.E.M., means of 3-5 values. Each individual log dose-response curve was obtained on a different cotyledon (Howard et al., 1986).

spontaneous baseline perfusion pressure and in preparations with $K^{+}$-elevated perfusion pressure.

### Responses to AI and AII

Injection of bolus doses of 1 nmole of AI and AII in the six cotyledons caused mean increases in perfusion pressure of 20.0 ± 1.8 mm Hg and 21.9 ± 2.2 mm Hg, respectively, which returned to basal levels within 5-12 minutes, depending on the cotyledon; within single cotyledons recovery times for both peptides varied by < 2 min. The pressor response to AI was reduced by 2.2 µM captopril, but the response to AII was unaffected by captopril. Results from three cotyledons showed that the antagonism by captopril was highly significant for AI ($p < 0.001$) and that captopril did not antagonize the AII response ($p > 0.05$) (Figure 3). After infusion of captopril was stopped pressor responses to AI were 87.0% of the pre-captopril response (Figure 3). Pressor responses to AI and AII were reversibly reduced by 94 nM saralasin. In three cotyledons, saralasin significantly inhibited the increase in perfusion pressure elicited by both AI ($p < 0.05$) and AII ($p < 0.001$) (Figure 4). After cessation of saralasin infusion, pressor responses to both AI and AII showed substantial recovery of the pre-saralasin responses, as indicated in Figure 4 ($p > 0.05$ for AI and AII; AII data were compared by the signed Wilcoxon rank test).

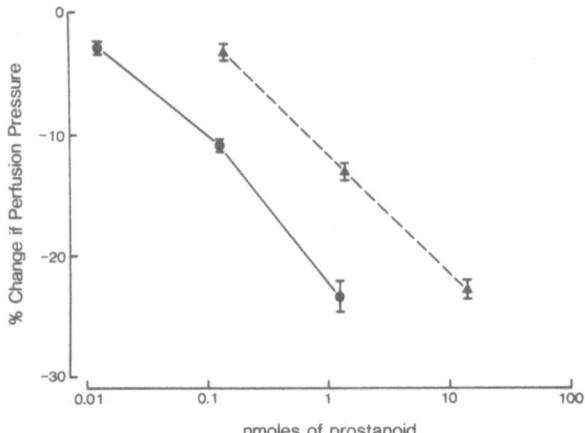

Figure 2. Log dose-response curves for the depressor actions of PGI$_2$ (o) and PGE$_1$ (Δ); curves are composites of 4 individual log dose-response curves for PGI$_2$ and of 3 for PGE$_1$. Each individual curve was obtained on a different cotyledon. Responses are shown as % change in perfusion pressure from baseline perfusion pressure which was taken as 100% (Howard et al., 1986).

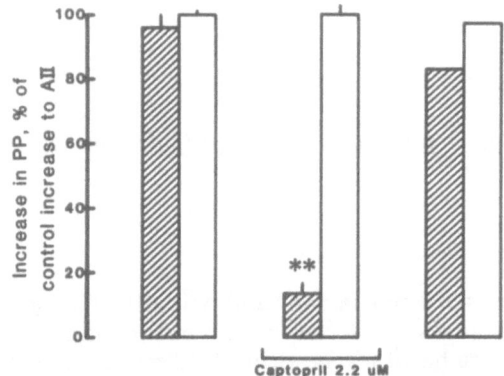

Figure 3. Effect of captopril on the increase in fetoplacental perfusion pressure elicited by AI and AII. Increases in perfusion pressure (PP) elicited by 1 nmole of AI (hatched bars) and 1 nmole of AII (open bars) before, during and after infusion of captopril (final concentration 2.2 μM) are expressed as a percentage of the average pre-captopril response to AII, which is taken as 100%; in each cotyledon responses were measured in triplicate). Bars represent means ± S.E.M. for 3 cotyledons before and during captopril infusion, and means for 2 cotyledons 30 minutes after cessation of the infusion. ** $p < 0.001$ for difference from the pre-captopril response to AI. (Actual increases in PP elicited by 1 nmole doses of AI and AII before captopril infusion were: AI, 17.4 ± 1.9 mm Hg; AII, 18.2 ± 2.5 mm Hg.) (Hosokawa et al., 1985).

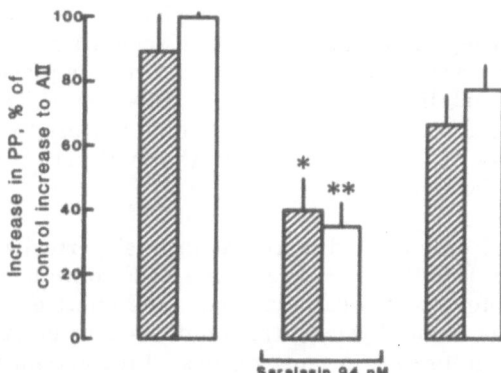

Figure 4. Effect of saralasin infusion on the increase in fetoplacental perfusion pressure elicited by AI and AII. Increase in perfusion pressure (PP) elicited by 1 nmole of AI (hatched bars) and 1 nmole of AII (open bars) before, during and after infusion of saralasin (final concentration 94 nM) are expressed as a percentage of the pre-saralasin response to AII, which is taken as 100%. Bars represent means ± S.E.M. for 3 cotyledons before, during, and 30 minutes after cessation of saralasin infusion; in each cotyledon responses were measured in triplicate. *p < 0.05 and ** p < 0.001 for difference from the pre-saralasin response to AI and AII, respectively (Hosokawa et al., 1985).

## Release of Renin

Analysis of fetal venous perfusates for the presence of renin was performed in four dual-perfused cotyledons. Fetal perfusate of one cotyledon was gassed with 95% oxygen-5% carbon dioxide; fetal perfusates of the other three cotyledons were gassed with 94% nitrogen-6% carbon dioxide. Cotyledon weights ranged from 7 g to 15 g (mean $11.75 \pm 1.6$ g). Gas and pH values of fetal venous perfusates of the four cotyledons were similar to the corresponding gas and pH values shown in Table 1. Renin was not detectable in the fetal venous perfusates of the four cotyledons, under baseline conditions, during or after pressor responses to maternal hypoxia, 1 nmole of AII or 57 nmoles of $PGD_2$, or during the depressor response to 54 nmoles of histamine. However, the samples of maternal venous perfusate collected concurrently with fetal venous samples contained renin in all cases. More than 95% of the renin was in the form of trypsin-activatable renin. Total renin levels under baseline conditions ranged from 0.11 to 10.6 μunits per ml of perfusate. To confirm the findings of maternal release of renin and of the range of biological variation in the renin levels, renin was measured in maternal perfusates of another four cotyledons, each from a different placenta. Levels of renin measured were 0.127, 2.33, 1.55 and 10.2 μU per ml. Again, more than 95% of the renin was trypsin-activated.

## DISCUSSION

The prostaglandins $PGE_2$, $PGF_{2\alpha}$, and the thromboxane mimetic U46619 elicited increases in perfusion pressure in the perfused fetoplacental vascular bed. $PGE_2$ exhibited considerable variation in potency between different cotyledons.

Differences in sensitivity to $PGE_2$ between cotyledons may reflect differences in receptor number, perhaps resulting from down-regulation by exposure to $PGE_2$ prior to delivery. The observation that umbilical venous plasma contains higher levels of iPGE than umbilical arterial plasma (Bibby et al., 1979) suggests that exposure to $PGE_2$ could occur. Moreover, the dual-perfused placental cotyledons released 57-170 fmoles of $iPGE_2$ $min^{-1}g^{-1}$ into the fetal perfusate (Howard, et al., unpublished observations).

$PGF_{2\alpha}$ induced dose-related increases in fetal perfusion pressure but was much less potent than U46619. Prostcyclin and $PGE_1$ were potent dose-dependent vasodilators in the fetoplacental vascular bed. The effect of $PGE_1$ is probably of pharmacological rather than physiological significance as prostaglandins of the 1-series are of minor significance in most tissues. Prostacyclin was shown to be a particularly potent depressor agent in the fetoplacental vascular bed. This finding, together with the observation (Howard et al., unpublished observations) that the perfused placental cotyledon releases 6-keto-$PGF_{1\alpha}$, 18 pmoles $min^{-1}g^{-1}$ into the fetal circuit, strongly suggest that endogenous $PGI_2$ could play a role in regulating resistance of the fetoplacental vasculature of term placenta. That thromboxane $A_2$ may also contribute to the regulation is also suggested by the potent dose-dependent pressor effects of the thromboxane $A_2$-mimetic U46619 in the fetoplacental vascular bed.

Pressor effects of AI are believed to be due almost entirely to its conversion to AII by angiotensin converting enzyme (ACE) (Peach, 1977). As AI had similar vasoconstrictor potency to AII in the fetal circuit of the dual-perfused placental cotyledon, AI must be rapidly converted to AII during transit through the fetoplacental vascular bed, indicating also that ACE is present in the fetoplacental vasculature. Captopril, a potent inhibitor of ACE, reduced the pressor response to AI by more than 80%, further supporting the conclusion that the pressor response to AI was due to its conversion to AII by ACE. Moreover, the pressor response to AII was not affected by captopril, indicating that the effect of captopril on the response to AI was not due to a non-specific diminution of vascular smooth muscle responsiveness. In addition, the vascular response to AI substantially recovered after cessation of captopril infusion, in accord with the reversible nature of the inhibition of ACE by captopril (Cushman et al., 1977).

Both AI and AII were similarly and reversibly antagonized by the AII receptor blocker, saralasin, which caused a rightward shift of the log dose-response curve for the pressor response to AII in the fetoplacental vascular bed (Howard et al., 1983). These findings indicate that the cotyledonary vascular bed of the human term placenta contains considerable ACE activity, and ipso facto that AII can be generated within the fetoplacental vascular bed. No fetal release of renin was detected by the perfused cotyledon, suggesting that placental renin may not contribute significantly to formation of AI within the fetal circuit of the placenta in vivo, and that AI in the fetal circuit may be primarily of fetal origin. In contrast, it was demonstrated that renin was released into the maternal circuit of the dual-perfused cotyledon, consistent with the findings of Skinner et al. (1968), who reported on the presence of renin in human placenta. These authors found that the maternal surface of the villous placenta had low concentrations of renin relative to the amount of renin in the fetal membrane (chorion laeve). However, these early studies did not differentiate between active and inactive renin since acid pretreatment was used prior to assay of renin and it is now known that this pretreatment activates an inactive form of renin. Renin in the villous placenta is mostly inactive (Poisner, unpublished observations), and has been localized by immunofluorescence to the cytotrophoblast (Poisner and Wood, unpublished observations). The cytotrophoblast may be the source of renin found in the maternal perfusates, which was shown to be primarily inactive renin. It is unlikely that the release of renin into the maternal circuit has any direct influence on the fetoplacental vasculature in vivo. However, some indirect effect via AII formed within the maternal circuit may be speculated upon, e.g., via prostanoid generation. It remains to be determined if there is conversion of the inactive to active renin in the maternal circuit of the in situ placenta and if the small amount of active renin released on the maternal side of the in vitro placental cotyledon has any physiological significance. The finding in the dual-perfused cotyledon of only small amounts of active renin in maternal perfusates, and the inability to detect any renin in fetal perfusates, do not appear to support an important role for placental renin in local regulation of fetoplacental blood flow, but the question of a contribution by placental renin remains open to further study.

In view of the potent pressor actions of AII and thromboxane (in the form of its mimetic U46619) and the potent depressor actions of prostacyclin, it is tempting to speculate that these substances generated within the fetoplacental vascular bed may contribute to local regulation of fetoplacental vascular resistance. The current studies show that the classic prostaglandins $PGE_2$ and $PGF_{2\alpha}$ are relatively weak vasoconstrictors, suggesting that these arachidonate metabolites may not have an important direct role in modulating resistance. However, other arachidonate metabolites such as leukotrienes may contribute. The placenta was shown to contain 5-lipoxygenase and the 5-lipoxygenase products $LTC_4$ and $LTD_4$ are potent pressor agents in the perfused cotyledon (Kitagawa et al., 1987). Furthermore, autacoids such as adenosine may also be involved in local regulation of fetoplacental vascular resistance. In support of this possibility the human term placenta contains adenosine (Maguire et al., 1986a; Maguire et al., 1986b), which is a pressor agent in the perfused cotyledon (Hosokawa and Maguire, unpublished observations), and the ischemic perfused placental cotyledon releases adenosine into the fetal perfusate concurrently with increase in fetoplacental perfusion pressure (Slegel et al., 1987).

## SUMMARY

Locally produced vasoactive autacoids such as prostanoids may play a role in local modulation of fetoplacental blood flow, or humoral agents such as angiotensin, could be involved. Dual-perfused cotyledons from human term placentae were used to evaluate effects of prostanoids and angiotensins on fetoplacental vascular resistance and to measure placental release of renin. Fetal arterial injections of $PGE_2$, $PGF_{2\alpha}$ and the thromboxane mimetic U46619 elicited reversible increases in fetal perfusion pressure. Pressor responses to $PGF_{2\alpha}$ and U46619 were dose-related. $PGI_2$ and $PGE_1$ elicited reversible dose-related decreases in perfusion pressure. Fetal arterial injections of 1 nmole doses of AI and AII caused similar marked increases in perfusion pressure. The angiotensin-converting enzyme inhibitor captopril at 2.2 $\mu M$ reversibly reduced the AI response to $13.7 \pm 5.2\%$ (mean $\pm$ SEM) of the AII response which was unaffected. Saralasin, an AII receptor blocker, at 94 nM reversibly antagonized both AI- and AII-induced increases in perfusion pressure. No renin was detected in fetal perfusates of 4 cotyledons, but a low level of renin was released into the maternal perfusate. It is concluded that in vivo AII can be generated within the umbilicoplacental circulation from AI of fetal origin, via the action of ACE. Given the potent effects of AII, thromboxane (as U46619) and $PGI_2$ on fetoplacental perfusion pressure, and evidence for their endogenous formation, our findings suggest that these agents may be important in the local regulation of fetoplacental vascular resistance.

## ACKNOWLEDGEMENTS

We wish to thank Dr. C.R. King and the staff of the delivery room of Bell Memorial Hospital for help in obtaining placentae. This work was supported by a National Institutes of Health Grant HD14888.

## REFERENCES

Bibby, J.G., Brunt, J.D., Hodgson, H., Mitchell, M.D. and Anderson, A.B.M. (1974) Prostaglandins in umbilical plasma at elective caesarian section. *Br.J. Obstet. Gynecol.* 86, 282-284.

Broughton Pipkin, F. and Symonds, E.M. (1977) Factors affecting angiotensin II concentrations in the human infant at birth. *Clin. Sci. Mol. Med.* 52, 449-456.

Cushman, D.W., Cheung, H.S., Sabo, E.F., and Ondetti, M.A. (1977) Design of potent competitive inhibitors of angiotensin-converting enzyme. Carboxyalkanoyl and mercaptoalkanoyl amino acids. *Biochem.* 16, 5484-5491.

Earle, W.R. (1943) Production of malignancy in vitro. IV. The mouse fibroblast cultures and changes seen in the living cells. *J. Natl. Canc. Inst.* 4, 165-212.

Granström, E., Dicfalusy, U. and Hamberg, M. (1983) The thromboxanes. In: *Prostaglandins and Related Substances*, (eds)., C. Pace-Asciak and E. Granström, New York: Elsevier, p. 45.

Harper, M.J.K., Khodr, G.S., and Valenzuela, G. (1983) Prostaglandin production by human term placentas in vitro. *Prost. Leuk. Med.* 11, 121-129.

Hosokawa, T., Howard, R.B., and Maguire, M.H. (1985) Conversion of angiotensin I to angiotensin II in the human fetoplacental vascular bed. *Br. J. Pharmacol.* 84, 237-241.

Howard, R.B., Hosokawa, T., and Maguire, M.H. (1983) Effects of drugs and autacoids on human fetoplacental vascular bed. *Fed. Proc.* 42, 468.

Howard, R.B., Hosokawa, T. and Maguire, M.H. (1986) Pressor and depressor actions of prostanoids in the intact human fetoplacental vascular bed. *Pros. Leuk. Med.* 21, 323-330.

Howard, R.B., Levy, J., Hosokawa, T., and Maguire, M.H. (1986) Interrelationships of perfusion parameters in the dual-perfused human placental cotyledon. *Trophoblast Research* 2, 585-596.

Kadowitz, P.G., Lippton, H.L., McNamara, D.B., Wolin, M.S., and Hyman, A.L. (1984) Cardiovascular actions of the prostaglandins. In: *Cardiovascular Pharmacology*. 2nd edition (ed.), M.H. Antonaccio, New York:Raven Press, p. 453.

Kitagawa, H., Howard, R.B., and Maguire, M.H. (1987) Effects of leukotrienes on human fetoplacental vascular resistance in vitro. *Fed. Proc.* 46,1142.

Lumbers, E.R. and Reid, G.C. (1977) Effects of vaginal delivery and caesarian section on plasma renin activity and angiotensin II levels in human umbilical cord blood. *Biol. Neonate* 31, 127-134.

Maguire, M.H., Westermeyer, F.A., and King, C.R. (1986) Measurement of adenosine, inosine and hypoxanthine in human term placenta by reversed-phase high performance liquid chromatography. *J. Chromatog.* 380, 55-66.

Maguire, M.H., Westermeyer, F.A., and King, C.R. (1986) HPLC determination of adenosine, inosine and hypoxanthine levels in human term placenta. In: *Purine and Pyrimidine Metabolism in Man V, Part A*, (eds.), W.L. Nyhan, L.F. Thompson. and R.W.W. Watts, New York:Plenum Publishing Corp, pp. 583-585.

Makila, U-M., Viinikka, L., and Ylikorkala, O. (1984) Increased thromboxane $A_2$ production but normal prostacyclin by the placenta in hypertensive pregnancies. *Prostaglandins* 27, 87-95.

Mitchell, M.D., Kraemer, D.L. and Strickland, D.M. (1982) The human placenta: A major source of prostaglandin $D_2$. *Prost. Leuk. Med.* 8, 383-387.

Peach, M.J. (1977) Renin-angiotensin system: Biochemistry and mechanisms of action. *Physiol. Rev.* 57, 313-370.

Poisner, A., Johnson, R.L., Hanna, G., and Poisner, R.B. (1981a) Activation of renin in human amniotic fluid and placental membranes. In: *Heterogeneity of Renin and Renin-Substrate* (ed.), M. Sambhi, Amsterdam:Elsevier/North Holland, pp. 335-347.

Poisner, A.M. and Poisner, R. (1987) The use of human chorionic membranes and isolated trophoblasts for studying renin secretion. In: *In Vitro Methods for Studying Secretion*, (eds.), A.M. Poisner and J.M. Trifaro, Amsterdam: Elsevier/North Holland (in press).

Poisner, A.M., Wood, G.W., and Poisner, R. (1982) Release of inactive renin from human fetal membranes and isolated trophoblasts. *Clin. Exp. Hypertension* A4, 2007-2017.

Poisner, A.M., Wood, G.W., Poisner, R., and Inagami, T. (1981b) Localization of renin in trophoblasts in human chorion laeve at term pregnancy. *Endocrinol.* 109, 1150-1155.

Schneider, H., Panigel, M., and Dancis, J. (1972) Transfer across the perfused human placenta of antipyrine, sodium, and leucine. *Am. J. Obstet. Gynecol.* 114, 822-828.

Skinner, S.L., Lumbers, E.R., and Symonds, E.M. (1968) Renin concentration in human fetal and maternal tissues. *Am. J. Obstet. Gynecol.* 101, 529-533.

Slegel, P., Kitagawa, H. and Maguire, M.H. (1987) Effect of ischemia on fetal release of adenosine in perfused human placental cotyledons: Measurement of adenosine by fluorescence derivatization and HPLC. *Fed. Proc.* 46, 804.

Symonds, E.M. (1979) The placenta and the renin-angiotensin system. *J. Reprod. Med.* 23, 129-133.

Whittle, B.J.R. and Moncada, S. (1984) Prostacyclin-thromboxane interactions in hemostasis. In: *Cardiovascular Pharmacology*, 2nd edition, (ed.), M.J. Antonaccio, New York:Raven Press, p. 519-534.

# MATERNAL/FETAL
# INTERRELATIONS

Trophoblast Research 3:217-233, 1988

# PLACENTAL VASCULATURE AND CIRCULATION IN PRIMATES

## - A Review -

Elizabeth M. Ramsey[1,3] and Martin W. Donner[2]

[1]Carnegie Institution of Washington
Department of Embryology
Baltimore, Maryland

[2]Department of Radiology and Radiological Science
Johns Hopkins Medical Institutions
Baltimore, Maryland

## INTRODUCTION

When the fertilized primate ovum, whether of human, monkey, baboon, or mangabey, comes to rest on the lining epithelium of the uterus, the trophoblast of its wall promptly begins to invade the endometrium over an ever widening base (Heuser and Streeter, 1941; Enders, 1976; Houston, 1969, 1975; Enders et al., 1983). This usually occurs in the immediate vicinity of a capillary (Figure 1). In the human the whole blastocyst sinks into the endometrial stroma while in nonhuman primates the implantation remains superficial (compare Figures 2 and 3). As the trophoblast encounters maternal capillaries in the course of its penetration of the endometrium it surrounds them, and they thus become one source of the lacunae which appear in the trophoblastic shell. The tissue spaces which develop between trophoblastic cells constitute the second source (Figures 3 and 4). These lacunae enlarge and intercommunicate. Further communication between them and the maternal vascular system is established as progressive trophoblastic invasion erodes maternal vessel walls. Maternal blood in the lacunae, propelled at first only by capillary pressure, moves sluggishly. With deeper penetration of the trophoblast endometrial spiral arteries are tapped. Blood from them enters the lacunae under higher pressure and thus the first stage of placental circulation is established.

Further trophoblastic invasion is in the form of finger-like processes which project from the trophoblastic shell. The chorionic villi develop and rapidly interlace. The spaces between them, replacing the lacunae, become the intervillous space of the placenta (Figure 4). The cores of the chorionic villi are soon replaced by mesoderm contiguous with that which forms the chorion proper, or roof of the placenta (Figure 5). Within this mesoderm, fetal capillaries develop.

[3]To Whom Correspondence Should Be Addressed: 3420 Que Street, NW, Washington, DC 20007 USA

The trophoblast itself, meanwhile, has evolved into a two layered tissue. The layer adjacent to the mesodermal core is the cytotrophoblast, characterized by discrete cells with single, uniformly stained nuclei. The layer outside the cytotrophoblast and lining the intervillous space is the syncytiotrophoblast which lacks cell boundaries and in which the nuclei are multiple and pleomorphic and irregularly stained. Recent work, especially immunohistochemical studies (Kurman et al., 1984), demonstrates a third layer, the intermediate trophoblast, in which the morphology partakes in part of the features of both cyto- and syncytiotrophoblast (Figure 4). The cytotrophoblast can be recognized as the seminal layer, giving rise to the syncytium, which is the secretory layer. The intermediate trophoblast shows transitional stages in the genesis of the syncytium and the maturing of its secretory activity.

By the start of the fourth week all the features of the mature organ are beginning to show (Figure 5): the intervillous space, anchoring and floating villi, mesodermal cores in the villi, fetal vessels in the villi containing fetal blood cells, connection of sprial arteries and venous drainage channels with the intervillous space, and presence of blood in the latter. By the sixth week, these features are fully established (Figure 6). Quantitative changes will, of course, develop as the placenta grows to its maximum size around the end of the first trimester.

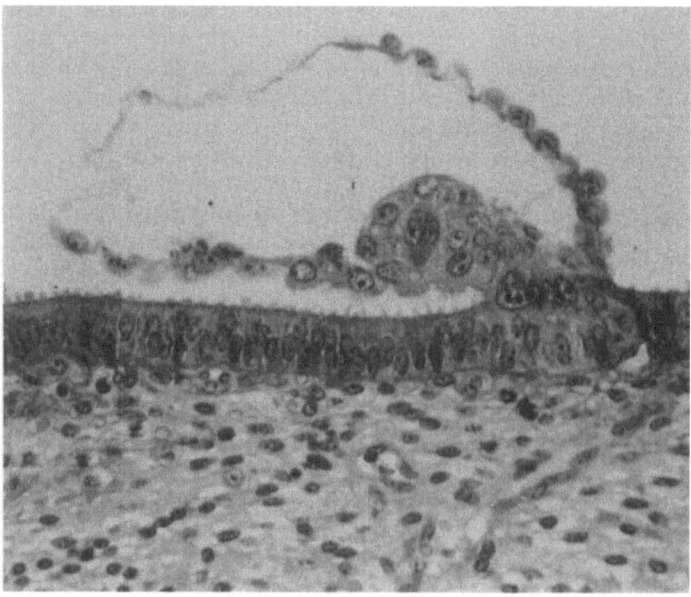

Figure 1. Photograph of a section showing the attachment of a monkey ovum to the endometrium on the 9th day after fertilization. A single trophoblast cell is seen inserting between two endometrial epithelial cells on the right. This is occurring in the immediate vicinity of a maternal capillary. This stage has not yet been seen in the human. Carnegie C-560; 2-4-7.

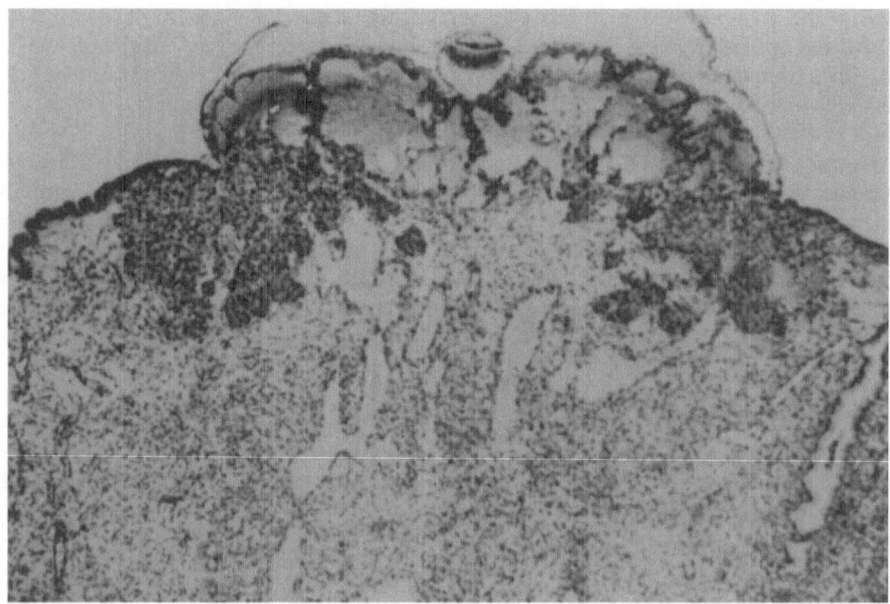

Figure 2.  Photomicrograph showing superficial implantation in rhesus.  Carnegie C-652. 13th day.

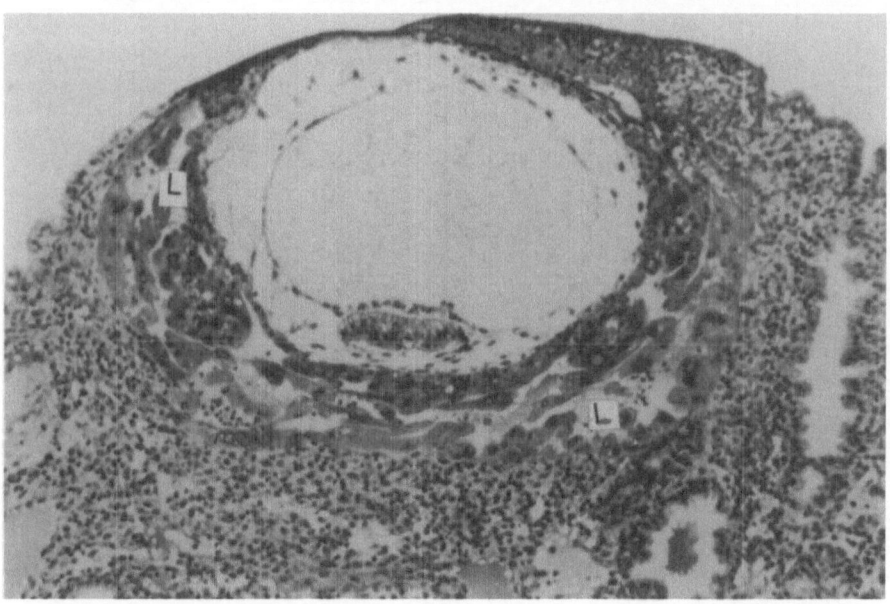

Figure 3.  Section through an implanted human ovum on the 12th day of pregnancy, showing interstitial implantation.  Early proliferation of trophoblast is seen and early forming lacunae.  L = lacunae.  Carnegie #7700.

The mechanisms of uteroplacental circulation may be clearly envisaged by following the progress of a bolus of radiopaque material, into and through the intervillous space, by rapid serial and cineradioangiography (Ramsey et al., 1963). Introduced into the femoral artery of the anesthesized rhesus monkey, the medium enters the aorta and rises to the level of the renal arteries. It returns through the hypogastrics to the uterine arteries. The endometrial spirals are filled, and the medium enters the intervillous space in fountain-like spurts. Figure 7 illustrates this sequence. Venous drainge from the intervillous space cannot be visualized in an arterial injection as the clearance time is so slow that the early arterial filling obscures the later venous stages of the cycle. Rather, the opaque medium is injected directly into the intervillous space by constant infusion pump (Ramsey et al., 1966). It slowly disperses through the intervillous space, and venous drainage channels appear in increasing numbers as the space fills (Figure 7).

The progress of the opaque medium in both arterial and venous injections is impeded or halted by uterine contractions throughout pregnancy, depending upon their strength as determined by continuous monitoring of uterine activity. Compare Figures 8A, 8B, 9A, and 9B.

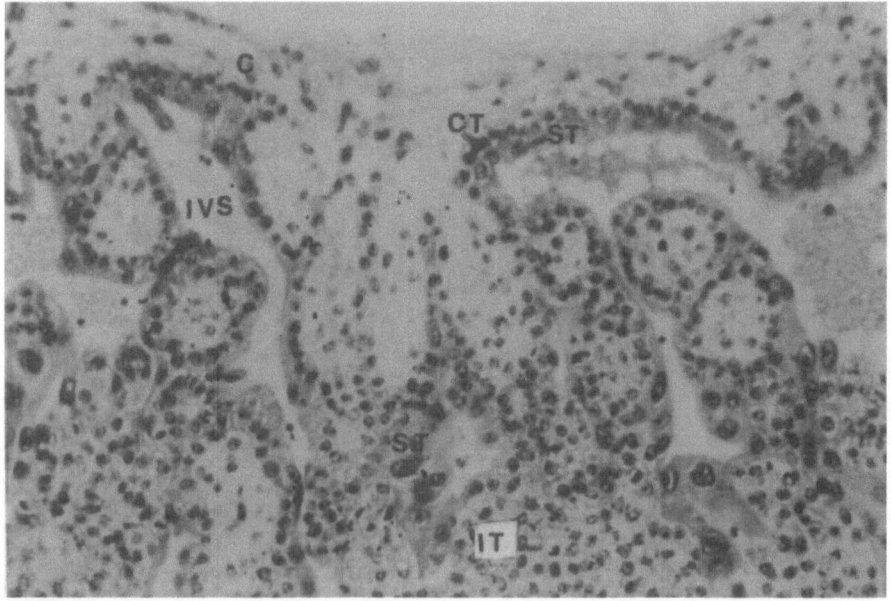

Figure 4. Section of a portion of the wall of the blastocyst of a human ovum on the 16th day of pregnancy showing early ramification of chorionic villi. C = Chorion; CT = Cytotrophoblast; ST = Syncytiotrophoblast; IT = Intermediate Trophoblast; IVS = Intervillous Space. Carnegie #7802.

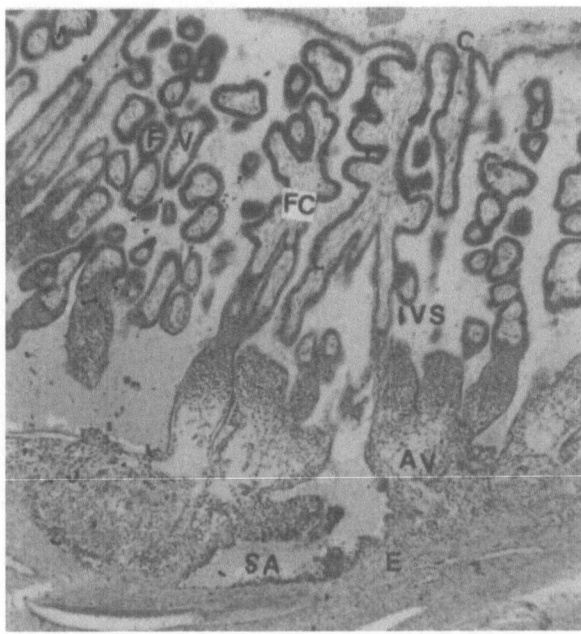

Figure 5. Section of the in situ placenta in a 29 day monkey specimen. E = Endometrium; AV = Anchoring Villi; FV = Floating Villi; FC = Fetal Capillaries; SA = Spiral Artery at point of connection with intervillous space; IVS = Intervillous Space. Carnegie C-477, Section B47.

The course of fetal circulation can be demonstrated by a similar technique (Martin et al., 1966). At laparotomy, the uterus is delivered and incised and a fetal leg brought out. The groin is opened, the femoral artery is exposed and a small polyethylene catheter is inserted. Through this, the opaque medium is injected. It returns to the fetal hypogastric and umbilical arteries rising to the level of the chorionic plate and diffusing into the subchorial vessels. The capillaries of the fetal lobules or cotyledons are filled and appear as cottony puffs (Figure 10A). From the cotyledons blood is drained into the umbilical vein and returned to the fetal circulation. Double injection may be achieved by immediately following a fetal injection with an arterial one (Ramsey et al., 1967). Spurts into the intervillous space occasioned by the arterial injection overlie the fetal cotyledons in the ratio of 1:1 (Figure 10B).

Two important clinical implications emerge from the radioangiographic studies: Firstly, during contractions inflow of oxygenated blood is impeded, resulting in a decreased oxygen supply to the fetus. Should uterine contractions be unduly prolonged or intensified by pathology or oxytocic drugs. This could be of serious consequence to the fetus. Secondly, and mitigating this under normal circumstances, is the fact that the pool of blood within the intervillous space is largely maintained during the contraction, thus assuring continued oxygenation, though at a reduced level.

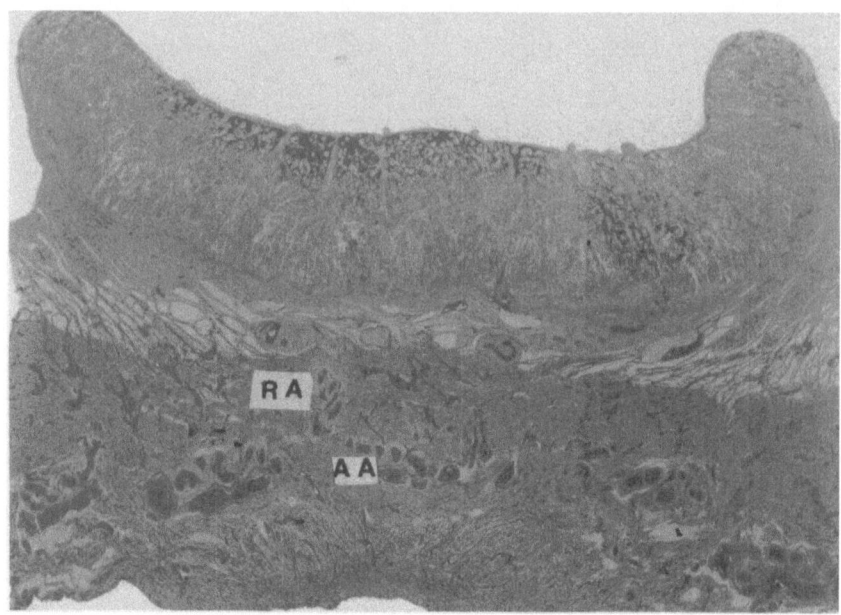

Figure 6. Full cross section of the uterine wall and attached placenta from a monkey on the 28th day of pregnancy. India ink injection in vivo. A spiral artery crosses the endometrium on the right. At its communication with the intervillous space, a spurt of ink rises almost to the subchorial lake. At center, ink from the intervillous space is entering an endometrial vein. The ink in the subchorial lake and that entering the vein are derived from two separate spiral arteries. Note radial (RA) and arcuate (AA) arteries. Carnegie C-658, Section 34.

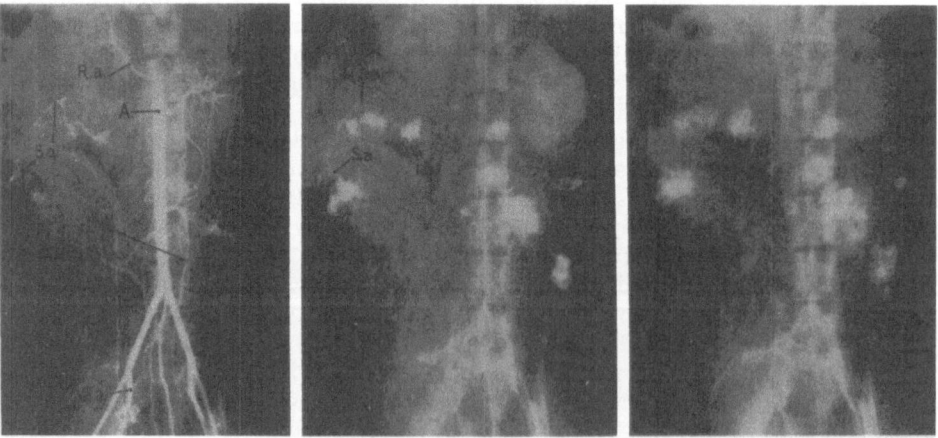

Figure 7. Three of a series of anteroposterior angiograms made at 3 second intervals after injection of contrast medium into the femoral artery of a monkey 100 days pregnant. Spurts of medium appear in both discs of the placenta. A = Aorta; Ra = Renal Artery; Sa = Spiral Artery; Ha = Hypogastric Artery; Ua = Uterine Artery. Arrows point to spurts. Carnegie #60-14.

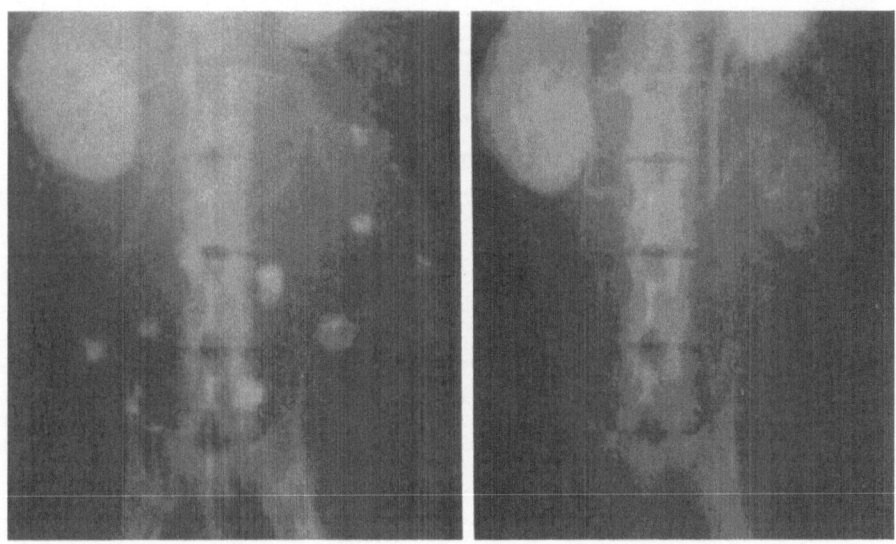

A                                    B

Figure 8A. Radiogram made 10 seconds after injection of contrast material into a maternal fetal artery in a monkey on the 87th day of pregnancy. Injection made during uterine relaxation. Numerous spurts of the medium into the intervillous space are seen. Carnegie #980. 8B). Injection, in the same animal, made during a strong uterine contraction. No spurts are seen.

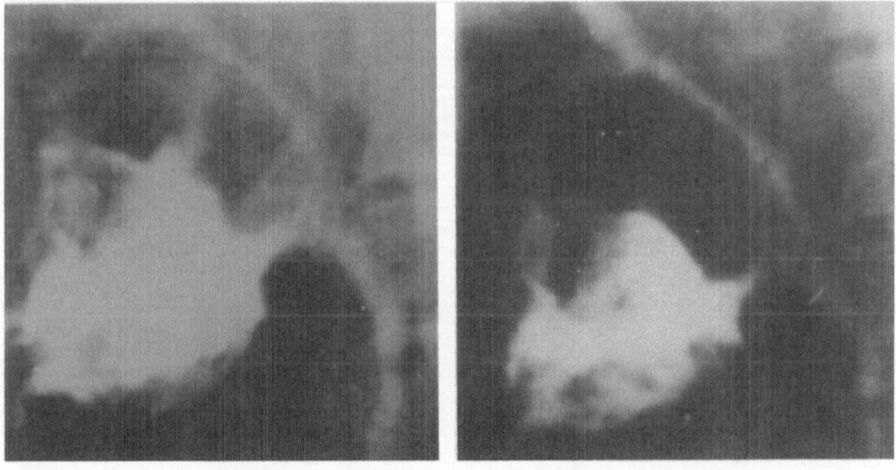

A                                    B

Figure 9A. Radioangiograms made during uterine relaxation immediately at the conclusion of a slow infusion of contrast material into the intervillous space in a monkey on the 99th day of pregnancy. Carnegie #62-29. 9B). Radioangiograms in the same animal made at the peak of the contraction following exposure in Figure 9A. Note disappearance or narrowing of drainage channels. Pool of blood in the intervillous space maintained throughout A and B.

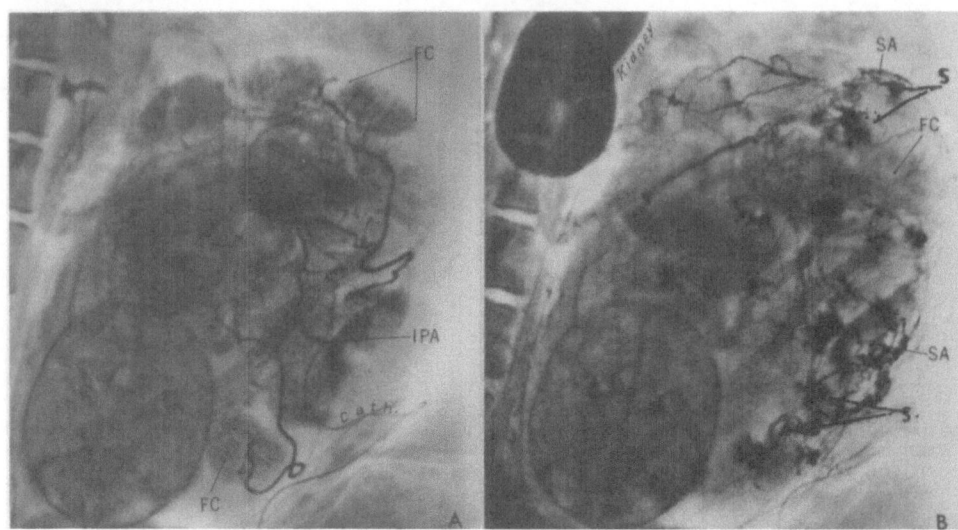

224                                                    **Ramsey and Donner**

Figure 10A. Radiogram made 3 seconds after a fetal injection of contrast material, introduced proximally into a interplacental vessel.  FC = Fetal Cotyledon; IPA = Interplacental Artery.  10B).  Radiogram made 2 seconds after injection of contrast material into the maternal femoral artery of the same animal.  This injection was performed immediately after the fetal injection recorded in 10A.  Maternal spurts overlie fetal cotyledons in the ratio of 1:1.  SA = Spiral Artery; S = Spurts. Carnegie#65-80.  152nd day of pregnancy.

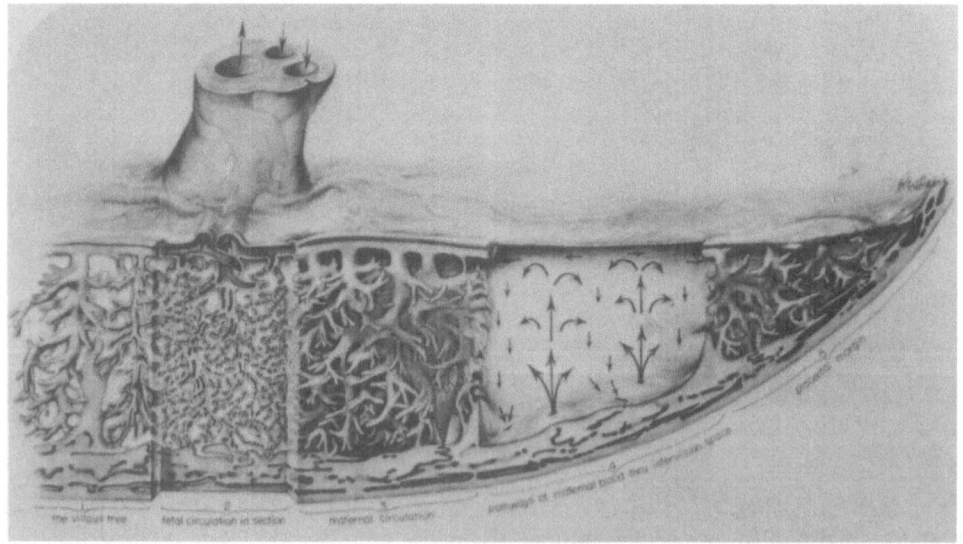

Figure 11.  A composite drawing of the primate placenta showing its structure and circulation.  Drawing by Ranice W. Crosby.  From Carnegie Year Book, 1961-1962.

The foregoing information about placental vasculature and circulation is graphically summarized in the drawing by Ranice Crosby shown in Figure 11. The placental constituents are as follows (Ramsey and Donner, 1980):

Panel 1: *The villous tree*: composed of two sorts of trophoblast and suspended in the intervillous space.
Panel 2: The *fetal arteries and veins* contained within the villi and communicating with the fetus through the two arteries and vein in the umbilical cord.
Panel 3: *Maternal blood* entering the intervillous space from the spiral arteries in fountainlike spurts and drained from it into the endometrial veins.
Panel 4. The *circulatory path* of maternal blood through the intervillous space is portrayed diagrammatically by arrows.
Panel 5. The *margin of the placenta* where the population of chorionic villi is sparse, but inflow and outflow of maternal blood are similar to that elsewhere in the placental base.

Two additional aspects of placental vasculature which have been recognized in the course of recent research must be added to the above basic pattern.

First, the phenomenon of intermittent functioning of the spiral arteries, i.e., the occurrence of intervals in which one or more arteries are constricted and fail to transmit maternal blood to the portions of placenta they supply (Martin et al., 1964). Figures 12 through 14 illustrate this in a monkey on the 123rd day of pregnancy. Figure 12 shows a cross section of the entire uterus with placenta in situ. The characteristic picture of a spiral artery crossing the endometrium is seen at the left. It connects with the intervillous space discharging blood in a spurt which reaches the subchorial lake with minimal lateral dispersion. On the right, a venous channel drains the adjacent portion of the intervillous space. The blood within it comes from an entirely different spurt from that seen on the right which, in its turn, drains into a vein in another part of the placenta. In Figure 13, a section, some millimeters deeper in the same tissue block, its accumulation of blood in the intervillous space on the right and in the endometrial and myometrial veins has come from a different spiral artery. Carnegie C-750. 123rd day of pregnancy.

Second, trophoblastic invasion of the walls and lumina of spiral arteries. This action has been demonstrated (Brosens et al., 1967) and abundantly confirmed by numerous investigators (Sheppard and Bonnar, 1974; Harris and Ramsey, 1966; Pijnenborg et al., 1980; Ramsey and Harris, 1966; Boyd and Hamilton, 1970). Referred to as "the physiological process" it is an entirely normal one, not to be confused with pathological changes such as are seen in hypertension. The contribution of the Carnegie Institution's group has consisted in describing the basic similarity of the process in various of the higher primates plus noting certain species differences among them (Ramsey et al., 1976).

To illustrate other differences between human and nonhuman primates, monkey, baboon, and mangabey are selected as representative of the nonhuman forms. Thus, as shown earlier (Figures 2 and 3), there is a difference in the type of implantation: interstitial in man; superficial in rhesus and baboon.

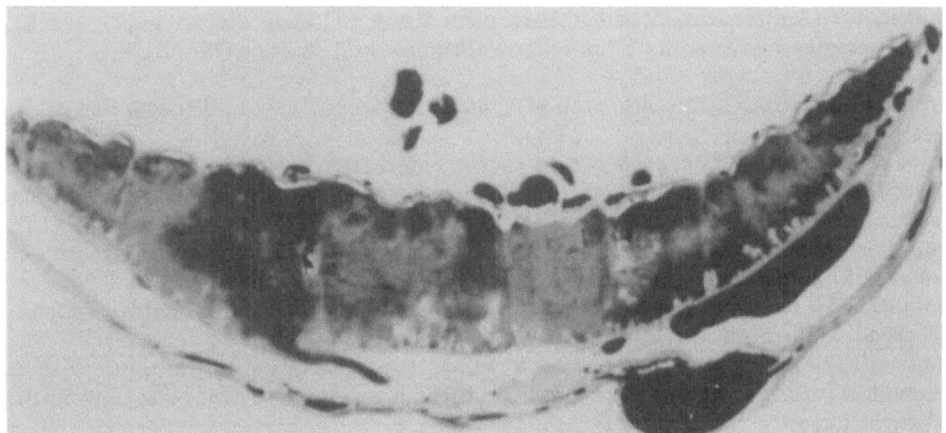

Figure 12. Cross section of a monkey uterus with placenta in situ. Blood is seen entering the intervillous space from a single spiral artery on the left. The fountain-like spurt with minimal lateral diffusion is apparent. The base. Figure 14 shows a section still deeper in the block in which a myometrial coil of the same artery is completely occluded without any obstruction in the lumen. The contraction of the vessel, apparently the result of intrinsic vasoconstriction, accounts for the bloodless area seen in the intervillous space. Radioangiography confirms these constrictions (Figure 15) (Ramsey et al., 1963), which occur at irregular time intervals and in heterogeneous locations in all specimens studied. Such constrictions last for about 12 seconds (Ramsey et al., 1979). It may be noted that these constrictions are continuations of the process occurring in the nonpregnant uterus which are responsible for the ischemia leading to the menstrual slough.

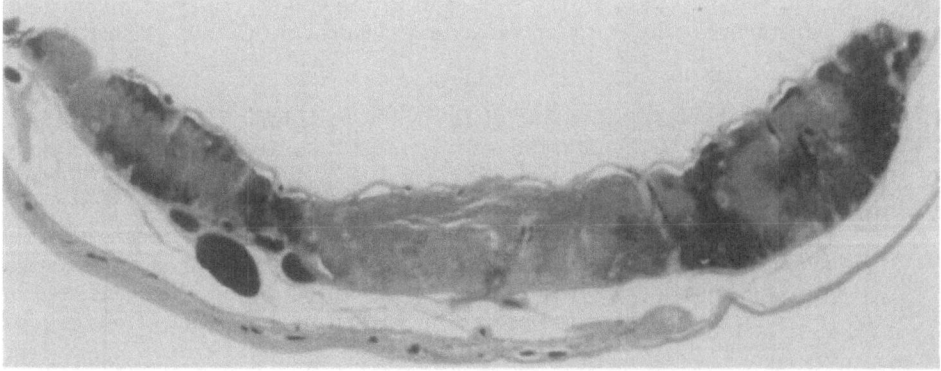

Figure 13. View of another section of the same artery as in Figure 12 some millimeters deeper in the tissue block. There is a bloodless area in the intervillous space. The spiral artery supplying it is patent but bloodless.

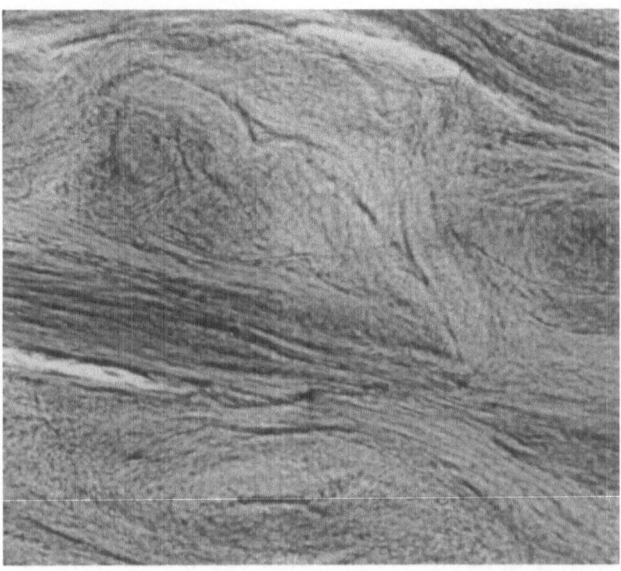

Figure 14. View of a section still deeper in the block of Figure 12. A myometrial coil of the same artery is contracted without any occluding plug. This intrinsic vasocontriction accounts for the bloodless area in the intervillous space.

Figure 16, taken from a human placenta in the 12th week of pregnancy, shows the growth of trophoblast into the lumen of a spiral artery producing an obstructing plug at the artery's point of communication with the intervillous space. From the area of obstruction, the invading trophoblast drips into the adjacent coils of the artery resembling the dripping of wax down the side of a candle. The process extends into the myometrial portion of the artery, deeply in the human but only just beyond the myometrial-endometrial junction in the other primates studied. The subsequent invasion of the vessel wall and replacement of normal muscle and elastic tissue, by trophoblast at first and eventually by fibrosis, is closely similar in all the primates studied (Ramsey et al., 1976). A "secondary wave" of trophoblastic invasion in the human described by Sheppard and Bonnar (1974) and Pijenborg et al. (1980) is not noted in nonhuman primates.

The junction between trophoblast and maternal tissue also varies: it is very irregular in man; smooth in rhesus and baboon. Note that the smooth junction does not constitute an impenetrable barrier. As seen in Figure 6, both arterial and venous connections with the intervillous space pierce it. A further difference lies in the type and extent of trophoblastic invasion. In the nonhuman primates this is restricted to the action upon the arteries, but in the human there is widespread dissemination of wandering trophoblastic giant cells in the decidua and into the myometrium (Figure 17).

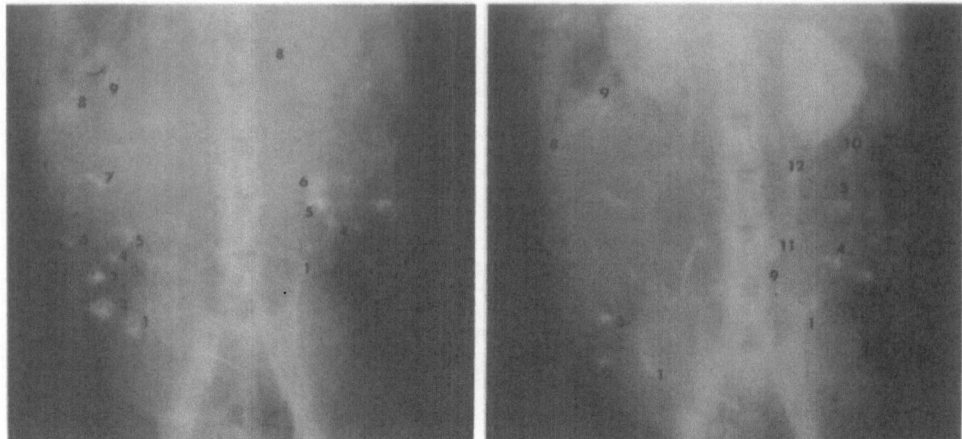

Figure 15.  Photograph of radiograms taken in successive periods of relaxation following injection of contrast material into a maternal femoral artery.  Different arteries are patent in different cycles.  This observation confirms radiologically the condition shown by histological studies in Figures 13 and 14.

Figure 18 shows the effect of the "physiological process" upon the arteries, in diagrammatic representations of the course and configuration of monkey and human uteroplacental arteries at comparable stages of pregnancy.  The changes resulting from replacement of muscle and elastic tissue in the vessel wall are basically the same in the two species qualitatively.  The quantitative differences are occasioned by the differences in myometrial thickness, etc. between them.  Physiologically, the end results are: 1) provision, by the vascular dilatation, of increased volumes of blood for the intervillous space and, 2) decreased pressure of entering blood occasioned both by the dilatation and by the extensive coiling of the arteries.

These examples of variations in trophoblastic activity, even between animals as closely related as the higher primates, buttressed by one or two other circumstances, for example, the lack of choriocarcinoma in nonhuman primates, point to a fundamental and significant difference in what may be called the "invasive potential" of the various sorts of trophoblast.

## ACKNOWLEDGEMENTS

The authors express their appreciation to the following Institutions for their kind permission to reproduce photographs of material in their collections: Carnegie Institution of Washington for Figures 11 and 18; Carnegie Laboratories of Embryology, University of California - Davis for Figures 1 through 6, 12 through 14, and 17; Department of Radiology and Radiological Sciences, Johns Hopkins

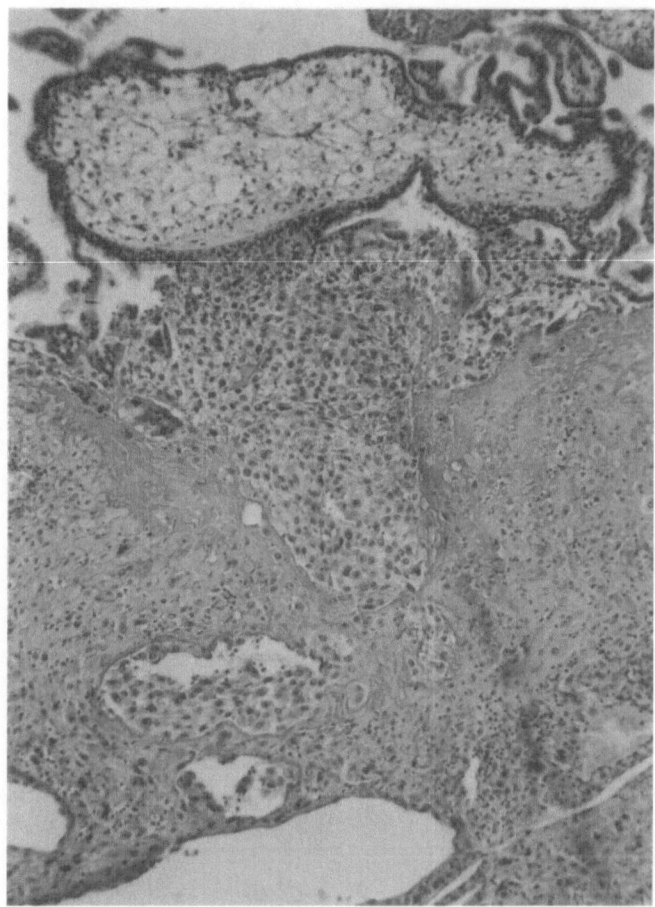

Figure 16. Arterial migration of trophoblast with plug formation in a human placenta. University of Virginia 32-2, 12th week.

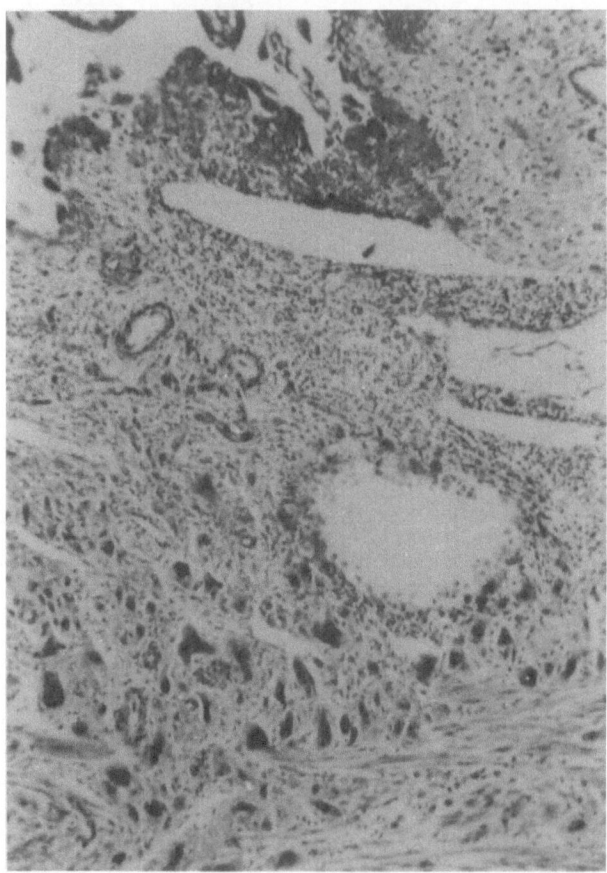

Figure 17.   Invasion of human endometrium by wandering trophoblastic giant cells. Carnegie D104, 17 weeks.

Monkey

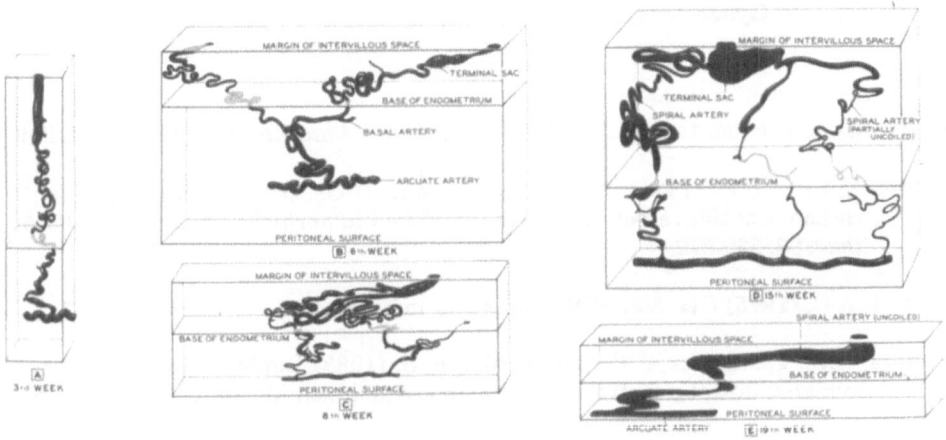

Human

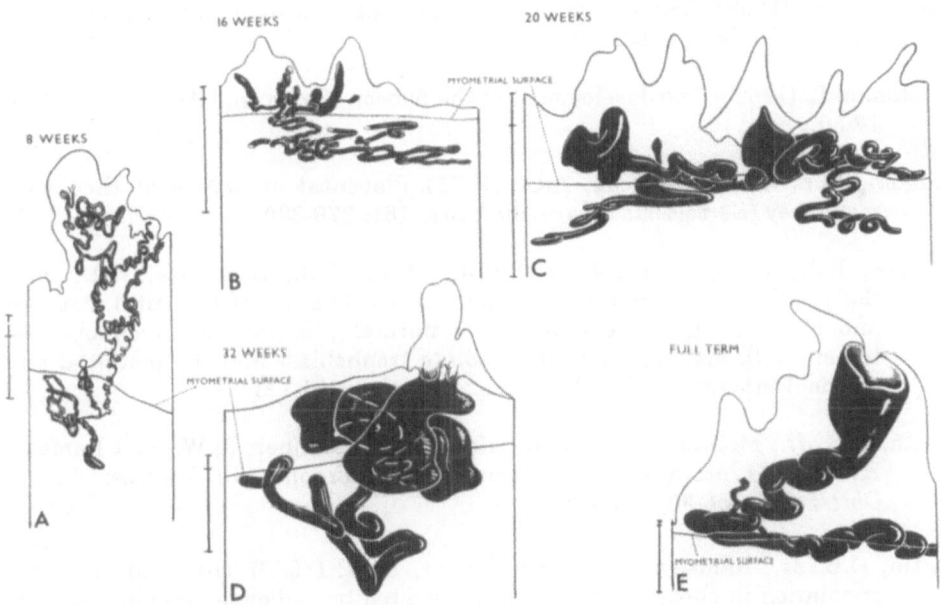

Figure 18. Effect of loss of muscle and elastic tissue in arterial walls as the result of trophoblastic action. Drawings based on graphic, three-dimensional recontructions of injected uteri at comparable stages of pregnancy. The changes are similar in monkey and man, qualitatively. The quantitative differences arise from diversity of myometrial thickness.

Medical Institutions for Figures 7 through 10, and 15, Department of Obstetrics and Gynecology, University of Virginia for Figure 16; Departments of Anatomy and of Obstetrics and Gynecology.

## REFERENCES

Boyd, J.D. and Hamilton, W.J. (1970) *The Human Placenta*, Cambridge, Heffer.

Brosens, I.A., Robertson, W.B., and Dixon, H.G. (1967) The physiological response of the vessels of the placental bed to normal pregnancy. *J. Pathol. Bact.* 93, 569-579.

Enders, A.C. (1976) Cytology of human early implantation. *Res. Reprod.* 8, 1-2.

Enders, A.C., Hendrickx, A.G., and Schlafke, S. (1983) Implantation in the rhesus monkey: initial penetration of endometrium. *Am. J. Anat.* 167, 275-298.

Harris, J.W.S. and Ramsey, E.M. (1966) The morphology of human uteroplacental vasculature. *Carnegie Contrib. Embryol.* 38, 43-58.

Heuser, C.H. and Streeter, G.L. (1941) Development of the macaque embryo. *Carnegie Contrib. Embryol.* 29, 15-55.

Houston, M.L. (1969a) The villous period of placentogenesis in the baboon (Papio sp). *Am. J. Anat.* 126, 1-16.

Houston, M.L. (1969b) The development of the baboon (Papio sp). *Am. J. Anat.* 126, 17-30.

Houston, M.L. and Hendrickx, A.G. (1975) Placental structure of the sooty mangabey (Cercocebus atys). *Anat. Rec.* 181, 379-380.

Kurman, R.J., Young, R.H., Norris, H.J., Main, C.S., Lawrence, W.D., and Sully, R.E. (1984) Immunocytochemical localization of placental lactogen and chorionic gonadotropin in the normal placenta and trophoblastic tumors with emphasis on intermediate trophoblast and the placental site trophoblastic tumor. *Int. J. Gynecol. Pathol.* 3, 101-121.

Martin, C.B. Jr., McGaughey, H.S. Jr., Kaiser, I.H., Donner, M.W., and Ramsey, E.M. (1964) Intermittent functioning of the uteroplacental arteries. *Am. J. Obstet. Gynecol.* 90, 819-823.

Martin, C.B. Jr., Ramsey, E.M., and Donner, M.W. (1966) The fetal placental circulation in rhesus monkeys demonstrated by radioangiography. *Am. J. Obstet. Gynecol.* 95, 943-947.

Pijnenborg, R., Dixon, G., Robertson, W.B., and Brosens, I. (1980) Trophoblastic invasion of human decidua from 8 to 18 weeks of pregnancy. *Placenta* 1, 3-19.

Ramsey, E.M., Chez, R.A., and Doppman, J.L. (1979) Radioangiographic measurement of the internal diameters of the uteroplacental arteries in rhesus monkeys. *Am. J. Obstet. Gynecol.* 135, 247-251.

Ramsey, E.M., Corner, G.W. Jr., and Donner, M.W. (1963) Serial and cineradioangiographic visualization of maternal circulation in the primate (hemochorial) placenta. *Am. J. Obstet. Gynecol.* 86, 213-225.

Ramsey, E.M. and Donner, M.W. (1980) *Placental Vasculature and Circulation*, Stuttgart, Thieme.

Ramsey, E.M. and Harris, J.W.S. (1966) Comparison of uteroplacental vasculature and circulation in the rhesus monkey and man. *Carnegie Contrib. Embryol.* 38, 59-70.

Ramsey, E.M., Houston, M.L., and Harris, J.W.S. (1976) Interactions of the trophoblast and maternal tissues in three closely related primate species. *Am. J. Obstet. Gynecol.* 124, 647-652.

Ramsey, E.M., Martin, C.B. Jr., and Donner, M.W. (1967) Fetal and maternal placental circulations. *Am. J. Obstet. Gynecol.* 98, 419-423.

Ramsey, E.M., Martin, C.B. Jr., McGaughey, H.S. Jr., Kaiser, I.W. and Donner, M.W. (1966) Venous drainge of the placenta in rhesus monkeys: radioangiographic studies. *Am. J. Obstet. Gynecol.* 95, 948-955.

Sheppard, B.L. and Bonnar, J. (1974) The ultrastructure of the arterial supply of the human placenta in early and late pregnancy. *J. Obstet. Gynecol. Br. Cmwlth.* 81, 497-511.

Trophoblast Research 3:235-260, 1988

# COMPARATIVE MORPHOLOGICAL ASPECTS OF PLACENTAL VASCULARIZATION*

Vibeke Dantzer[1], Rudolf Leiser[2], Peter Kaufmann,[3,5]
and Michael Luckhardt[4]

[1]Department of Anatomy
Royal Veterinary and Agricultural University
Bülowsvej 13
Dk 1870 Copenhagen V, Denmark

[2]Institut für Tieranatomie, Universität Bern
Länggassstrasse 120
Ch 3001 Bern, Switzerland

[3]Abt. Anatomie, RWTH Aachen
Melatener Strasse 211
D 5100 Aachen, West Germany

[4]Universitäts-Frauenklinik Hamburg
Martinistrasse 52
D 2000 Hamburg 20, West Germany

## INTRODUCTION

The placental vascular architecture is interesting not only from the morphological point of view, but also as a basis for functional interpretation. The materno-fetal vascular arrangement in the placental exchange areas is one important criterion for the effectiveness of transplacental transport.

The question arises whether materno-fetal vessel arrangements correlate better with neonatal/placental weight ratios than the hitherto used anatomical classification system.

There are very few comparative morphological studies of placental vascularization (Tsutsumi, 1962; Leiser et al., 1984). The disadvantage of most publications dealing with vascular architecture is that they are studies of single species, where different methods and criteria have been used. Thus, they are not comparable. To avoid such problems the same group of investigators studied several species using virtually identical methods. To establish a broad basis for the study species were selected with placentae differing in shape, materno-fetal interdigitation, and composition of the materno-fetal barrier (Table 1). The placentae of the human, the guinea pig, the chinchilla, the rabbit, the tupaia, the cat, the goat, and the pig, were investigated using standard methods, namely semithin serial sections and scanning electron microscopy of vessel casts.

[5]To Whom Correspondence Should Be Addressed
* Dedicated to Professor Theodor Heinrich Schiebler, Würzburg, on the occasion of his 65th birthday.

Table 1

Simplified Morphological Characterization of the Placentae Described in the Present Study

| Species | Placental Shape | Type of Feto-maternal Interdigitation | Placental Barrier | Feto-maternal Blood Flow Interrelations | Neonatal Placental Weight Ratios |
|---|---|---|---|---|---|
| Human | Discoidal | Villous | Hemomonochorial | Multivillous | 6:1 |
| Guinea Pig/Chinchilla | Discoidal | Labyrinthine | Hemomonochorial | Countercurrent | 20:1 |
| Rabbit | Bidiscoidal | Labyrinthine | Hemodichorial | Countercurrent | 6:1 |
| Tupaia | Bidiscoidal | Labyrinthine | Endotheliochorial | Radiate Crosscurrent | 18:1 |
| Cat | Zonary | Lamellar (Complexly Folded) | Endotheliochorial | One-way Crosscurrent | 8:1 |
| Goat/Sheep | Cotyledonary | Villous | Epitheliochorial | Multivillous to Countercurrent | 10:1 |
| Pig | Diffuse | Folded | Epitheliochorial | One-way Crosscurrent | 9:1 |

## MATERIALS AND METHODS

Placentae were studied from 9 humans, 8 guinea pigs (Pirbright-White), 10 chinchillas (Chinchilla laniger), 8 rabbits (different house races), 12 tupaias (Tupaia belangeri), 7 cats (domestic cats), 6 pygmy goats, and 7 domestic pigs (Danish landrace). Semithin sections were prepared following perfusion fixation of either the fetal or the maternal vessel system of the placentae. When possible, perfusion was performed during narcosis of the animal. The exceptions were the humans (freshly delivered placentae) and 3 pigs (immediately after slaughter).

A 2.2% phosphate-buffered glutaraldehyde (360 mosmol, pH 7.3) was used as a fixative for all animals except the pigs, in which 3% glutaraldehyde in the same buffer with 6% polyvinylpyrrolidone (mol wt 40000, 570 mosmol, pH 7.3) was used. Postfixation was done in 1% phosphate or cacodylate buffered $OsO_4$. Following dehydration in a graded series of ethanol, the material was embedded in Epon.

For the preparation of vessel casts, the reader is referred to Leiser and Kohler (1983) and Leiser (1985). The maternal or fetal placental vessels were rinsed with warm (37°C) physiological salt solution containing heparine and phentolamine to remove blood. The preparation was then cooled to 5°C by rinsing with the same solution. As plastic components Batson No. 17® corrosion compound (Polysciences) mixed with Sevriton® (33:12) was used. The injection with cooled and freshly prepared plastic via either maternal or fetal vessel systems was performed as close to the area chosen as possible. In some cases (cat, goat, pig), additional double injections into both fetal and maternal vessel systems were undertaken.

After the start of polymerization, the treated parts of the organs were excised. Final hardening of the plastic was achieved in water baths at 20°C for 0.5 hours, followed by heating to 80°C for 4 hours, remaining at 60°C overnight. The tissue was removed by alternating immersion of the specimens in 40% KOH and in distilled water at 60°C. To obtain suitable pieces for mounting, large pieces of the casts were embedded in 20% warm gelatin (50°C) and frozen to -5°C for cutting with a knife, or frozen in liquid nitrogen for cracking. After thawing, gelatin was removed by a second corrosion procedure. The cleaned and dried specimens were mounted with double tape or conductive carbon cement after Goecke and sputter-coated with gold, before scanning electron microscopy was performed.

## RESULTS

The human placenta is discoidal, villous, and hemomonochorial. Its fetal vascularization has been described elsewhere in this volume (Kaufmann et al., 1987).

The fetal capillaries of the terminal villi are supplied in such a way that 3 to 5 terminal villi are supplied by the same multicoiled capillary loop. The maternal intervillous blood space is not a stagnant pool but exhibits a flow pattern, as indicated by arrows in Figure 1, due to a flow in the tight intervillous space from maternal arteries to maternal veins via openings in the basal plate. The direction of maternal and fetal blood flows is indicated in Figure 1.

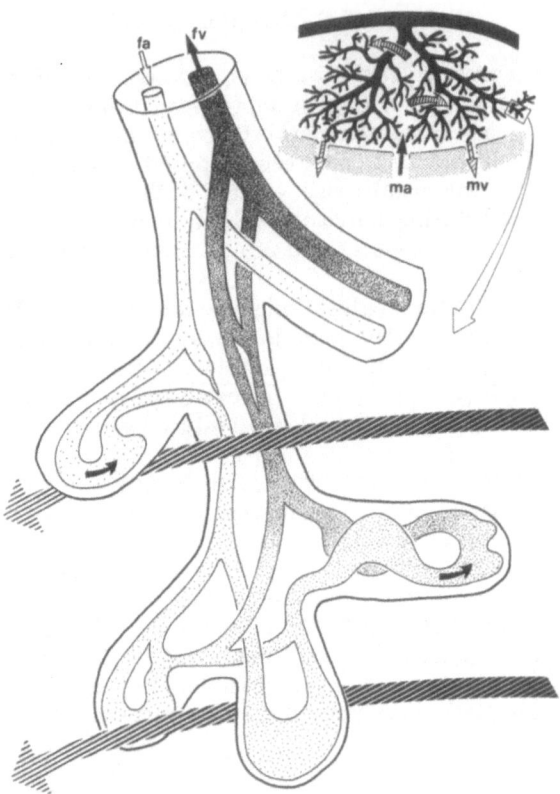

Figure 1. Schematic representation of materno-fetal blood flow relations in the human placenta. The inset demonstrates a vertical section across a single fetal cotyledon. The maternal, i.e., intervillous blood stream is indicated by arrows. Higher magnification of a small group of terminal villi illustrates the arrangement of the fetal capillaries (dotted) as compared with the maternal blood stream (line shaded arrows). Note that the capillary loops of the neighboring terminal villi are arranged mainly in series. Dilated capillary segments, so-called sinusoids, are situated mainly at the top of the villus. This vessel arrangement represents the multivillous condition. ma = maternal artery; mv = maternal vein; fa = fetal artery; fv = fetal vein.

      The guinea pig and the chinchilla placentae are discoidal, labyrinthine, and hemomonochorial. Because there are only minor differences between the vascular architecture and placental structure of the placentas of these two species they will be described together. The placenta is subdivided into several lobules supplied with fetal capillaries and maternal lacunae. A labyrinth is formed at the early stage, when a voluminous bulk of trophoblast is penetrated by channels, which alternately contain maternal blood or fetal capillaries. Each lobule is surrounded by septa, the interlobium, consisting of trophoblast supplied with the maternal lacunae only. The results described below are depicted in schematic drawings in Figures 2A and 2B. The fetal arteries branch at the level of the umbilical cord. The branches give off small arteries running parallel to the interlobar labyrinthine borderline. Along their passage they give off a capillary network, which radiates almost centripetally towards the fetal vein located centrally in the labyrinth of each lobule. The central veins from the individual lobules first are connected by collecting perpendicular veins and subsequentially are connected with the umbilical vein. The maternal arteriolar lacunae can be followed to the centers of the lobules, where they branch into a maternal lacunar network. This network is continuous with several maternal venous lacunae at the periphery of the lobules as indicated in Figure 2B. Thus the fetal capillary blood streams from the periphery of a lobule to the center, and the maternal blood is directed from the central to the peripheral part of the lobules.

The rabbit placenta is bidiscoidal, labyrinthine, and hemodichorial. The placental discs are subdivided into numerous cylindrically shaped lobules. The vascular pattern is depicted in schematic form in Figure 3. The fetal arteries give off branches, which run between the lobules from the fetal (allantoic) to the maternal (uterine) side of the placenta. Here they enter the lobules centrally and continue into a capillary network, which is connected with the fetal venule at the fetal pole of the lobules. The arrangement of the maternal lacunae is almost the same as that of the fetal capillaries. Maternal stem arteries run from the maternal to the fetal side of the placenta between the lobules. At the top of the lobules they branch into an intralobular capillary-like lacunal network which is connected with a maternal venous lacuna at the maternal side. The branching pattern on the arterial side is more regular than on the venous side. The maternal lacunae are located centrally in folds bordered by syncytiotrophoblast and cytotrophoblast, which in turn are surrounded by fetal capillaries and mesenchyme. The maternal lacunar network is thus enclosed by the fetal capillary network. The fetal blood flows from the maternal to the fetal side of an elongated lobule, and the maternal, vice versa, from the fetal to the maternal side.

The tupaia placenta is bidiscoidal, labyrinthine, and endotheliochorial. The two placental discs show a characteristic division into three broadly fused main lobules on the mesometrial side and some very small accessory lobules on the antimesometrial side (Figure 4A, inset). The main branching patterns of the maternal vessels can be seen in a schematic drawing (Figure 4A). The maternal arterioles enter the lobules from the maternal side at its center. About half way towards the fetal side, they continue into capillary networks. At the periphery of the lobules, the networks continue into 7 to 10 venules. Each lobule with one radiate maternal capillary net incorporates 7 to 10 smaller fetal circulatory units. The fetal arteries on the lobular surface branch into about 10 arterioles, which can be followed to the maternal side. During their course, capillaries are given off. These capillaries spread centrifugally or radiate over a short distance to be collected by several fetal venules. The venules collect blood from two to three surrounding fetal circular units, except for the ones at the periphery of the lobules (Figures 4A and 4B). The vascular architecture of the tupaia placenta indicates a maternal blood flow from the center of a lobule to its periphery, exchanging with about 10 fetal units that exhibit the same arrangement but are smaller.

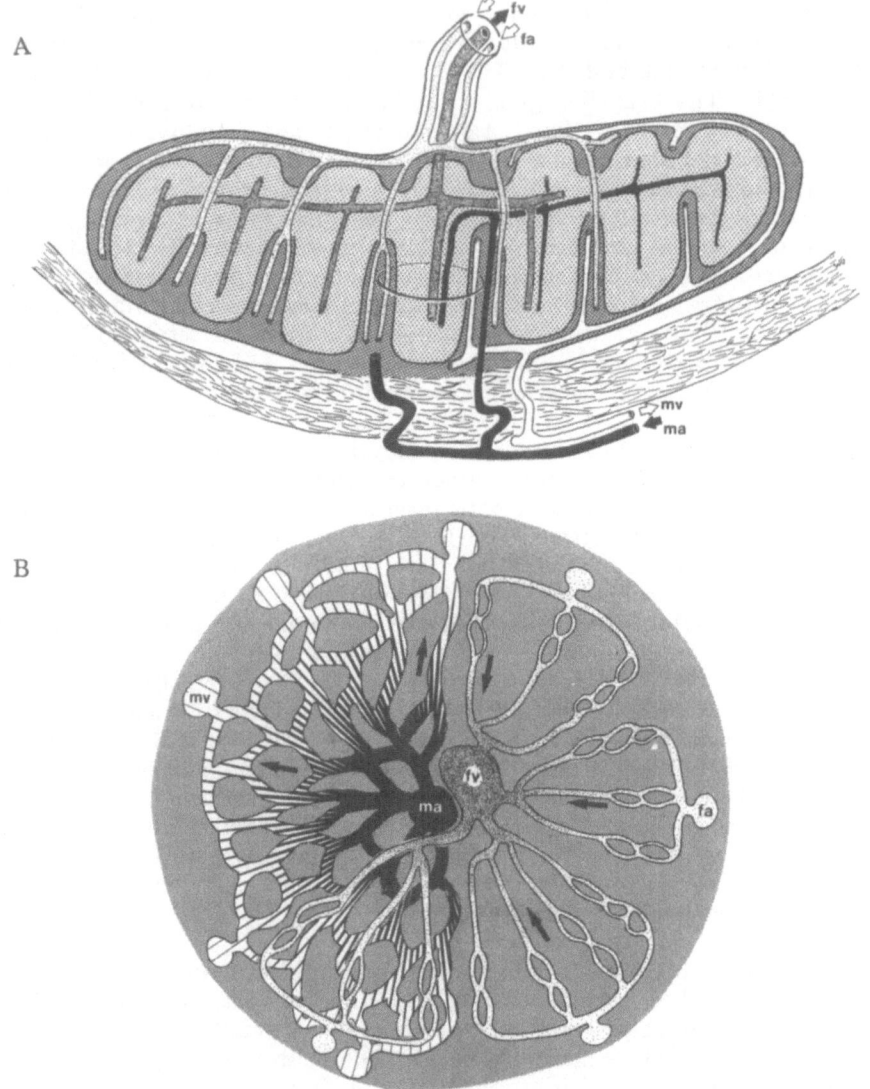

Figure 2. A) Vertical section across the nearly mature guinea pig or chincilla placenta with adjacent parts of the uterine wall (line shading). The organ is composed of cylindrical lobules with maternal and fetal capillaries (light stippling) which are surrounded by the interlobium (dense stippling), which has only maternal lacunae. Whereas maternal arterial lacunae (black) and fetal veins (densely dotted) run together in the center of the lobules, maternal venous lacunae (white) and fetal arteries run into the interlobium parallel to the lobular surface. B) Simplified cross section of one placental lobule. Maternal blood lacunae (line shading, left half) and fetal capillaries (dotted) have a predominantly radial arrangement, the maternal blood flowing centrifugally and the fetal blood flowing centripetally. Thus, the placentae of the guinea pig and the chinchilla provide nearly ideal conditions for countercurrent flow. ma - maternal artery; mv = maternal vein; fa = fetal artery; fv = fetal vein.

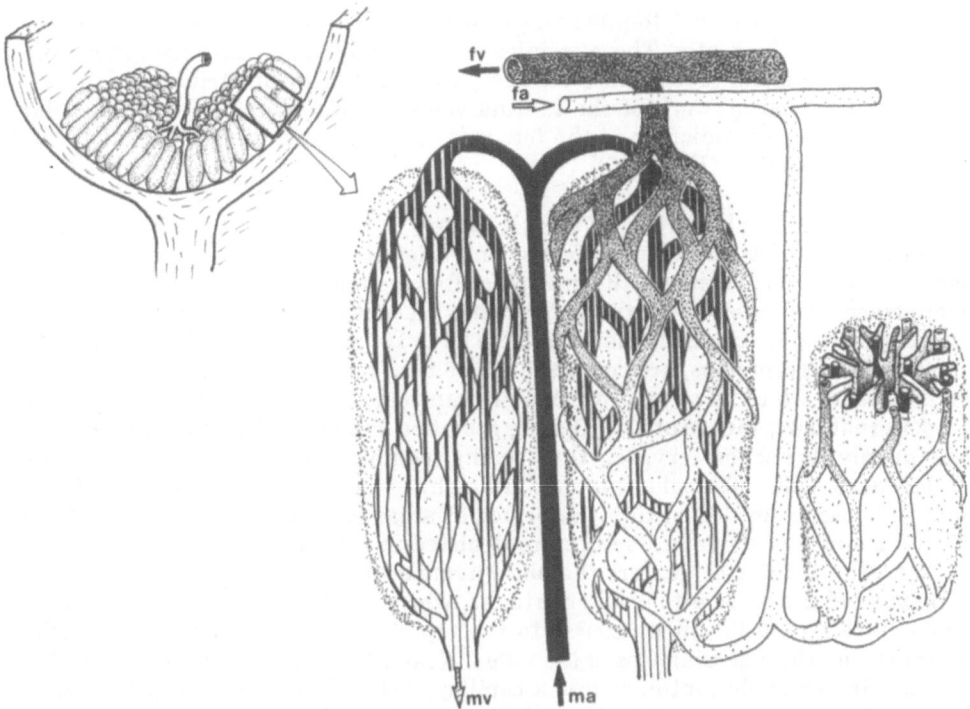

Figure 3. The bidiscoidal placenta of the rabbit (inset) is composed of numerous cylindrical lobules. The maternal lacunae (line shaded) are arranged inside the folded trophoblastic walls of the lobules, the maternal blood flowing in allanto-uterine direction. The fetal capillaries (dotted) surround the maternal capillary network and the folded trophoblastic covering, the fetal blood flowing mainly in utero-allantoic direction. This results in a clearly defined countercurrent flow system. ma = maternal artery; mv = maternal vein; fa = fetal artery; fv = fetal vein.

The cat placenta is zonary, lamellar or complexly folded, and endotheliochorial. On the fetal side of the allantochorionic placenta the branches from both umbilical arteries and veins follow a course parallel to the placental girdle. They join the double-layered fetal capillary network on different locations along the chorionic lamellae which generally exhibit a chorio-uterine orientation. On the maternal side this capillary network forms peduncular or tuft-like endings of capillary loops. The fetal venules arise from different levels of the capillary network inside the lamellar system. The vascular arrangement related to placental shape and interdigitation is illustrated in schematic form in Figure 5. On the maternal side the placenta is supplied by stem arteries, each crossing the myometrial and placental layers straight and branching several times before forming a funnel-shaped area on the fetal side of the placenta (cf. Leiser and Kohler, 1983). Arterioles ramifying from this system enter the maternal capillary network of the septa, parallel to the chorionic lamellae. These septa grow progressively complex in shape during pregnancy. The maternal capillary network is oriented in a feto-maternal direction as the venules originate on the maternal side of the septa. These venules continue into stem veins connected with the deep endometrial layers with venous plexus in the myometrium and finally join the superficial network of the uterine veins. The flow in the fetal vascular configuration is perpendicular to the feto-maternal direction seen in the maternal vascular organization (Figure 5).

The goat placenta is cotyledonary or multiplex, villous, and epitheliochorial. Because shape, type of interdigitation, and barrier of the sheep placenta are similar to that of the goat placenta, one may assume that the vascular arrangement, as observed in the pygmy goat placenta, is similar to the vascular interrelationship in the sheep placenta. The 80 to 100 materno-fetal placental units, the so-called placentomes, are composed of the fetal part, the chorion frondosum or the cotyledon, which is an aggregation of branched fetally vascularized villi, and the maternal part, the caruncle. During gestation the caruncles grow and develop into deeply branched crypts, thus being complementary to the opposing cotyledonary villi. The placentomes are richly vascularized by both fetal and maternal vessels and constitute the principal areas of placental exchange. Their structure and vascular architecture are depicted in schematic form in Figures 6A and 6B. The fetal artery enters the placentome at its central depression from the fetal side and branches into smaller arteries, which are located in the center of the fetal villi (Figure 6B). In its course to the top of the villus it may send smaller arterioles into the side branches of the villus. Near the villous tip or at the end of its branches the arteriole continues into a capillary network, which via capillary loops provides the entire villus with a capillary network. At the base of the villus the capillary network continues into fetal venules. The maternal arteriole follows a course through the septa lining and the caruncular crypts towards the top of the septa. Here, at the fetal side of the caruncle, it branches into a capillary network following the irregular contours of the branched maternal crypts to the maternal side, where the network converges into maternal veins of the caruncular stalk.

---

Figure 4. A) The placenta of the tupaia is bidiscoidal, each disc consisting of three larger lobules (inset). A vertical section across two lobules according to the inset illustrates the maternal vessel arrangement (left lobule) as well as the fetal vessel arrangement (right lobule). Several radially arranged fetal circulatory units are incorporated into one radially arranged maternal circulatory unit occupying the entire lobule. B) The horizontal section (maternal vessels depicted in the left half, fetal ones in the right half) across one single lobule reveals very complex materno-fetal vessel interrelations corresponding mainly to a one-way crosscurrent system, which is completed locally by vessels arranged following concurrent or even countercurrent conditions. This unusual situation is summarized as a radiate crosscurrent system. ma = maternal artery; mv = maternal vein; fa = fetal artery; fv = fetal vein.

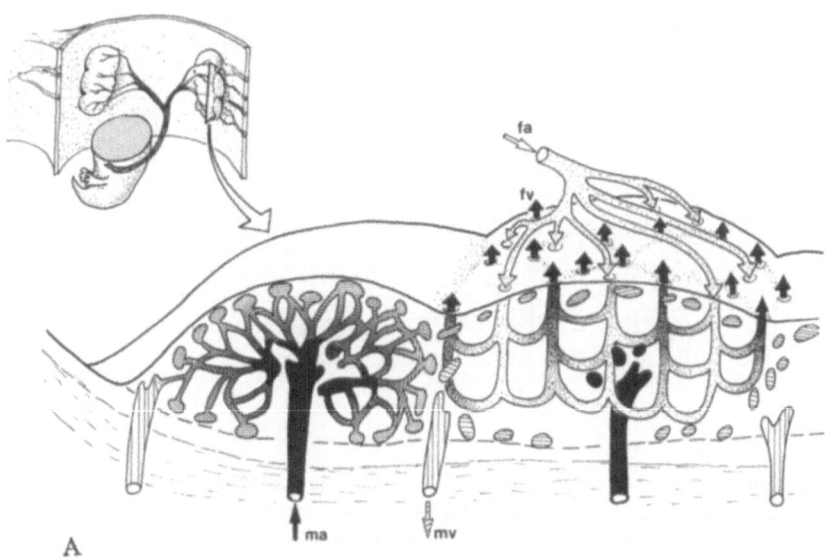

A

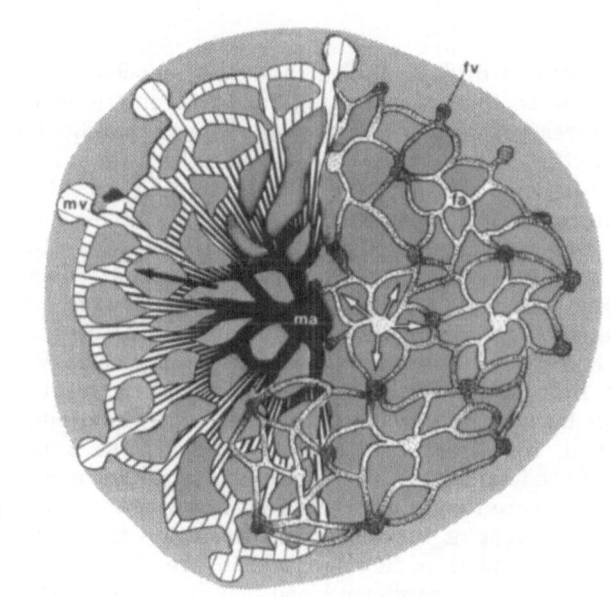

B

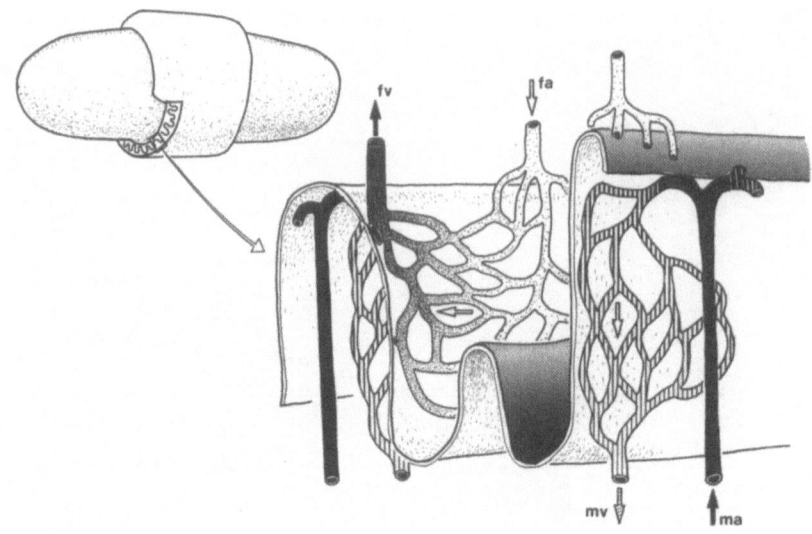

Figure 5. The zonary, lamellar placenta of the cat is composed of adjacent two-dimensional maternal or septal (line shading) and fetal or chorionic (point shading) capillary networks which are separated from each other by a folded trophoblastic lamella. The capillary networks are arranged in such a way that the blood flow within the fetal capillaries largely crosses that in the maternal capillaries at a right angle. This can be summarized as an one-way crosscurrent system. ma = maternal artery; mv = maternal vein; fa = fetal artery; fv = fetal vein.

The pig placenta is diffuse, folded, and epitheliochorial. The circular macroscopic folds of the endometrium are provided with microscopic folds, rugae, going in the same direction. During gestation short perpendicular folds arise, thereby subdividing the maternal fossae between the rugae into a series of continuous basket-like structures. The closely related fetal side shows a complimentary pattern, which, in the late stages, appears as rows of bulbous protrusions fitting into the complementary maternal "baskets" (Dantzer, 1984). This configuration and the vascular architecture depicted in schematic drawings (Figures 7A and 7B). The fetal arterioles enter the fetal rugae or bulbous pro-trusions on the fetal side, giving off branches during their course to the maternal side. At the top of the rugae, they continue into the capillary network. The capillary network converges into fetal venules at the sides of the fetal fossae. This arrangement evolves because the fetal fossae are lined by columnar trophoblast, not having a so-called "intraepithelial" capillary network, as is the case at the sides and at the top of the fetal rugae. The maternal arterioles can be followed to the top of maternal rugae, where they branch and continue into the maternal capillary network; the latter converges at the maternal fossae into the maternal venules. The maternal capillary blood thus flows mainly in the chorio-uterine direction. The reverse is valid for the fetal capillary blood flow. However, due to the arterial side branches to the capillary network during their course to the top of fetal and maternal rugae, respectively, maternal and fetal blood flow partly cross each other.

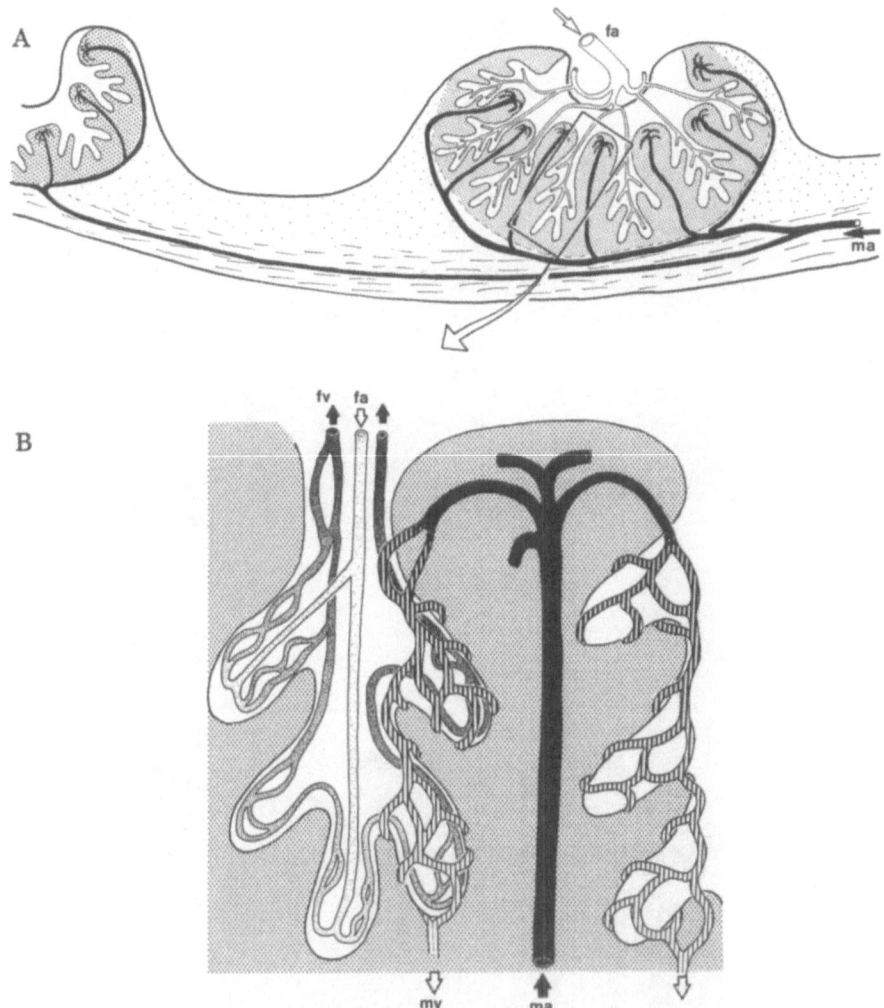

Figure 6. A) Each single cotyledon of the goat placenta consists of numerous fetal villi dipping into crypts formed by the maternal tissue (dotted). The course of the fetal (white) as well as the maternal (black) arteries and arterioles is indicated. B) Higher magnification of two of the fetal villi reveals a fetal vessel arrangement that roughly resembles that of the villous human placenta. However, most of the capillary loops are asymmetrically arranged with a shorter, more centrally positioned arterial capillary limb and longer superficial venous capillary limb. The fetal villi are surrounded by basket-like maternal capillaries (line shading), which on average exhibit a vertical, i.e., amnio-uterine, direction of blood flow. Anatomically the decision cannot be made whether this should be called a multivillous flow system with a certain countercurrent component or a random blood flow. ma = maternal artery; mv = maternal vein; fa = fetal artery; fv = fetal vein.

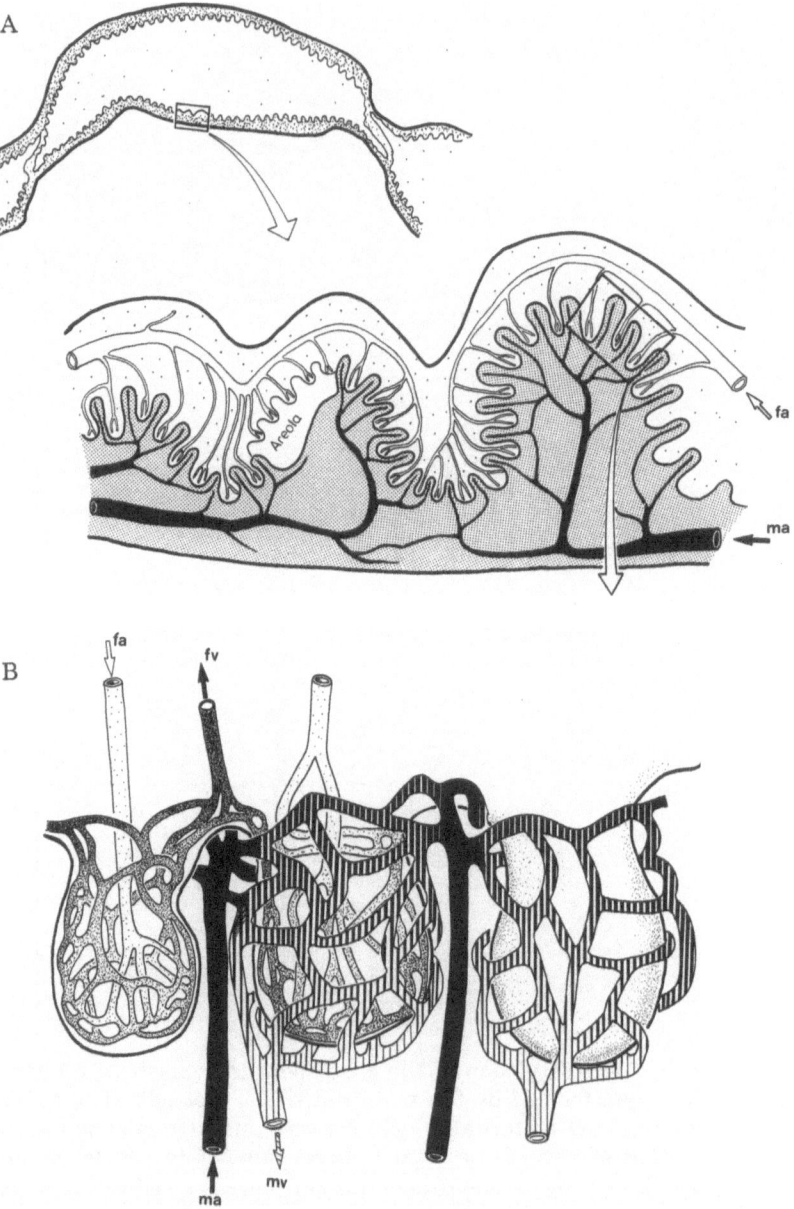

Figure 7. A) The diffuse, folded placenta of the pig (inset) displays greatly interdigitating maternal and fetal vessel systems arranged in larger macroscopic and smaller microscopic folds. B) Such microscopic folds, or rugae, seen at higher magnification consist of a bulbous fetal capillary net (dotted) inside a trophoblastic bulbous protrusion (left side), surrounded by a basket-like maternal capillary net (middle and right side), the maternal capillaries mainly crossing the fetal ones. On the basis of length and direction of the single capillary segment, this roughly resembles a one-way crosscurrent system. ma = maternal artery; mv = maternal vein; fa = fetal artery; fv = fetal vein.

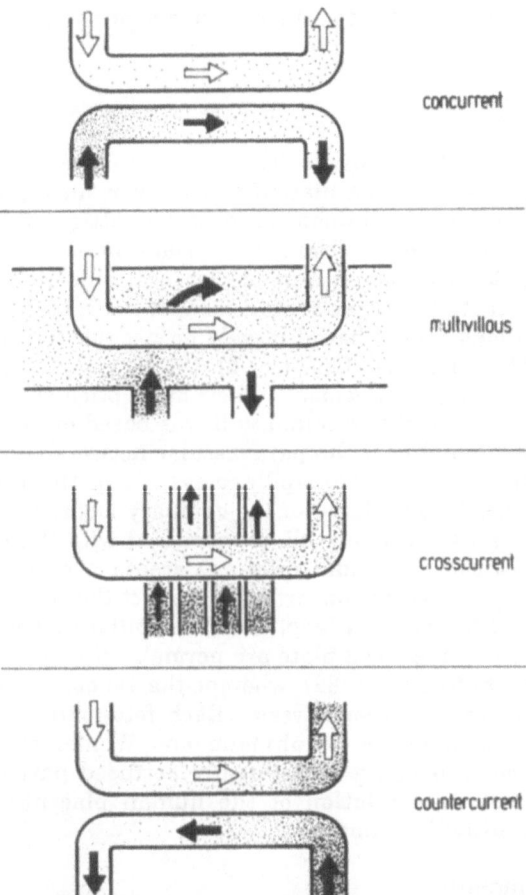

Figure 8. Idealized arrangement of the fetal (white arrows) and maternal (black arrows) blood stream of different types of exchange according to Moll (1972), Faber (1977), and Martin (1981). The density of dots in the venous limb of the fetal vessel loop (upper right) illustrates the efficiency of the various exchangers in diffusional exchange.


## DISCUSSION

For many years it has been recognized that the anatomical arrangement of placental vascular pathways differs from species to species, and that these different interrelations affect the efficiency of placental exchange. Physiologists have therefore proposed theoretical models of exchange systems (Figure 8) and calculated the relative efficiency of transfer of readily diffusible inert substances (Bartels and Moll, 1964; Faber, 1969, 1977; Moll, 1972; Martin, 1981; Schröder, 1982). The blood flow principles - multivillous (human, goat), countercurrent (rabbit, guinea pig), and several modifications of the one-way crosscurrent flow (cat, tupaia, pig) - are represented in the placentae studied (Table 1 and Figure 9).

However, no anatomical evidence for the concurrent or the pool flow interrelation have been observed.

## The Human

The fundamental studies by Boe (1953, 1969) and Arts (1961) clarified the fetal vascularization of the human placenta. However, during the last few years the fetal vascularization of the human placenta has attracted renewed attention (Thiriot and Panigel, 1978; Goyri O'Neill, 1983; Habashi et al., 1983; Lee and Yeh, 1983). According to classification of human placental villi (Kaufmann et al. 1979; Sen et al., 1979) further studies of the arrangement of the vessels were needed, as the subdivision of the villous tree is based largely on pecularities of the fetal vessels (cf. Kaufmann, 1985). Therefore, Leiser et al. (1985) and Kaufmann et al. (1985) reinvestigated the vascular arrangement. Their description of the stem villi, of the mature intermediate, and of the terminal villi was based on the same methods as were used here. They found that the paravascular network (Boe, 1953, 1969) has very few communications with the capillary system of the terminal villi. The determination of sinusoids, as related to the capillary loops, one of which provides the capillary system of 3-4 terminal villi, is consistent with the theory of Boyd and Hamilton (1970) that the sinusoidal dilations create a reduction in blood flow resistance. This theory is further supported by the fact that the extent of sinusoidal dilations multiplies with increased length of the capillary loops. On the maternal side, the arterial inlets in the basal plate are normally situated close to the centers of the villous trees (Schuhmann, 1982), whereas the venous openings are arranged around the periphery of the villous trees. Each feto-maternal circulatory unit, which is called a placentone by Schuhmann and Wehler (1971), consists of a villous tree with a corresponding centrifugally perfused part of the intervillous space. The blood flow interrelation of the human placenta can therefore be characterized as a multivillous flow.

## Guinea Pig and Chinchilla

The vascular arrangement in the guinea pig placenta has been described in detail by light and electron microscopy (Fischer, 1968; Kaufmann, 1969; Bailey, 1974; Kaufmann and Davidoff, 1977; Kaufmann, 1981 a,b). From these observations it was concluded that the labyrinthine placenta of the guinea pig has a nearly ideal countercurrent blood flow system although earlier anatomical and physiological considerations (Mueller and Fischer, 1968) have suggested a less efficient blood flow system, i.e., a "multi-capillary flow". The results of physiological experiments are largely in agreement with our views. Martin (1981) concluded from the investigations of Schröder and Leichtweiss (1977) that the blood flow in the guinea pig placenta showed a countercurrent blood flow. This has been stated by Moll and Kastendieck (1977) also. In their monograph on placental physiology, Faber and Thornburg (1983) came to the conclusion that the physiological and anatomical evidence agree on a countercurrent pattern of exchange. The present results confirm this statement. On the other hand, Schröder (1982) concluded, using reversed fetal blood flow, that there was a non-ideal countercurrent exchanger. This discrepancy may be due in part to biological variety and to arterio-venous shunts between fetal interlobar arteries and collecting veins (Kaufmann and Davidoff, 1977).

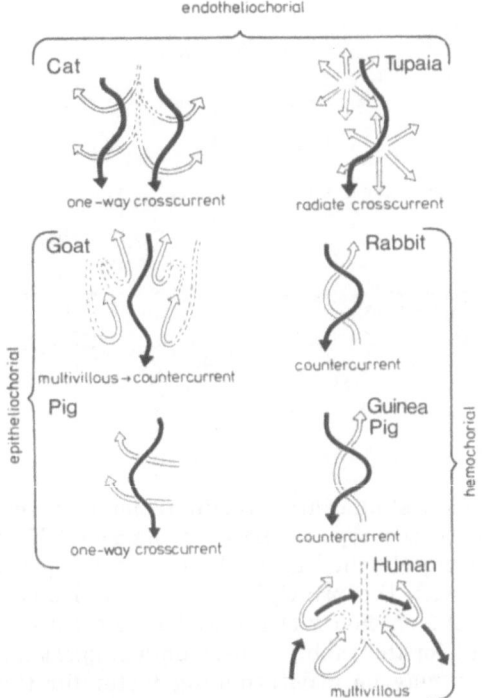

Figure 9. Synoptic representation of the vessel arrangement in 7 different types of placentae. The dotted parts of the arrows represent those arteriolar segments of the vessel loops participating in materno-fetal exchange to a lesser extent. Maternal blood flow = black arrows. Fetal blood flow = point-shaded arrows.

## Rabbit

In his classical study of the rabbit placenta, Mossman (1926) used pigmented gelatin to clarify the vessel arrangement. Based on these studies the vascular interrelation has been described as countercurrent. Tsutsumi (1962) using neopren latex and ink to study the vascular pattern of this organ has confirmed Mossman's results. The studies of the maternal vasculature of the rabbit placenta by Carter (1975), using angiographic techniques, resulted in only minor modifications of the original diagram from Mossman. Our plastic vessel casts studied by scanning electron microscopy have led us to the same basic conclusions. However, concerning the vascular arrangement inside the lobules there is some discrepancy. It has been assumed by Mossman (1926) that the maternal blood lacunae surround the fetal capillary network, whereas from our studies it becomes evident that the fetal capillary network is surrounding the maternal lacunar network (Figure 3). This difference probably is important only from the morphological point of view since it clarifies the three dimensional arrangement of both vessel systems. Physiologically it may be unimportant. Physiological experiments, too, show a countercurrent flow system in the rabbit (Barron and Battaglia, 1955; Faber and Hart, 1966; Bartels et al., 1967). The anatomical and physiological observations are therefore in good agreement.

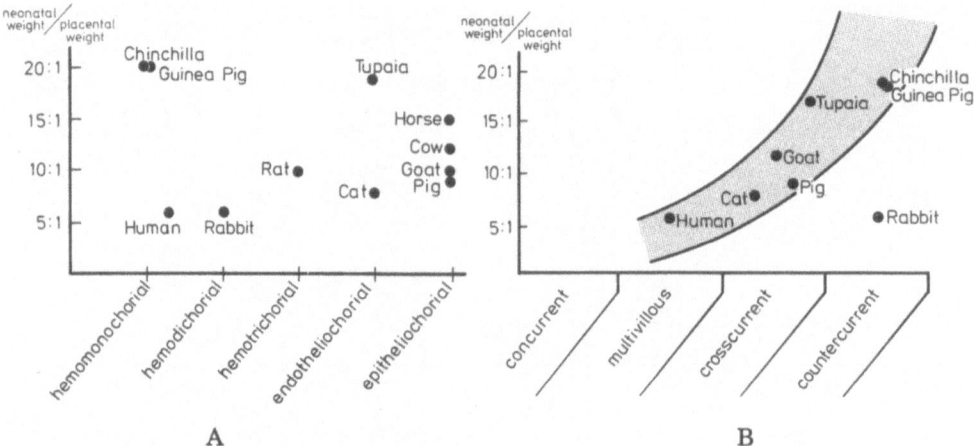

Figure 10. A) The neonatal/placental weight ratios at term of different species show no correlation with the type of placental barrier. Neonatal and placental weights following own unpublished data. B) If comparing the neonatal/placental weight ratios at term with the principle feto-maternal blood flow interrelations arranged according to the efficiency of the exchange system, a certain correlation becomes evident, except for the rabbit. These data suggest that placental capacity for diffusional transfer may be a determining factor for the neonatal/placental weight ratio.

## Tupaia

The vascularization of the tupaia placenta has recently been studied by Luckhardt et al. (1985). These authors discussed in detail the discrepancy with an earlier investigation by Luckett (1968), who concluded from his observations of intraplacental vascular arrangement that the tupaia has a countercurrent exchange pattern. From the investigation by Luckhardt et al. (1985), using almost the same methods as in the current comparative study, it was demonstrated that the flow interrelation could not be countercurrent; on the basis of the anatomy of feto-maternal vessel interrelation it was suggested that the tupaia placenta exhibited a kind of one-way crosscurrent system as the dominating feature. This reinvestigation of the vessel architecture of the tupaia placenta has confirmed that view. However, a more descriptive expression is suggested, namely radiate crosscurrent type of feto-maternal blood flow. Correlative physiological experiments are still missing.

## Cat

Some features of maternal vessels, such as their location in the tissue, luminal shape, and the type of endothelium, as well as the differences from fetal chorioallantoic vessels on histological sections have been previously described (Amoroso, 1952; Bjoerkman, 1970; Malassine, 1974). The vascular architecture on the maternal side (Leiser and Kohler, 1983) as well as on the fetal side (Leiser and

Kohler, 1984) of the zonary cat placenta have been studied in detail recently. These investigations are part of our comparative study, supplemented by double injections of maternal and fetal vessels in the same cast preparation. The general organization is that the maternal blood pathway has a distinct allantochorionic-uterine direction, via a two-dimensional capillary network within the septa of the feline placenta. The fetal blood flow in the capillary network of the chorionic lamellae can be described as more or less horizontally crossing the maternal blood flow. Therefore, it is concluded that the predominant blood flow interrelation is of the one-way crosscurrent type. The interhemal membrane surface in the lamellar zone increases during gestation. The lamellae become even more densely packed towards the end of pregnancy (Malassine, 1974). This situation may increase the efficiency of the system when the fetal demand is high. For further details see Leiser and Kohler (1983, 1984).

### Goat

Based on anatomical studies several theories of the blood flow interrelation in the cotyledonary villous sheep placenta have been suggested. Barcroft and Barron (1946) found that the fetal capillary blood flows from the tip to the base of the villus, whereas the maternal capillary blood pursued an opposite direction, thus performing a countercurrent exchange system. This could not be confirmed by physiological experiments using reverse direction of fetal blood flow (Metcalfe et al., 1965). Steven (1966) considered the mean direction of flow in the fetal capillaries to be at right angles to the long axis of the villi, thus giving a crosscurrent flow interrelation. This conclusion was also drawn by Makowski (1968) but based on the opposite anatomical situation, namely a fetal blood flow parallel to the long axis of the villi and the maternal blood at right angles to it. Referring to this controversy Carter (1975) suggested that the maternal and fetal capillaries are more or less randomly arranged, thereby explaining why a reverse fetal blood flow would give no change in overall efficiency. Tsutsumi (1962) described the vascular arrangement in the placentomes of the sheep and found that it was quite different from that seen in the cow, whereas it was comparable to the vascular arrangement in the microplacentomes of the diffuse placenta of the horse. The current results derived from vascular casts from the placentomes of the pygmy goat of fetal, maternal, and combined preparations supplemented by serial sections have provided new aspects of this topic since the vascular pattern of the goat placenta is similar to that of the sheep (Makowski, 1968). Fetal arterioles were found to supply the small villous trees. The capillaries branch off, near the top of the villous trees, forming loops following the surface of the branched villi towards the basis of the villous trees. Thus the configuration is comparable to the vascular arrangement in the distal part of the villous tree of the human placenta. The maternal arterioles located in the septa separating the crypts of the caruncle can be followed to its fetal side, where they continue into the capillary network, the latter underlying the surfaces of the branched crypts. This network converges into veins on the maternal side. Therefore, it is suggested that the blood flow interrelation of the goat placenta is of a combined type, in some areas multivillous to countercurrent, in others more or less crosscurrent (Leiser, 1987). One may summarize these complex results as a random vessel relationship. Because the sheep and the goat are frequently used animals for studies of fetal physiology a considerable volume of data is available (see Silver, 1981; Longo, 1981; Faber and Thornburg, 1983). The results of physiological experiments would largely fit a concurrent vascular arrangement. Such an anatomical situation has not been observed in the placentae investigated. This is not necessarily a conflict between physiological and morphological findings since the experimental results are compatible with more efficient arrangements, too, if the latter are burdened for example by inhomogeneous perfusion.

## Pig

The maternal and fetal vessels of the diffuse folded porcine placenta have been studied by light microscopy of neoprene latex corrosion casts (Tsutsumi, 1962) and later by scanning electron microscopy of colored methyl methacrylate cement casts of the maternal (MacDonald, 1976) and fetal (MacDonald, 1981) vessels of the placenta. MacDonald (1976) interpreted the vascular interrelations in the pig placenta on the basis of his own as well as previous investigations to be concurrent. The current investigation, which has been preliminarily reported (Leiser and Dantzer, 1986), has led us to another interpretation. A different type of methylmethacrylate was used to study maternal, fetal, and feto-maternal cast preparations combined with semithin serial sections of Epon embedded material. From these observations, it was concluded that the blood flow interrelation in the porcine placenta was predominantly one-way crosscurrent. However, the predominant arrangement of fetal arteriolar-venular axes and maternal arteriolar-venular axes, their branching into the capillary network may indicate even a countercurrent component. Physiological experiments with different aims (Flexner and Gellhorn, 1942; Comline and Silver, 1974; Faber, 1977; Randall, 1977; Caton and Bazer, 1978; Silver, 1980, 1981; Silver et al., 1982) have not led to any conclusion concerning the vascular arrangement in the pig. The data, however, on oxygen tension, indicate that the pig placenta has a rather poor exchange capacity, although it seems to increase during the last third of gestation.

## GENERAL DISCUSSION AND CONCLUDING REMARKS

The assessment of the principal feto-maternal blood flow interrelation of different placental types has shown that there is no correlation between the classical morphological classification (Grosser, 1909) and the blood flow interrelation. The multivillous flow system exists in the discoidal hemochorial human placenta as well as in the cotyledonary epitheliochorial goat placenta. Crosscurrent conditions are found in the zonary endotheliochorial cat placenta and in the diffuse epitheliochorial pig placenta etc. (cf. Table 1 and Figure 9).

However, there is some correlation between feto-maternal blood flow interrelation and the type of feto-maternal interdigitation (Table 1). The villous placentae of human and goat have multivillous flow conditions. Three of the four labyrinthine placentae studied, i.e., guinea pig, chinchilla, and rabbit, are characterized by countercurrent conditions. The lamellar or folded placentae, cat and pig, display an one-way crosscurrent vessel arrangement. This correlation probably occurs because the geometry of feto-maternal interdigitation influences the vascular architecture.

The weight ratios of neonate and placenta (Table 1) may reflect to some extent the effectiveness of placental transfer. If we compare these weight ratios with the generally used anatomical classifications regarding shape, interdigitation (Table 1) and interhemal barrier (Figure 10A) there is no correlation. These criteria do not seem to be decisive factors for placental transfer, although an increase in complexity of interdigitation and a decreasing thickness of the interhemal barrier should facilitate placental transfer of diffusible components. It is worth mentioning that in the hemomonochorial human placenta (Sen et al., 1979), in the endotheliochorial cat placenta (Leiser, 1982), and in the epitheliochorial pig placenta (Friess et al., 1980) the thickness of the interhemal barrier at term are almost the same, i.e., about 2 μm in minimal barrier thickness. The effectiveness of placental transfer may therefore be due predominantly to other factors, e.g., blood flow interrelation. In a recent review, Jones et al. (1985) stated that there is a close relationship between placental weight, uterine blood flow and fetal growth, thereby indicating that placental capacity may determine prenatal growth. However, concerning man, Carter (1975) stated that there is no reliable information on the relation between fetal weight, placental weight, and maternal placental blood flow, or, as emphasized by Garrow (1970), the weight of the placenta is a poor indicator of its functional capacity.

If the weight ratios of neonate and placenta are compared with the principal feto-maternal blood flow interrelation (Figure 10B), as determined by this anatomical study, there is a certain correlation, except for the rabbit. The placentae with the most efficient exchange system, the countercurrent blood flow interrelation, have a higher neonatal/placental weight ratio than do placentae with a less efficient blood flow interrelation, such as crosscurrent or multivillous. In this system the rabbit is far out of range. However, this seems to be in agreement with the experience of physiologists (Faber and Thornburg, 1983), who found that the rabbit placenta is special in many ways.

There are, of course, two problems with the use of placental weight as an index of placental exchange function. Firstly, the exchange efficiency as related to the materno-fetal vascular interrelations primarily benefits oxygen transfer. However, it is very likely that oxygen consumption depends not only on fetal weight but also on the fetal growth rate. This, however, is not exactly determined for most of the species dealt with in this study. It should be the subject of future research. Secondly, the true correlation of permeability is with the ratio of surface area over barrier thickness. We assume that the barrier thickness does not differ so very much from species to species, as this is valid for example for the human (Sen et al., 1979), the guinea pig (Kaufmann and Davidoff, 1977), the cat (Leiser, 1982), and the pig (Friess et al., 1980). If we neglect, moreover, differences in the share of connective tissue, one can follow, that to some extent, an increase of placental weight reflects an increase of surface area. If these assumptions are correct the correlation of placental weight with blood flow conditions as demonstrated in Figure 10B makes sense.

Many factors influence the effectiveness of exchange between mother and fetus and hence fetal development, e.g., growth hormones, estrogens, insulin-like factors, stage of gestation, umbilical and uterine blood flows, transfer capacity for glucose and oxygen, etc. (Allen, 1975; Caton and Bazer, 1978; Peeters et al., 1979; Faber and Thornburg, 1983; Heap et al., 1983; Goplerud and Delivoria-Papadopoulos, 1985; Jones et al., 1985; Longo, 1985; Owens et al., 1985a, b; Bell et al., 1986; Dantzer and Svenstrup, 1986). The maternal and fetal organisms thus interact using a variety of regulatory mechanisms to adjust the placental transfer or exchange capacity to guarantee appropriate fetal development. Nevertheless, the determination of the principal feto-maternal blood flow interrelation in placenta from different species with quite different placental types and the subsequent correlation with neonatal/placental weight ratios may therefore be an useful criterion for the discussion of some aspects of placental efficiency.

## SUMMARY

The materno-fetal vascular interrelations in the placental exchange area largely influence diffusional transfer across the placenta. Many controversies regarding this subject arise because in most cases the single species have been studied by different authors using various methods. The aim of this study is to achieve comparable morphological data of representative placental types by having the same group of investigators use largely identical methods: SEM of vessel casts, semithin histology, and TEM of the placental barrier.

The diffuse, folded, epitheliochorial placenta of the pig displays rather effective crosscurrent flow conditions. The cotyledonary, villous, epitheliochorial placenta of the goat has predominantly a multivillous flow system, sometimes complicated by crosscurrent and countercurrent components. Therefore, this variable arrangement may be described as random flow also. The cat placenta belonging to the zonary, folded, endotheliochorial type, offers a nearly ideal one-way crosscurrent condition. The complicated vascular arrangement of the bidiscoidal, labyrinthine, endotheliochorial placenta of the prosimian tupaia is best described as a modified, radially arranged crosscurrent system. The labyrinthine, hemodichorial rabbit placenta, is well known as a prototype of a countercurrent flow system. The same vascular arrangement can be demonstrated in the discoidal, labyrinthine, hemomonochorial placenta of the guinea pig and of the chinchilla. The discoidal, villous, hemomonochorial placenta of the human represents multivillous flow conditions. The comparison of the neonatal/placental weight ratios with the materno-fetal blood flow interrelations, arranged according to the exchange efficiency, shows a certain correlation except in the case of the rabbit.

## ACKNOWLEDGEMENTS

Parts of this study were supported by The Danish Agricultural and Veterinary Research Council (No. 13-3500) and by the Deutsche Forschungsgemeinschaft (No. Ka 360/6-4).

## REFERENCES

Allen, W.R. (1975) Endocrine functions of the placenta. In: *Comparative Placentation. Essays in Structure and Function*, (ed.), D.H. Steven, New York: Academic Press, pp. 214-267.

Amoroso, E.C. (1952) Placentation. In: *Marshall's Physiology of Reproduction*, (ed.), A.S. Parkes, vol. 2, chpt. 15, London: Longmans Green and Co., pp. 127-311.

Arts, N.F.T. (1961) Investigations on the vascular system of the placenta. Part 1. *Am. J. Obstet. Gynecol.* 82, 147-158.

Bailey, D.J. (1974) Counter-current flow of maternal and fetal bloodstreams of guinea pig placenta. *J. Physiol.* (Paris) 242, 104P.

Barcroft, J. and Barron, D.H. (1946) Observations upon the form and relations of the maternal and fetal vessels in the placenta of the sheep. *Am. J. Anat.* 94, 569-595.

Barron, D.M. and Battaglia, F.C. (1955) The oxygen concentration gradient between the plasmas in the maternal and fetal capillaries of the placenta of the rabbit. *Yale J. Biol. Med.* 28, 197-207.

Bartels, H. and Moll, W. (1964) Passage of inert substances and oxygen in the human placenta. *Pflügers Arch.* 280, 165-177.

Bartels, H., El Yassin, D., and Reinhardt, W. (1967) Comparative studies of placental gas exchange in guinea pigs, rabbits and goats. *Resp. Physiol.* 2, 149-162.

Bell, A.W., Kennaugh , J.M., Battaglia, F.C., Makowski, E.L., and Meschia, G. (1986) Metabolic and circulatory studies of fetal lamb at midgestation. *Am. J. Physiol.* 250, E538-E544.

Bjoerkman, N. (1970) *An Atlas of Placental Fine Structure.* London: Bailliere, Tindall & Cassell.

Boe, F. (1953) Studies on the vascularization of the human placenta. *Acta Obstet. Gynecol. Scand.* (Suppl. 5) 32, 7-92.

Boe, F. (1969) Studies on the human placenta. *Acta Obstet. Gynecol. Scand.* 48, 159-166.

Boyd, J.D. and Hamilton, W.J. (1970) *The Human Placenta.* Cambridge: Heffer.

Carter, A. M. (1975) Placental circulation. In : *Comparative Placentation. Essays in Structure and Function,* (ed.), D.H. Steven, New York: Academic Press, pp. 108-160.

Caton, D. and Bazer, F.W. (1978) Respiratory gases in uterine circulation of pregnant domestic swine as sampled by indwelling catheters. *Am. J. Physiol.* 234, R25-R28.

Comline, R.S. and Silver, M. (1974) A comparative study of blood gas tensions, oxygen affinity and red cell 2,3 DPG concentrations in foetal and maternal blood in the mare, cow and sow. *J. Physiol.* (London) 242, 805-826.

Dantzer, V. (1984) Scanning electron microscopy of exposed surfaces of the porcine placenta. *Acta Anat.* 118, 96-106.

Dantzer, V. and Svenstrup, B. (1986) Relationship between ultrastructure and oestrogen levels in the porcine placenta. *Anim. Reprod. Sci.* 11, 139-150.

Faber, J.J. (1969) Application of the theory of heat exchangers to the transfer of inert materials in placentas. *Circ. Res.* 24, 221-234.

Faber, J.J. (1977) Steady-state methods for the study of placental exchange. *Fed. Proc.* 36, 2640-2646.

Faber, J. J. and Hart, F.M. (1966) The rabbit placenta as an organ of diffusional exchange. *Circ. Res.* 19, 816-833.

Faber, J.J. and Thornburg, K.L. (1983) *Placental Physiology. Structure and Function of Fetomaternal Exchange.* New York: Raven.

Fischer, W.M. (1968) Das Strombahnsystem und der Austausch der Atemgase in der Meerschweinchenplazenta. *Verh. Anat. Ges. 62, Anat. Anz.* 121 (Suppl.) 241-248.

Flexner, L.B. and Gellhorn, A. (1942) The comparative physiology of placental transfer. *Am. J. Obstet. Gynecol.* 43, 965-974.

Friess, A.E., Sinowatz, F., Skolek-Winnisch, R. and Traeutner, W. (1980) The placenta of the pig. I. Finestructural changes of the placental barrier during pregnancy. *Anat. Embryol.* 158, 179-191.

Garrow, J.S. (1970) The relationship of foetal growth to size and composition of the placenta. *Proc. Royal Soc. Med.* 63, 498-500.

Goplerud, J.M. and Delivoria-Papadopoulos, M. (1985) Physiology of the placenta-gas exchange. *Ann. Clin. Lab. Sci.* 15, 270-278.

Goyri O'Neill, J.E. (1983) Vascularizacao da placenta humana. *Dissertacao Universidade Nova de Lisboa/Portugal.*

Grosser, O. (1909) *Vergleichende Anatomie und Entwicklungsgeschichte der Eihaeute und der Placenta mit besonderer Beruecksichtigung des Menschen.* Wien: Braumueller.

Habashi, S., Burton, G.J., and Steven, D.H. (1983) Morphological study of the fetal vasculature of the human term placenta: scanning electron microscopy of corrosion casts. *Placenta* 4, 41-56.

Heap, R.B., Flint, A.P.F., and Staples, L.D. (1983) Endocrinology of trophoblast in farm animals. In: *Biology of Trophoblast*, (eds.), Y.W. Loke and A. Whyte, Amsterdam, New York, Oxford: Elsevier, pp. 353-409.

Jones, C.T., Rolph, T.P., Lafeber, H.N., Gu, W., Harding, J.E., and Parer, J.T. (1985) Experimental studies on the control of fetal growth. In: *The Physiological Development of the Fetus and Newborn*, (eds.), C.T. Jones and P.W. Nathanielsz, New York: Academic Press, pp. 11-20.

Kaufmann, P. (1969) Die Meerschweinchenplacenta und ihre Entwicklung. *Anat. Entwickl.-Gesch.* 129, 83-101.

Kaufmann, P. (1981a) Functional anatomy of the non-primate placenta. *Placenta* (Suppl. 1), 13-28.

Kaufmann, P. (1981b) Electron microscopy of the guinea-pig placental membranes. *Placenta* (Suppl. 2), 3-10.

Kaufmann, P. (1985) Basic morphology of the fetal and maternal circuits in the human placenta. *Contr. Gynecol. Obstet.* 13, 5-17.

Kaufmann, P. and Davidoff, M. (1977) The guinea-pig placenta. *Adv. Anat. Embryol.* Vol 53, Fasc 2, Berlin, Heidelberg, New York: Springer.

Kaufmann, P., Sen, D.K., and Schweikhart, G. (1979) Classification of human placental villi. I. Histology. *Cell Tiss. Res.* 200, 409-423.

Kaufmann, P., Bruns, U., Leiser, R., Luckhardt, M., and Winterhager, E. (1985) The fetal vascularisation of term human placental villi. II. Intermediate and terminal villi. *Anat. Embryol.* 173, 203-214.

Kaufmann, P., Luckhardt, M., and Leiser, R. (1988) Three-dimensional representation of the fetal vessel system in the human placenta. *Trophoblast Research* 3, 113-137.

Lee, M.M.L. and Yeh, M.N. (1983) Fetal circulation of the placenta: a comparative study of human and baboon placenta by scanning electron microscopy of microvascular casts. *Placenta* 4, 515-526.

Leiser, R. (1982) Development of the trophoblast in the early carnivore placenta of the cat. *Biblthca Anat.* 22, 93-107.

Leiser, R. (1985) Fetal vasculature of the human placenta: Scanning electron microscopy of microvascular casts. *Contr. Gynecol. Obstet.* 13, 27-31.

Leiser, R. (1987) Mikrovaskularisation der Ziegenplazenta dargestellt mit rasterelektronisch untersuchten Gefaessausguessen. *Schw. Arch. Tierheilk.* 129, 59-74.

Leiser, R. and Kohler, T. (1983) The blood vessels of the cat girdle placenta. Observations on corrosion casts, scanning electron microscopical and histological studies. I. Maternal vasculature. *Anat. Embryol.* 167, 85-93.

Leiser, R. and Kohler, T. (1984) The blood vessels of the cat girdle placenta. Observations on corrosion casts, scanning electron microscopical and histological studies. II. Fetal vasculature. *Anat. Embryol.* 170, 209-216.

Leiser, R. and Dantzer, V. (1986) New aspects of microvasculature on the mature pig placenta. Congr. Europ. Ass. Vet. Anat., 24.-29. 8. 1986, Budapest. *Abstract in Anat. Hist. Embryol.* (in press).

Leiser, R., Kaufmann, P., and Luckhardt, M. (1984) Materno-fetal vessel interrelationship in different types of placenta. *Abstract. Ist Meeting of the European Placenta Group*, Sept. 10/11, Cambridge.

Leiser, R., Luckhardt, M., Kaufmann, P., Winterhager, E., and Bruns, U. (1985) The fetal vascularisation of term human placental villi I. Peripheral stem villi. *Anat. Embryol.* 173, 71-80.

Longo, L.D. (1981) The interrelations of maternal-fetal transfer and placental blood flow. *Placenta* (Suppl. 2), 45-64.

Longo, L.D. (1985) The role of the placenta in the development of the embryo and fetus. In: *The Physiological Development of the Fetus and Newborn*, (eds.), C.T. Jones, and P.W. Nathanielsz, New York: Academic Press, pp. 1-9.

Luckett, W.P. (1968) Morphogenesis of the placenta and fetal membranes of the tree shrews (Family Tupaiidae). *Am. J. Anat.* 123, 385-428.

Luckhardt, M., Kaufmann, P., and Elger, W. (1985) The structure of the tupaia placenta. I. Histology and vascularisation. *Anat. Embryol.* 171, 201-210.

MacDonald, A.A. (1976) Uterine vasculature of the pregnant pig: A scanning electron microscope study. *Anat. Rec.* 184, 689-698.

MacDonald, A.A. (1981) The vascular anatomy of the pig placenta: A scanning electron microscope study. *Acta Morph. Neerl. Scand.* 19, 171-172.

Makowski, E.L. (1968) Maternal and fetal vascular nets in placentas of sheep and goats. *Am. J. Obstet. Gynecol.* 100, 283-288.

Malassine, A. (1974) Evolution ultrastructurale du labyrinthe de placenta de chatte. *Anat. Embryol.* 146, 1-20.

Martin, C.B., Jr. (1981) Models of placental blood flow. *Placenta* (Suppl. 1) 65-80.

Metcalfe, J., Moll, W., Bartels, H., Hilpert, P., and Parer, J.T. (1965) Transfer of carbon monoxide and nitrous oxide in the artificially perfused sheep placenta. *Circ. Res.* 16, 95-101.

Moll, W. (1972) Gas exchange in concurrent, countercurrent and cross current flow systems. The concept of the fetoplacental unit. In: *Respiratory Gas Exchange and Blood Flow in the Placenta*, (eds.), L.D. Longo and H. Bartels, U.S. DHEW Pub. No. (NIH) 73-361, Bethesda (Maryland), pp. 281-294.

Moll, W. and Kastendieck, E. (1977) Transfer of $N_2O$, CO, and $H_2O$ in the artificially perfused guinea pig placenta. *Resp. Physiol.* 29, 283-302.

Mossman, H.W. (1926) The rabbit placenta and the problem of placental transmission. *Am. J. Anat.* 37, 433-497.

Mueller, G. and Fischer, W.M. (1968) Ueber den fetalen und maternen Blutkreislauf in der Meerschweinchenplazenta. *Verh. Anat. Ges. 62, Anat. Anz.* (Suppl.) 121, 231-239.

Owens, J.A., Allotta, E., Falconer, J., and Robinson, J.S. (1985a) Effect of restricted placental growth upon oxygen and glucose delivery to the fetus. In: *The Physiological Development of the Fetus and Newborn,* (eds.), C.T. Jones and P.W. Nathanielsz, New York: Academic Press, pp. 33-36.

Owens, J.A., Allotta, E., Falconer, J., and Robinson, J.S. (1985b) Effect of restricted placental growth upon umbilical and uterine blood flows. In: *The Physiological Development of the Fetus and Newborn,* (eds.), C.T. Jones and P.W. Nathanielsz, New York, Academic Press, pp. 51-54.

Peeters, L.L., Sheldon, R.E., Jones, M.D.Jr., Makowski, E.L., and Meschia, G. (1979) Blood flow to fetal organs as a function of arterial oxygen content. *Am J. Obstet. Gynecol.* 135, 637-646.

Randall, G.C.B. (1977) Daily changes in the blood of conscious pigs with catheters in fetal and uterine vessels during late gestation. *J. Physiol.* 270, 719-731.

Schröder, H. (1982) Structural and functional organization of the placenta from the physiological point of view. *Biblthca Anat.* 22, 4-12.

Schröder, H. and Leichtweiss, H.P. (1977) Perfusion rates and the transfer of water across isolated guinea-pig placenta. *Am. J. Physiol.* 232, H666-H670.

Schuhmann, R.A. (1982) Placentone structure of the human placenta. *Biblthca Anat.* 22, 46-57.

Schuhmann, R. and Wehler, V. (1971) Histologische Unterschiede an Plazentazotten innerhalb der maternofetalen Stroemungseinheit. Ein Beitrag zur funktionellen Morphologie der Plazenta. *Arch. Gynaek.* 210, 425-439.

Sen, D.K., Kaufmann, P., and Schweikhart, G. (1979) Classification of human placental villi. II. Morphometry. *Cell Tiss. Res.* 200, 425-434.

Silver, M. (1980) Intravascular catheterization and other chronic fetal preparations in the mare and the sow. In: *Animal Models in Fetal Medicine,* (ed.), P.W. Nathanielsz, Amsterdam: Elsevier Press, pp. 173-193.

Silver, M. (1981) An assessment of the chronically catheterized fetal preparation in sheep and other species. *Placenta* (Suppl. 2), 89-108.

Silver, M., Barnes, R.J., Comline, R.S., and Burton, G.J. (1982) Placental blood flow: some fetal and maternal cardiovascular adjustments during gestation. *J. Reprod. Fert. Suppl.* 31, 139-160.

Steven, D.H. (1966) Further observations on placental circulation in the sheep. *J. Physiol.* (London) 183, 13.

Thiriot, M. and Panigel, M. (1978) Microcirculation. La microvascularisation des villosites placentaires humaines. *CR Acad. Sci. Paris Ser. D.* 287, 709-712.

Tsutsumi, Y. (1962) The vascular pattern of the placenta in farm animals. *J. Facul. Agr., Hokkaido Univ, Sapporo,* 52, 372-482.

Trophoblast Research 3:261-268, 1988

# A THEORETICAL ANALYSIS OF THE INFLUENCE OF MATERNAL AND FETAL BLOOD FLOW ON PLACENTAL GAS EXCHANGE IN THE GUINEA PIG

Anthony M. Carter, Poul Christensen, and Jørgen Grønlund


Department of Physiology
University of Odense
Campusvej 55
DK-5230 Odense M, Denmark

## INTRODUCTION

In the guinea pig it is difficult to maintain a viable fetus during the three day period required for maternal metabolites to stabilize following anesthesia and surgery (Sparks et al., 1981). Therefore, it is necessary to study fetal respiration in the anesthetized animal (Moll & Kastendieck, 1978; Grønlund and Carter, 1982; Girard et al., 1983; Christensen et al., 1986). Maternal placental blood flow is reduced during anesthesia and surgery. In unanesthetized guinea pigs with chronically implanted catheters, Peeters et al. (1982) found a placental blood flow of 15 ml/min, approximately twice as high as that determined after fetal surgery during pentobarbital anesthesia (Grønlund and Carter, 1982). This reduction in flow is due to hypotension produced by a reduction in cardiac output (Peeters et al., 1982).

To evaluate the consequences for fetal oxygenation, a theoretical analysis of the influence of alterations in maternal or fetal placental perfusion on the transplacental exchange of respiratory gases was undertaken. The analysis used a mathematical model of placental gas exchange in the guinea pig (Christensen et al., 1986) based upon a rigid treatment of the oxygen and carbon dioxide binding properties of blood (Grønlund et al., 1986). The input parameters of the model include the blood flow on the two sides of the placenta and the pH, $PCO_2$, $PO_2$, hematocrit, and intraerythrocytic concentration of 2,3-diphosphoglycerate (DPG) in uterine and umbilical arterial blood. The predictions of the model were made using the simplifying assumption that end venous equilibration is achieved between fetal and maternal blood with respect to the partial pressure of oxygen and carbon dioxide. This approximation appears to be valid for placental types with a large countercurrent component such as those of the mare (Comline and Silver, 1974) and the guinea pig (Fischer, 1968).

## MATERIALS AND METHODS

The analysis depends upon a detailed knowledge of the blood interaction coefficients $\Delta\log PO_2/\Delta pH$, $\Delta\log PO_2/\Delta\log PCO_2$ and $\Delta\log PO_2/\Delta\log cDPG$ as functions of pH, concentration of DPG (cDPG) and oxygen saturation ($SO_2$), and of the relation between intracellular and extracellular pH as a function of $SO_2$ and cDPG. This information is not available for the guinea pig, and therefore data from adult human blood has been used. As shown elsewhere (Christensen et al., 1986), the binding of oxygen and carbon dioxide in adult guinea pig blood under standard conditions is known in sufficient detail to justify this approach. The guinea pig does not have a fetal hemoglobin, the difference in oxygen affinity between fetal and maternal blood being brought about by a difference in the red cell concentration of DPG (Bard and Shapiro, 1979). It is, therefore, possible to use data from adult human blood to simulate the binding of oxygen and carbon dioxide in fetal blood, provided that the observations extend to low levels of DPG. This requirement is met by the data of Winslow et al. (1983), which covers red cell concentrations in the range 0.2-2.7 mol DPG per mol hemoglobin tetramer.

The conservation equation for oxygen in the maternal and fetal blood of the placenta is given by:

$$\Delta cO_2(mother) \cdot PBF(mother) = - \Delta cO_2(fetus) \cdot PBF(fetus) - VO_2(placenta), \qquad (1)$$

where $\Delta cO_2$ is the arteriovenous difference in oxygen content, PBF is placental blood flow, and $VO_2(placenta)$ is the placental oxygen consumption. Similarly, the conservation equation for carbon dioxide is:

$$\Delta cCO_2(mother) \cdot PBF(mother) = - \Delta cCO_2(fetus) \cdot PBF(fetus) + VCO_2 (placenta), \quad (2)$$

where $\Delta cCO_2$ is the arteriovenous difference in carbon dioxide content, and $VCO_2$ (placenta) is the placental carbon dioxide production. Theoretically, the exchange of respiratory gases between maternal and fetal blood may be accompanied by changes in the concentration of buffer base. If it is assumed that the net exchange of acid or base across the placenta is negligible the conservation equations for the buffer base in the blood on the maternal and fetal sides of the placenta are given by:

$$\Delta cBB \text{ (mother)} = 0, \text{ and} \qquad (3)$$

$$\Delta cBB \text{ (fetus)} = 0, \qquad (4)$$

where $\Delta cBB$ is the arteriovenous difference in the concentration of buffer bases.

In a previous study (Grønlund et al., 1986), numerical expressions for $\Delta cO_2$, $\Delta cCO_2$ and $\Delta cBB$ as functions of arterial and venous $PO_2$, $PCO_2$ and pH at given values of hematocrit and red cell DPG concentration have been derived. If the $PO_2$, $PCO_2$, and pH of the umbilical and uterine arterial blood are known, substitution of these expressions into eq. (1-4) gives a system of four equations with six independent variables: the $PO_2$, $PCO_2$, and pH of fetal and maternal venous blood. If end venous equilibration is assumed, there are only four unknowns: the common $PO_2$ and $PCO_2$ values in the umbilical and uterine veins, the pH in the umbilical vein, and the pH in the uterine vein. The equations were solved using an iterative technique (Powell, 1970). The rate of oxygen transfer to the fetus was then calculated from:

$$VO_2(\text{fetus}) = \Delta cO_2(\text{fetus}) \cdot PBF(\text{fetus}), \tag{5}$$

using the estimated values for $PO_2$, $PCO_2$, and pH in the umbilical vein and the numerical expression for $\Delta cO_2$ (Grønlund et al., 1986).

The input variables of the model were assigned numerical values derived from measurements made in anesthetized guinea pigs under standardized experimental conditions. Published data (Table 1) on the values of $PO_2$, $PCO_2$, pH, and hematocrit in maternal and fetal arterial blood (Carter and Grønlund, 1982) and on the DPG content of maternal and fetal red cells (Carter and Grønlund, 1985) were used. Placental oxygen consumption, which has not been determined in the guinea pig, was set at 8 µmol/min. This value is commensurate with a placental weight of 7 g and equivalent to the oxygen consumption of the ovine placenta (Gu and Jones, 1986). Unless otherwise stated, maternal placental blood flow was 7.4 ml/min (Grønlund and Carter, 1982), and fetal placental blood flow was 7.5 ml/min (Carter, 1984).

This set of data has previously been used to test the validity of the model (Christensen et al., 1986). In a simulation of placental gas transfer, the predicted

Table 1

Input Parameters of the Placenta Model

| Parameter | Numerical value |
|---|---|
| **Maternal Artery** | |
| pH | 7.38 |
| $PCO_2$ (Torr) | 39.10 |
| $PO_2$ (Torr) | 114.20 |
| Hematocrit | 0.34 |
| cDPG (mole/mole Hb) | 1.28 |
| **Fetal Artery** | |
| pH | 7.27 |
| $PCO_2$ (Torr) | 53.40 |
| $PO_2$ (Torr) | 18.60 |
| Hematocrit | 0.39 |
| cDPG (mole/mole Hb) | 0.26 |
| **Placenta** | |
| Oxygen consumption ($\mu mol \cdot min^{-1} \cdot g^{-1}$) | 1.14 |

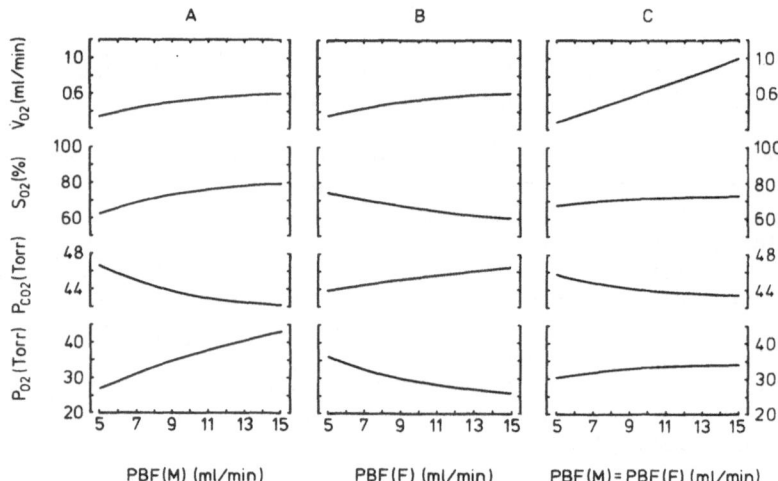

Figure 1. The influence of placental blood flow on the partial pressures of oxygen (PO$_2$) and carbon dioxide (PCO$_2$) and oxygen saturation (SO$_2$) in umbilical venous blood and on the placental transfer of oxygen (VO$_2$). A. Maternal placental blood flow (PBF(M)) altered at constant fetal placental perfusion. B. Fetal placental blood flow (PBF(F)) altered at constant maternal placental perfusion. C. Maternal and fetal placental blood flows altered concomitantly at a perfusion ratio of unity.

pH, PO$_2$, and PCO$_2$ of umbilical venous blood were in good agreement with measured values from the study that provided the data on arterial blood. Placental oxygen transfer derived from eq. (5) was 0.46 ml/min compared to a value of 0.47 ml/min computed from the measured arteriovenous difference in oxygen saturation, fetal hematocrit, and a fetal placental blood flow of 7.5 ml/min. This simulation was made on the assumption that there is no net transport of acid or base across the placenta. Placental transfer of the bicarbonate ion is currently thought to be negligible (Faber and Thornburg, 1983), but there is an apparent transfer of lactic acid from fetal to maternal blood during fetal acidosis (Moll et al., 1980). However, if the maximal rate of proton transfer is derived from data for the guinea pig (Moll et al., 1980) and incorporated into eq. (3) and eq. (4), the predicted rate of oxygen transfer is affected by less than 1%.

## RESULTS

Altered maternal and fetal placental perfusion does change umbilical venous PO$_2$, PCO$_2$, SO$_2$, and placental oxygen transfer (Figure 1). As the maternal placental blood flow is increased (Figure 1A), the amount of oxygen and carbon dioxide extracted from and delivered per unit volume of maternal blood decreases. Therefore PO$_2$ rises and PCO$_2$ falls both in the uterine vein and in the umbilical vein, assuming end venous equilibration. There is a corresponding increase in umbilical venous SO$_2$ and in placental oxygen transfer. When fetal placental blood flow is increased and maternal perfusion is kept constant (Figure 1B), the amount of oxygen and carbon dioxide extracted from and delivered per unit volume of maternal blood increases. As a result, $PO_2$ falls and $PCO_2$ rises in the uterine and umbilical veins. However, despite the fall in oxygen saturation, the net effect of increasing fetal placental perfusion is an increase in oxygen transfer. As discussed below, the ratio between maternal and fetal blood flows may be close to unity over a wide range of values. When the flow rates are increased in parallel at this flow ratio, the increase in placental oxygen transfer is almost linear (Figure 1C). The slight increase in umbilical $PO_2$ and $SO_2$ occurs because placental oxygen transfer becomes progressively larger than the oxygen consumption of the placental tissue (cf. eq. (1)). Similarly, the decrease in $PCO_2$ reflects the relatively smaller importance of placental carbon dioxide production (eq. (2)).

## DISCUSSION

This analysis enables an evaluation for the guinea pig of the restrictions placed on placental oxygen transfer by perturbations in placental perfusion due to anesthesia and surgery. Maternal placental blood flow was 7.4 ml/min in acute experiments (Grønlund and Carter, 1982) as opposed to 15 ml/min in the unanesthetized animal (Peeters et al., 1982). The corresponding values for placental oxygen transfer (Figure 1A) are 0.46 and 0.60 ml/min (19 and 25 µmol/min), a difference of 32%. Fetal placental blood flow has not been measured in the unanesthetized guinea pig. An increase in flow by a factor of two from the level of 7.5 ml/min reported for anesthetized animals (Carter, 1984) would result in an increase in oxygen transfer from 0.46 to 0.63 ml/min (Figure 1B), i.e. from 19 to 26 µmol/min. An alternative estimate of fetal placental blood flow during anesthesia was obtained in experiments where the maternal placenta was perfused through an extracorporeal circuit (Girard et al., 1983). When the hemoglobin flow rate was adjusted to a level corresponding to that measured in unanesthetized guinea pigs, fetal placental blood flow was 13 ml/min, which suggests that the perfusion ratio is kept close to unity. A simulation of placental gas exchange based on this assumption (Figure 1C) indicates that an increase in both flows from 7.5 to 15 ml/min would result in an increase in placental oxygen transfer from 0.46 to 1.00 ml/min (19 to 42 µmol/min). It should, however, be recognized that gas partial pressures and oxygen saturation in the umbilical artery were given constant values, implying that an increment in oxygen delivery would be matched by an increment in fetal oxygen consumption. This is unlikely to hold over the full range of flow. Girard et al. (1983) were able to vary the rate of hemoglobin flow on the maternal side of the placenta, and found that uteroplacental oxygen consumption rose to a maximum value of 35 µmol/min. This figure seems to include placental oxygen consumption, which we have set at 8 µmol/min.

Longo et al. (1972) simulated gas exchange in the ovine placenta between capillaries with ideal concurrent flow and at defined placental diffusing capacity. The approach adopted was to assume fetal compensation for any change in placental blood flow and to find the value of umbilical arterial $PO_2$ necessary to maintain constant placental $O_2$ transfer. It was concluded that, if the rate of blood flow on either side of the placenta fell below a critical level, normal fetal oxygenation could not be maintained. In recent experiments on the fetal lamb, umbilical blood flow has been manipulated by occluding the umbilical vein (Itskovitz et al., 1983) or by inflating a balloon in the descending aorta (Edelstone et al., 1985). In the sheep experiments, low flow rates were accompanied by an increase in oxygen extraction by the fetal tissues that was reflected in a reduced umbilical arterial oxygen content, with the oxygen content of the umbilical vein remaining constant (Itskovitz et al., 1983; Edelstone et al., 1985).

## SUMMARY

The influence of perturbations in placental blood flow on oxygen transfer to the guinea pig fetus was examined, using a mathematical model describing the exchange properties of the guinea pig placenta for defined conditions, including fetal-maternal venous equilibration and constant fetal arterial blood gas composition.  An increase in maternal placental perfusion from the level measured during pentobarbital anesthesia to that measured in the unanesthetized animal, with fetal placental blood flow kept constant, resulted in a 32% increase in placental oxygen transfer from 19 to 25 μmol/min.  A similar change occurred when fetal placental perfusion was doubled at a constant maternal placental blood flow.  When both flows were raised, at a perfusion ratio of unity, the increase in placental oxygen transfer was almost linear.  The predicted rise in oxygen transfer in the blood flow range 7.5 - 15 ml/min was from 19 to 42 μmol/min.  The latter value is regarded as an overestimate as fetal oxygen consumption is not expected to parallel oxygen delivery above the maximum experimental value of ca. 30 μmol/min.

## ACKNOWLEDGEMENT

This work was supported by grants from the Danish Medical Research Council.

## REFERENCES

Bard, H. and Shapiro, M. (1979) Perinatal changes of 2,3-diphosphoglycerate and oxygen affinity in mammals not having fetal type hemoglobins. *Pediatr. Res.* 13, 167-169.

Carter, A.M. (1984) The blood supply to the abdominal organs of the fetal guinea pig. *J. Develop. Physiol.* 6, 407-416.

Carter, A.M. and Grønlund, J. (1982) Blood gas tensions and acid-base status in the fetal guinea pig. *J. Develop. Physiol.* 4, 257-263.

Carter, A.M., and Grønlund, J. (1985) Influence of 2,3 diphosphoglycerate (DPG) concentration in maternal red cells on the transplacental exchange of respiratory gases. In: *The Physiological Development of the Fetus and Newborn,* (eds.) C.T. Jones and P.W. Nathanielsz, London: Academic Press, pp. 47-50.

Christensen, P., Grønlund, J., and Carter, A.M. (1986) Placental gas exchange in the guinea pig: fetal blood gas tensions following the reduction of maternal oxygen capacity with carbon monoxide. *J. Develop. Physiol.* 8, 1-9.

Comline, R.S. and Silver, M. (1974) A comparative study of blood gas tensions, oxygen affinity and red cell 2,3 DPG concentrations in foetal and maternal blood in the mare, cow and sow. *J. Physiol. (Lond.)* 242, 805-826.

Edelstone, D.I., Peticca, B.B., and Goldblum, L.J. (1985) Effects of maternal oxygen administration on fetal oxygenation during reductions in umbilical blood flow in fetal lambs. *Am. J. Obstet. Gynecol.* 152, 351-358.

Faber, J.J. and Thornburg, K.L. (1983) *Placental Physiology,* New York: Raven Press, pp. 75-78.

Fischer, W.M. (1968) Das Strombahnsystem und der Austausch der Atemgase in der Meerschweinchenplazenta. *Verh. Anat. Ges.* 62, 241-248.

Girard, H., Klappstein, S., Bartag, I., and Moll, W. (1983) Blood circulation and oxygen transport in the fetal guinea pig. *J. Develop. Physiol.* 5, 181-193.

Grønlund, J., and Carter, A.M. (1982) Continuous measurement of blood gas tensions in the fetal guinea pig by mass spectrometry. *J. Perinat. Med.* 10, 226-232.

Grønlund, J., Garby, L., Lorenzen, A.G., and Carter, A.M. (1986) An improved algorithm and a computer program for the analysis of capillary gas exchange. *Acta Physiol. Scand.* 126, 259-270.

Gu, W. and Jones, C.T. (1986) The effect of elevation of maternal plasma catecholamines on the fetus and placenta of the pregnant sheep. *J. Develop. Physiol.* 8, 173-186.

Itskovitz, J., LaGamma, E.F., and Rudolph, A.M. (1983) The effect of reducing umbilical blood flow on fetal oxygenation. *Am. J. Obstet. Gynecol.* 145, 813-818.

Longo, L.D., Hill, E.S. and Power, G.G. (1972) Theoretical analysis of factors affecting placental $O_2$ transfer. *Am J. Physiol.* 222, 730-739.

Moll, W., Girard, H., and Gros, G. (1980) Facilitated diffusion of lactic acid in the guinea pig placenta. *Pflügers Arch.* 385, 229-238.

Moll, W. and Kastendieck, E. (1978) Accumulation and disappearance of lactate in a fetus with a hemochorial placenta. The role of placental transfer and fetal metabolism. *J. Perinat. Med.* 6, 246-254.

Peeters, L.L.H., Sparks, J.W., Grutters, G., Girard, J., and Battaglia, F.C. (1982) Uteroplacental blood flow during pregnancy in chronically catheterized guinea pigs. *Pediatr. Res.* 16, 716-720.

Powell, M.J.D. (1970) A hybrid method for nonlinear algebraic equations. In: *Numerical Methods for Nonlinear Algebraic Equations,* (ed.) P. Rabinowitz, Gordon and Breach.

Sparks, J.W., Pegorier, J.P., Girard, J., and Battaglia, F.C. (1981) Substrate concentration changes during pregnancy in the guinea pig studied under unstressed steady state conditions. *Pediatr. Res.* 15, 1340-1344.

Winslow, R.M., Samaja, M., Winslow, N.J., Rossi-Bernardi, L., and Shrager, R.L. (1983) Simulation of continuous $O_2$ equilibrium curve over physiological pH, DPG and $PCO_2$ range. *J. Appl. Physiol.* 54, 524-529.

# DIAGNOSTIC METHODS

Trophoblast Research 3:271-282, 1988

# MAGNETIC RESONANCE IMAGING (MRI) OF THE PLACENTAL CIRCULATION USING GADOLINIUM-DTPA AS A PARAMAGNETIC MARKER IN THE RHESUS MONKEY IN VIVO AND THE PERFUSED HUMAN PLACENTA IN VITRO

Maurice Panigel[1,3], Carolyn Coulam[2], Gerald Wolf[2],
Anthony Zeleznik[2], Frank Leone[2], and Celia Podesta[2]

[1]Reproductive Biology
University P. and M. Curie
Paris, France

[2]Magee-Womens Hospital and
Pittsburgh Nuclear Magnetic Resonance Institute
Pittsburgh, Pennsylvania, USA

## INTRODUCTION

Imaging the placenta during its intrauterine development and maturation can be performed using various "non invasive" methods: femoral retrograde angiography, computer assisted x-ray tomography, radionuclide scintigraphy, ultrasonography, and magnetic resonance imaging. All can localize the placental site and, to a valuable degree, image the placental architecture in situ and in vitro post partum (Panigel, 1986b; Panigel et al., 1986a).

MRI promises to be a useful technique in the antenatal care of pregnant women. Several publications already deal with MRI of the human fetus in utero (Johnson et al., 1984; Smith et al., 1985; McCarthy et al., 1985; Powell et al., 1986). Unfortunately, MRI is sensitive to motion; movement of the fetus together with uterine contractions, can explain that some of the pictures obtained from the human fetus are not satisfactory. The movement of the placenta however, is quite limited and therefore better inherent contrast of placental tissues should be attained and maximized either in spatial or temporal resolution. Advances in MRI for animal research, have provided head and body coils appropriate for the species in question, as optimal resolution depends upon an appropriate "filling" factor (Bydder et al., 1985; Fisher et al., 1985). Temporal resolution has been improved by new fast-imaging sequences ("FLASH" "GRASS") (Haase, 1986; Frahm et al., 1986; Matthaei et al., 1985; Utz et al., 1986). Finally, a form of Cine MR uses gated sequences and fast imaging to create motion pictures of moving structures, a method primarily used for cardiovascular research. For readers not generally familiar with MRI the following references may be valuable (Smith et al., 1981; Crooks et al., 1980; Edelstein et al., 1983; Wehrli et al., 1985). These improved methods of resolution for MRI are an excellent way to study the dynamics of placental blood circulation.

[3]To Whom Correspondence Should Be Addressed: 4 Villa Patrice Boudard, 75016 Paris, France

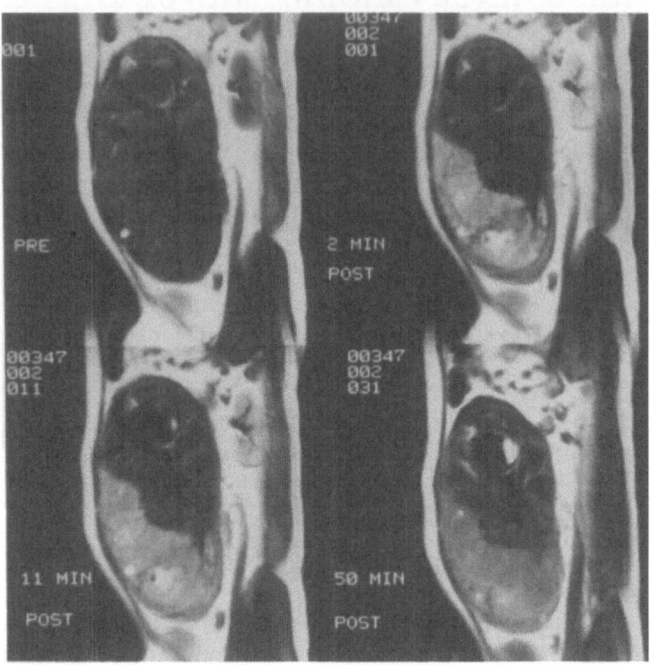

Figure 1. Sagittal images before and after Gd-DTPA, 100 micromoles/kg. The precontrast image is shown with one of the placental disc and the maternal kidney. Two, eleven, and fifty minute images are shown in the same slice with fetal urine enhancement identified at eleven and fifty minutes. When followed for up to four hours, the placental enhancement slowly faded to barely detectable on the fast image. TR = 600, TE = 25.

The purpose of the present investigation is to image the placental circulation observing the distribution of a paramagnetic contrast medium, Gadolinium-DPTA (Gd-DTPA) first examined in vivo for the detection of Gd with high field proton MRI in the maternal and fetal placental circulations of Rhesus monkeys. Then, the MRI of the placental vasculature in vivo of pregnant monkeys was compared to MRI of dually perfused isolated term human placental lobules in vitro.

## MATERIALS AND METHODS

Eight pregnant Rhesus monkeys were used, weighing 6 to 10 kg with gestational ages of 136-150 days for one series near term, 90-130 days for a second series. The animals were anesthetized with Pentobarbital (20 mg/kg), intubated, and studied in a body coil of 1.5 Signa MRI (General Electric, Milwaukee).

In the first series (4 monkeys, 136-150 days gestation), abdominal images were usually taken in both sagittal and axial planes using multislice spin-echo msec images with TR 600 msec, TE 25 msec, 128 x 256 matrix, two excitations and 5

mm thick slices. These imaging parameters allow multislice scanning to provide
6 slices in 3 minutes and are considered T1 weighed sequence (T1 is a time for
proton relaxation, a basic NMR phenomenon). Following precontrast images, 100
micromoles/kg Gd-DTPA was administered intravenously in the saphenous vein.
Serial images with the same imaging parameters were obtained from a few
minutes to 4 hours after the injections (Figure 1). In one case, amniocentesis was
performed and a large dose (up to 500 micromoles) of Gd-DTPA (supplied as the
sodium salt at 0.6 M by Mallinckrodt, St. Louis) was injected intraamniotically
(Figure 2). In some cases, maternal blood and urine samples were obtained to
estimate Gd-DTPA concentration from complete NMRD (Nuclear Magnetic
Relaxation Dispersion) curves of T1 relaxation rate at fields from 0.01-60 MHz.

In the second series of experiments (4 animals, 90-130 days gestation), the
monkeys at earlier stages of gestation were used under similar conditions using
the same intravenous dose of Gd-DTPA (100 micromoles/kg) except for one case in
which the dose was trebled in order to obtain a better contrast of the fetal placental
circulation with cine NMR. To study the circulatory dynamics in this second
series of experiments, we have used new imaging sequences: Fast Low Angle Shot
(or FLASH) and Gradient Recalled Acquisition in a Steady State (or GRASS)
(General Electric, Milwaukee). These methods involve complex NMR computed
analyses which are still in progress at the Pittsburgh NMR Institute. A
preliminary series of images for which an optimum plane is selected for the
scanning sequences with a one second internal at 5.6 seconds acquisition time
(Figure 4) is presented. These times have been chosen to be sufficiently short to
image changes in the blood stream carrying the paramagnetic contrast agent to
and from the placenta in both the maternal and fetal circulatory channels (Figures
3 and 4).

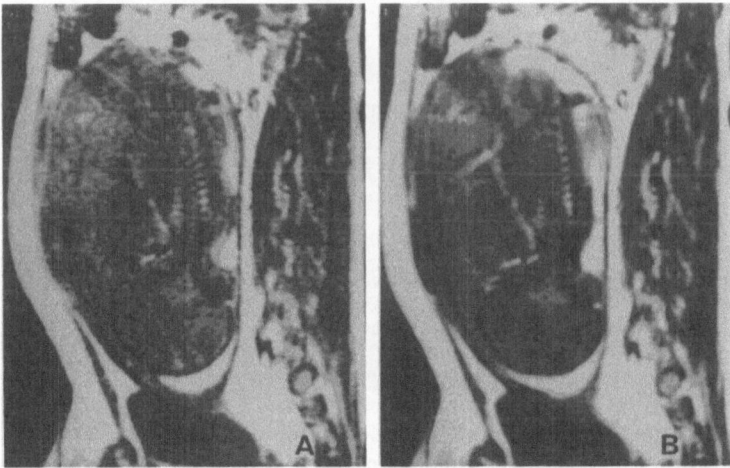

Figure 2. Sagittal MRI of the uterine contents after injecting Gd-DTPA into the
amniotic cavity which becomes apparent as well as the external shape of the fetus.

## MRI OF THE IN VITRO PERFUSED HUMAN PLACENTA

Magnetic resonance images were obtained in dually perfused human placental lobules using equilibrated salt solutions (Hanks' or Earle's) as perfusion medium while controlling pH and respiratory gases $O_2 + CO_2$ equilibrium and monitoring perfusion pressure and flow in maternal and fetal circuits as detailed in previous papers (Panigel, 1962, 1968; Schneider et al., 1972). Doses of 100 micromoles Gd-DPTA were added either to the maternal or to the fetal inflow of perfusion medium to the placenta; as maternal and fetal placental circulations were separately perfused (any leakage of perfusion fluid being controlled) one can obtain sequence of images imaging the transit of the paramagnetic agent across the placenta. MRI was performed in the course of perfusion using an 8 cm circular surface coil under the catheterized placenta. MRI thus follows the maternal inflow of perfusate through the catheter placed in the arterial opening into the intervillous space or the circulation of perfusate in the fetal vessels or capillaries in the cotyledonary villous tree at different times (a few minutes to 45 minutes after addition of Gd-DPTA in the perfusion circuit) T1 relaxation time measurements were performed with a Radx and an NMRD Relaxometer (Burnett et al., 1985; Koenig et al., 1986).

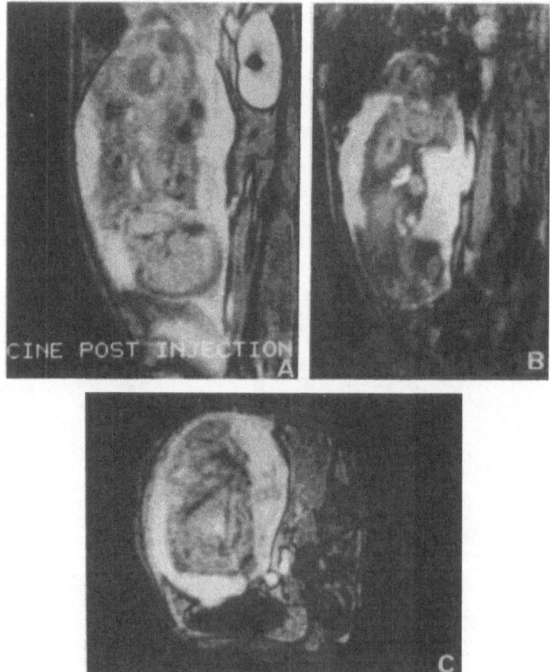

Figure 3. Cine magnetic resonance after injection of Gd-DTPA. The fetus with its different organs (heart, intestine, urinary bladder) is observed with a well contrasted placental disc on each side. Maternal kidney and urinary bladder also contain the paramagnetic contrast agent (A, B, and C sagittal and transverse planes).

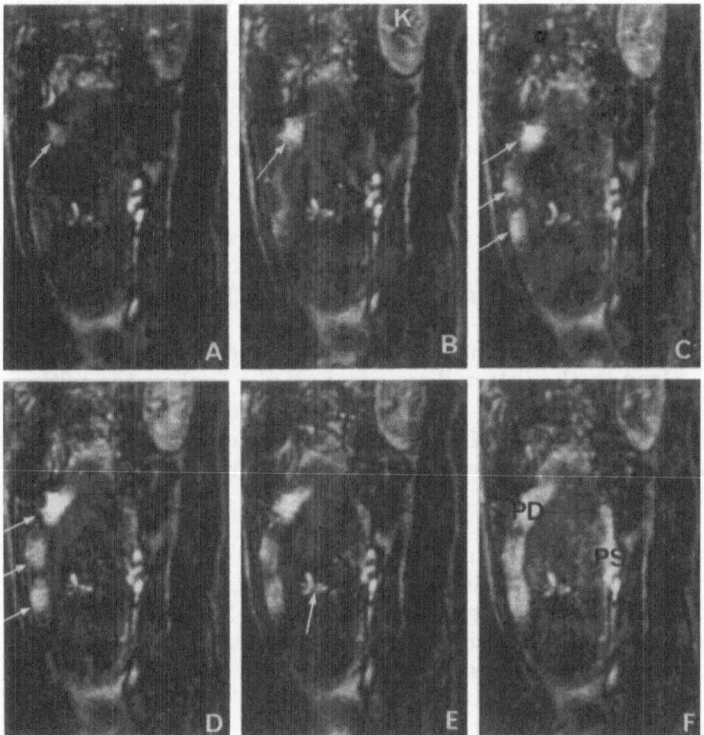

Figure 4. Fast scan MRI Post Gd-DTPA sequence of images = 5.6 second data collection with a 1 second delay between each - contrast (Gd-DTPA) injected at the same time that the first data collection was initiated (see text). The sequence uses serial GRASS images with TR = 22 msec, TE = 12 msec, and 1 excitation. There was a one second wait period between consecutive images.A - Arrow points to the maternal blood carrying the contrast beginning to spurt into the intervillous space.B, C, D - Arrows show the different placental lobules injected with contrast.E - Arrow points to the fetal heart which has high signal intensity characteristic of moving blood in GRASS images.F - PD = primary placental disc; PS = secondary placental disc.

## RESULTS

### Rhesus Monkey - Experiments In Vivo

1.      In part due to anesthesia, maternal motion and fetal movements were minimal allowing satisfactory and accurate imaging of the uterine contents and the maternal kidney (Figures 2 and 3).

2.      Within one minute after injection of Gd-DTPA, the bidiscoid placenta showed rapid contrast enhancement, more intense and faster than the intensity change in the maternal kidney.

3.      In each placental disc, maternal intervillous space and then fetal placental blood circulation have been imaged. The main disc and the accessory disc appear contrasted one after the other.

4.      Fast scan (GRASS) sequences permitted imaging the penetration, circulation and washout of the paramagnetic contrast agent a few seconds to a few minutes after its intravenous administration (Figure 4A).

        The arterial supply of the uterus already appears together with the first spurt of maternal blood in the intervillous space on the first image within 5.6 seconds acquisition time, the sequence having begun before the Gd-DTPA is administered intravenously.   The secondary placental disc appears several images later although the uterine arteries are apparent in the part of the uterine wall on which it is inserted.

        In the primary placental disc, a second spurt appears next to the first one during the following 6 second intervals from another spiral artery opening into the maternal intervillous space (Figure 4B). It is only 12 and 24 seconds later the other spurts become conspicuous in the main placental disc in the optimum place selected for pregnant uterus scanning sequences.

        The maternal kidney becomes contrasted during the same period, but it remains less conspicuous than the placental discs (Figure 4).

        The fetal heart is recognized because moving blood has high signal on GRASS images.

        Determination of contrast intensity which is proportional to paramagnetic concentration shows a heterogeneous distribution of Gd-DTPA in the different lobules as well as in different locations of each placental lobule.

5.      Post injection, cine NMR, as well as prolonged MRI scanning, 2 minutes, 11 minutes, and 50 minutes post intravenous injection of Gd-DTPA (Figure 1), shows that Gd-DTPA enhancement of maternal circulation begins after 11 minutes. The washout of the paramagnetic agent is not completed in the placenta 50 minutes later.

6.      Within 15 minutes, contrast enhancement of fetal urine is evident (Figure 1).  Maternal urinary excretion of Gd-DTPA is also visualized.  The fetal urinary bladder enhancement takes place within 12 to 15 minutes, becomes complete in an hour, and may persist for at least four hours.

7.      Gd-DTPA injected directly intraamniotically in the fetus (100 to 500 micromoles) immediately images the contours of the amniotic cavity, the fetus becoming very apparent. The contrast of paramagnetic Gd-DTPA remains in the amnion for a long period (more than one hour).

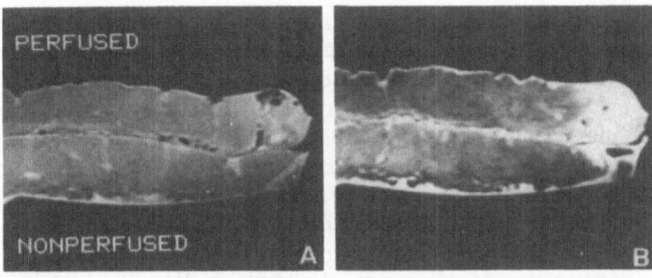

Figure 5. MRI of two post partum human placentae - one lobule of the upper disc is dually perfused with physiological solution (A) and then with Gd-DTPA added to the perfusate (B).

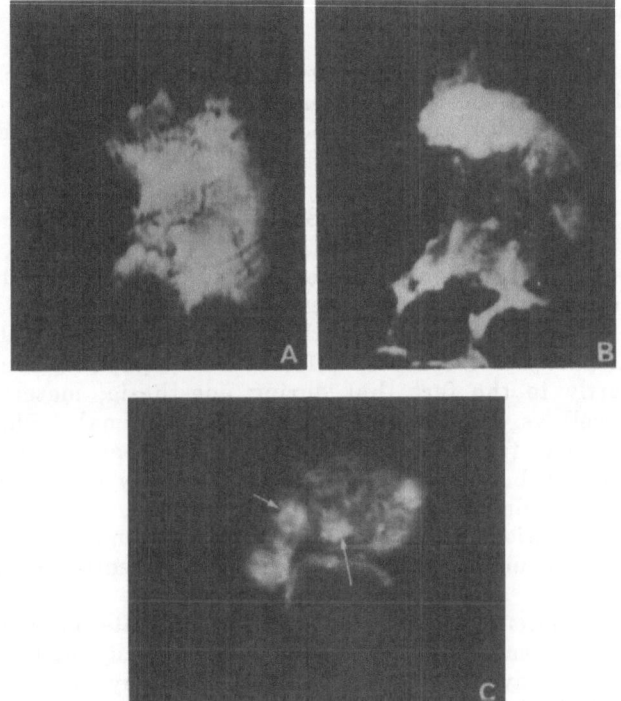

Figure 6. MRI of the maternal circuit in the isolated post partum placenta perfused with Gd-DTPA. A) The interseptal lobular intervillous compartment fills with paramagnetic contrast which spurts from the inflow cannula ("Borell's jet"). B) The perfusate containing the paramagnetic contrast Gd-DTPA, washes out to the periphery of the lobule as the perfusion continues. C) The Gd-DTPA passes across the placenta into the fetal blood capillary network of the cotyledonary villous tree (contrasted "puffs" on the fetal side of the perfusion circuit [arrows]).

## IN VITRO HUMAN PLACENTAL PERFUSION EXPERIMENTS

Measurements of T1 relaxation times under these in vitro conditions of artificial survival of the human placental lobule, demonstrated transfer of Gd-DTPA from maternal to fetal circuit, detected by lowering of the T1 in the fetal placental vein perfusate after injecting Gd-DTPA in the maternal arterial side as a bolus of 100 µmoles. It is to be understood that this preliminary MR scanning on the human placenta surviving in vitro was done only to establish the relationships between maternal and fetal vasculature and not to obtain quantitative data on placental tissues uptake and transfer of the paramagnetic ion. Other papers provide quantitative data on the placental transfer in vitro of another paramagnetic, manganese (Mattison et al., 1986; Miller et al., 1987). Magnetic resonance images of Borell's jets of maternal blood diffusing in the intervillous space were observed (Figure 6). The maternal perfusate carrying the paramagnetic ion was washed from the interlobular intervillous compartment in the heterogenous way as a "smoke ring" centered by the tip of the inflow arterial catheter (Figures 6A and 6B).

On the other side of the placenta, fetal capillary "puffs" were observed in the cotyledonary villous tree once the paramagnetic ion was "washed out" from the maternal intervillous space, part of it being transferred to the fetal perfusion circuit (Figure 6C).

## DISCUSSION

The present MRI of the uterine contents of the pregnant Rhesus monkey appears more accurate than some pictures of the human fetus already published (Johnson et al., 1984; Smith, 1985; McCarthy et al., 1985; Powell et al., 1986). This seems to be due partly to the use of different MRI equipment and sequence of images, and partly to the fact that during anesthesia, maternal and fetal movements as well as uterine contractions, are minimal. Pharmacological sedation of the human fetus has been discussed (it is part of the safety of the diagnostic procedure), but it appears possible especially with fast scans while monitoring blood circulation and uterine contractions, to obtain satisfactory images at the proper period when the fetus does not move and the myometrium does not contrast. Better pictures of the nonmobile inserted placenta are thus obtained.

The MRI of placental blood circulation on both maternal and fetal sides of the placenta does confirm some of the observations already published using cine radioangiography and dynamic radionuclide scintigraphy i.e., the intermittent inflow of maternal blood as spurts (or Borell's jets) into the intervillous space, the heterogenous distribution of blood in the placenta marked with radiopaque or paramagnetic media in the different compartments of the maternal intervillous space as well as at different levels of the cotyledonary fetal vascular tree. As for femoral radioangiography, many problems concerning details of maternal and fetal placental circulations remain to be solved (Ramsey and Donner, 1984; Panigel, 1986). The great advantage of the MR method over conventional radiology and nuclear medicine is the fact that like for ultrasound echosounding, there are no ionizing radiation hazards to the fetus. A good protocol established on an animal model like the pregnant Rhesus monkey, may be used for maternal or fetal blood flow monitoring in pregnant women. The NMR images presented here provide anatomo-physiological foundation for this research. The sequence of images obtained in the dually perfused isolated term placental lobule using Gd-DTPA as a paramagnetic agent is also preliminary to future studies in vivo.

Gadolinium DTPA (Gadolinium diethylene triamine pentaacetic acid) has been tested as a potential agent for MRI. This complex appears to be efficient and stable at intravenous doses of 100 micromoles/kg body weight. It is cleared by glomerular filtration and urinary excretion both in the mother and in the fetus and its pharmacokinetics mimic water soluble iodinated contrast media used in x-ray or in nuclear medicine. The present study has shown that the use of this paramagnetic agent is efficient and apparently safe for pregnant Rhesus monkeys as well as for their progeny (as monitored acutely). This fact does not preclude further research on other paramagnetic and super paramagnetic contrast media which may appear satisfactory for placental circulation research.

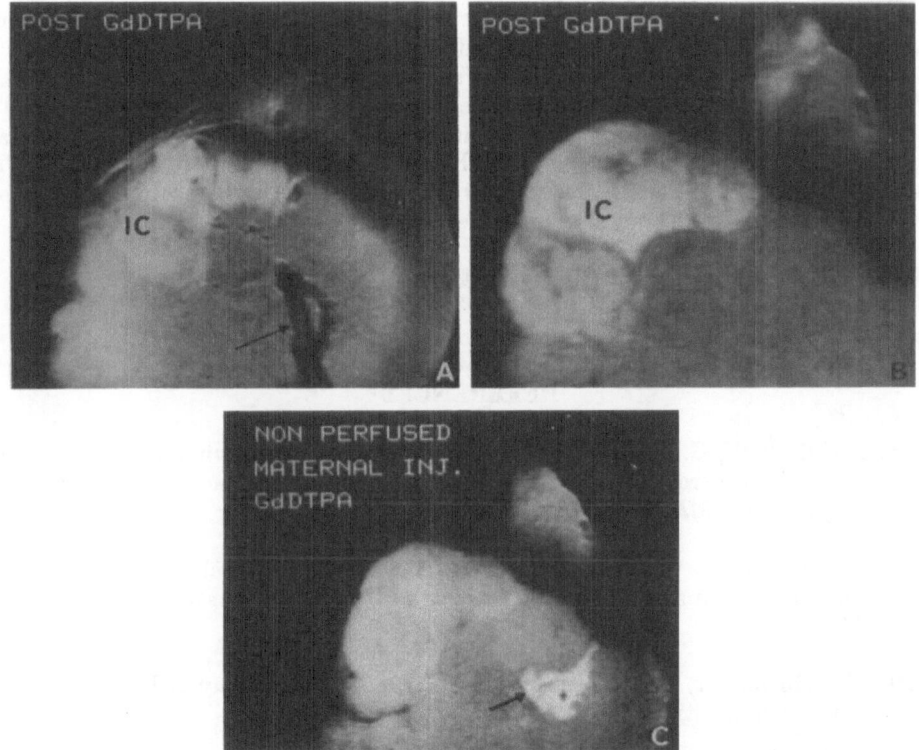

Figure 7. MRI of the fetal circuit in the isolated post partum placenta dually perfused with equilibrated physiological solution. A and B) The umbilical vessels insertion on the placenta is apparent (arrow) together with the placental cotyledons the fetal vasculature of which get filled with Gd-DTPA (IC). C) Gd-DTPA is injected on the maternal side of the nonperfused part of the isolated placenta. The contrast does not circulate and remains as such near the injection hole (arrow).

## SUMMARY

Maternal intervillous as well as fetal placental blood circulations have been imaged using MR. In vivo images were obtained in a 1.5 T Signa MRI using T1-weighed pulsing sequences before and after IV injection of Gd-DTPA (100 micromoles/kg). MR images of the perfused placenta were obtained using an 8 cm circular surface coil. As both maternal and fetal placental circulations were separately perfused, it was possible to add Gd-DTPA to each circulation and follow its transit through the placenta with serial MR images. Penetration, circulation, transfer, and washout of paramagnetic MR contrast agent, gadolinium DTPA, has been detected at different concentrations in vivo in the term Macaque placenta as well as in vitro in the dually perfused term human placental lobules. Placental tissues in both instances, show a significant contrast enhancement. In vivo, the rapid appearance and fading of the Gd-DTPA reflects the high uteroplacental blood flow. Gd-DTPA enhancement does not, however, disappear completely for hours both in the mother and fetus in which clearance of the paramagnetic compound demonstrates maternal fetal transfer.

In vitro, Gd-DTPA passes also across the perfused human placenta from maternal to fetal side as demonstrated by MR images and confirmed by T1 relaxation time measurements of the perfusates. The temporal distribution of Gd-DTPA mimics that of iodinated or isotopes tagged media. MR images of Borrell's jets of maternal blood diffusing in the intervillous space were observed. Fetal capillary "puffs" were seen in the cotyledonary villous tree. Thus, Gd-DTPA visualized using MRI, constitutes a high sensitivity and high resolution detector for human placental hemodynamic studies.

## ACKNOWLEDGEMENT

This work was supported partly by NIH Grant HD08610.

## REFERENCES

Burnett, K.R., Wolf, G.L., and Goldstein, E.J. (1985) NMR in vitro measurements: a quality control study of the RADX table-top spectrometer. *Phys. Chem. Phys. Med. NMR* 17, 123-129.

Bydder, G.M., Curati, W.L., and Hall, A.S. (1985) Use of closely coupled receiver coils in MR imaging: practical aspects. *J. Comput. Assist. Tomogr.* 9(5), 987-996.

Crooks, L., Hoenniger, J., and Arakawa, M. (1980) Tomography of hydrogen with nuclear magnetic resonance. *Radiol.* 136, 701-706.

Edelstein, W.A., Bottomley, P.A., Hart, H.R., and Smith L.S. (1983) Signal, noise and contrast in Nuclear Magnetic Resonance (NMR) Imaging. *J. Comput. Assist. Tomogr.* 7, 391-401.

Fisher, M.R., Barker, B., and Amparo, E.G. (1985) MR imaging using specialized coils. *Radiology* 157, 443-447.

Fobben, E. and Wolf, G.L. (1983) Gadolinium DTPA - a potential NMR contrast agent. Effects upon tissue proton relaxation and cardiovascular function in the rabbit. *Invest. Radiol.* 18, 55.

Frahm, J. Haase, A., and Matthaei, D. (1986) Rapid NMR imaging of dynamic processes using the FLASH technique. *Magn. Reson. Med.* 3, 321-327.

Haase, A., Frahm, J., Matthaei, D., Hänicke, W., and Merboldt, K.D. (1986) FLASH Imaging. Rapid NMR imaging using low flip-angle pulses. *J. Magn. Reson.* 67, 258-266.

Johnson, I.R., Symonds, E.M., Kean, D.M., Worthington, B.S., Broughton-Pipkin, F., Hawkes, R.C., and Gyngell, M. (1984) Imaging the pregnant human uterus with nuclear magentic resonance. *Am. J. Obstet. Gynecol.* 148, 1136-1139.

Koenig, S.H., Spiller, M., Brown, R.D., and Wolf, G.L. (1986) Magnetic field dependence (NMRD profile) of 1/tl of rabbit kidney medulla and urine after intravenous injection of Gd (DTPA). *Invest. Radiol.* 26, 697-704.

McCarthy, S.P., Stark, D.D., Filly, R.A., Callen, P.W., Hricak, H., and Higgins, C.B. (1985) Obstetrical magnetic resonance imaging maternal anatomy. *Radiol.* 154, 421-427.

Matthaei, D., Frahm, J., Haase, A., and Hänicke, W. (1985) Regional physiological functions depicted by sequence of rapid magnetic resonance images. *Lancet* 2, 893.

Mattison, D.R., Miller, R.K., Panigel, M., Bryant, R., and Merril, K. (1986) Magnetic resonance imaging (MRI) of the human placenta: kinetics and distribution of Manganese (Mn) in the perfused lobule. *33rd Meeting of the Society for Gynecologic Investigation,* Toronto, Canada, Abstract 420, p. 245.

Miller, R.K., Mattison, D.R., Panigel, M., Ceckler, T., Bryant, R., and Thomford, P. (1987) Kinetic Assessment of manganese using magnetic resonance imaging (MRI) in the dually perfused human placenta in vitro. *Environ. Hlth Persp.* 74, 81-91.

Panigel, M. (1962) Placental perfusion experiments. *Am. J. Obstet. Gynecol.* 84, 1664-1683.

Panigel, M. (1968) Placental perfusion. In: *Fetal Homeostasis,* Vol. 4 (4th Conference - NY Academy of Science), ed., R.M. Wynn, Appleton Century Crofts, New York, pp. 15-25.

Panigel, M. (1986) Anatomy and morphology. In: *The Human Placenta,* (ed.), T. Chard, Clinics in Obstetrics and Gynecology 13, Saunders, London, pp. 421-445.

Panigel, M., Coulam, C., Wolf, G., Zeleznik, A., Leone, F., and DePodesta, C.V. (1986) Placental transfer and fetal excretion of GdDTPA in pregnant rhesus monkeys. *Soc. Magn. Reson. Med.* 4, 1504-1505.

Podesta, C., Zeleznik, A., Leone, F., Coulam, C., Wolf, G., and Panigel, M. (1986) Fetal magnetic resonance imaging in pregnant macaques: localization of the urinary bladder with Gadolinium-DTPA. *Surgical Forum,* New Orleans, in press.

Powell, M.C., Worthington, B.S., and Symonds, E.M. (1986) MRI a new milestone in modern OB care. *Diagn. Imag.* 8, 86-91.

Ramsey, E.M. and Donner, M.W. (1980) *Placental Vasculature and Circulation.* Georg Thieme, Stuttgart.

Schneider, H., Panigel, M., and Dancis, J. (1972) Transfer across the perfused human placental of antipyrine, sodium and leucine. *Am. J. Obstet. Gynecol.* 113, 822-828.

Smith, F.M. (1985) Magnetic resonance imaging of human pregnancy. *Soc. Magn Reson. Med* 14, 214-215.

Smith, F.W., Mallard, J.R., and Hutchinson, J.M.S. (1981) Clinical application of nuclear magnetic resonance. *Lancet* 1, 78-79.

Utz, J., Herfkens, R.J., Glover, G., and Pelc, N. (1986) Three second clinical NMR images using a gradient recalled acquisition in a steady state mode (GRASS). *Magn. Reson. Imag.* 4, 106.

Wehrli, F., MacFall, J., and Newton, T. (1985) Parameters determining the NMR appearance, etc. *Advanced Imaging Techniques, Vol. 2, Modern Neuroradiology.*

Wolf, G.L. (1984) Contrast enhancement in biomedical NMR. *Phys. Chem. Phys. Med. NMR.* 16, 93-95.

Wolf, G.L., Burnett, K.R., Goldstein, E.J., and Joseph, P.M. (1985) Contrast agents for magnetic resonance imaging. In: *Magnetic Resonance Annual,* (ed.), H.Y. Kressel, Raven Press, New York, pp. 231-266.

Trophoblast Research 3:283-289, 1988

# HEMODYNAMIC CONTROL OF END-DIASTOLIC VELOCITY: AN IN VITRO STUDY

Dev Maulik and Prasad Yarlagadda

Department of Obstetrics and Gynecology
University of Missouri
Kansas City School of Medicine
Kansas City, Missouri, 64108 USA

## INTRODUCTION

In recent years, analysis of Doppler Frequency Shift Waveform has been used extensively in assessing peripheral hemodynamics (Woodcock, 1972; Pourcelot, 1974; Gosling and King, 1975; Blackshear et al., 1980). In the perinatal area, the use of normalized End-Diastolic Velocity (EDV) has been proposed as an index of adequacy of placental circulation (Maulik, 1982). In pediatric practice, neonatal cerebral perfusion has been assessed using the various Doppler indices including the EDV, and the efficacy of the technique has been compared against the [133]Xenon clearance method for measuring perfusion (Greisen, 1984). More recently, the absence of EDV in the umbilical artery has been shown to be an important predictor of fetal compromise (Rochelson et al., in press). The assumption underlying the use of these analytic techniques proposes that they can unravel the hemodynamic factors in the target circulation that control the shape of the Doppler waveform. This assumption, which is supported by empiric data, has not been subjected to in depth hemodynamic validation. Obviously, providing evidence of a reasonable hypothesis cannot act as a substitute for experimental verification. This ongoing project has been undertaken in order to address the above issue and to clarify the fundamental hemodynamic concepts which form the basis for using the Doppler waveform analysis to assess circulatory adequacy. Specifically, this paper presents the results from a preliminary study in which the effects of up and downstream hemodynamic alterations on the Doppler derived EDV were investigated in an in vitro circulatory system.

## MATERIALS AND METHODS

### Instrumentation

The schematic of the in vitro system is depicted in Figure 1. The ventricular chamber was made of a rubber bulb encased in an air chamber. Pressure changes in the latter chamber produce ventricular contractions and relaxations. The unidirectionality of ventricular in and out flows was maintained by a check valve between the atrial reservoir and the ventricular chamber, and by a prosthetic cardiac valve (St. Jude's tilting disc, St. Jude's Medical, Inc., St. Paul, MN) between the ventricle and the systemic circuit. Ventricular contractility, stroke rate, systolic/diastolic phase ratio, end diastolic pressure, and maximum systolic pressure were controlled with a custom built electronic pulse duplicator system. The compliance test section was a length of gouche tubing encased in an air chamber, pressure in which was experimentally controlled. The multiple branching test section consisted of a variable number of multiple polythethylene semi-rigid tubings encased in a plexiglass cassette, which could be changed, thus allowing variations in branching. The perfusion fluid was 25% glycerin in water solution, (a viscocity of 3.5 cp) with 0.5% v/v suspension of starch particles.

A continuous and pulsewave Doppler instrument with a 2 mHz transducer and a real time FFT spectral analyzer (Model SD 100, Vingmed, Inc., Allendale, NJ) was used. An electromagnetic flowmeter (Model 500A, Carolina Medical Products, Inc., King, NC) and a pressure transducer (Model CD12, Volidyne Engineering Corp., Northridge, CA) were incorporated in the circuit. The flow meter was calibrated by comparing the analog signals with the directly measured volumetric flow rates. The accuracy of the flow meter readings were within plus or minus 5% of the volumetric flow rates for pulsatile flows, and within plus or minus 1% for study flows. The pressure transducer was calibrated by connecting it to a water manometer and recording the analog signals for known pressure gradients. Both the flow and pressure transducers generated linear signals with zero signals at zero flow and pressure gradients, respectively. An on-line microcomputer (PC AT, International Business Machines Corp., Boca Raton, FL) was used for data acquisition and analysis.

**Procedure**

Experiments were conducted to measure the instantaneous flow, pressure, and the maximum Doppler frequency shift waveforms from the test locations. Initially, the different components of the in vitro circulatory system were manipulated in order to produce flow velocity waveforms resembling those encountered in umbilical and uteroplacental circulations. Two sets of experiments were then conducted. In the first set, the compliance of the upstream flow section was altered, and the variations in the Doppler frequency shift signals at the test location (T) were measured. In the second set of experiments, the downstream branching section was changed and variations in the flow, pressure, and Doppler signals were measured at the test location. In each experiment, the system was allowed to reach a steady state that was monitored by observing the flow waveform in an oscilliscope. All of the three analog signals from the flowmeter, pressure transducer, and the Doppler equipment were directly entered into a computer with an analog to digital conversion capability. The connections, the null position, and the calibration signals were verified first by running a customized data acquisition program in real time mode, and monitoring the waveforms on the computer graphics screen. The actual data recording was performed in the high speed mode, collecting samples at a rate of 2000/second for each channel, over a period of 10 seconds. The data were stored on a 30 megabyte hard disk.

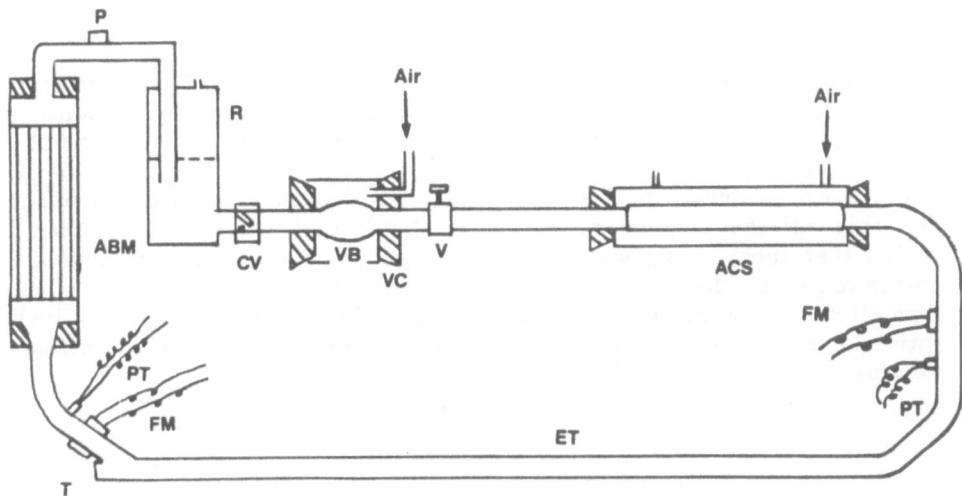

Figure 1. In Vitro Circulation Model: PT, Pressure Transducer; ACS, Aortic Compliance Section; CV, Check Valve; ABM, Arterial Branching Model; ET, Elastic Tubing; FM, Electromagnetic Flow Meter; R, Arterial Reservoir; T, Test Location; V, Valve; VB, Ventricular Bulb; VC, Ventricular Chamber; and P, Pressure Tap.

The compliance (C) of the upstream test section, between the aortic valve and the rest of the systemic circuit was indirectly measured from the volumetric expansion of the test section at different steady pressures (Noordergraaf, 1978). Three assumptions were made in these calculations: (1) The compressability of the test fluid was negligible, (2) that the compliance of the test section (4 cm diameter elastic tubing) was independent of the frequency, since the complex Young's modulus for larger arteries (example: aorta) reaches a plateau (Westerhof and Noordergraaf, 1970), and (3) that the systolic/diastolic pressure differences attained in these experiments were of the order 20-30 mm Hg, and therefore the compliance could be assumed to be constant, independent of the pressure. The compliance (C) is related to the systolic and diastolic volumes according to the formula: $C \propto (V_s - V_d)$ where $V_s$ is the systolic volume and $V_d$ is the diastolic volume.

In relation to the downstream hemodynamic alterations, the peripheral resistance, which is the input impedance at zero frequency, in relation to each of the branching section alterations were measured. The digitized information of the 10 cycles was used to calculate the average pressure and flow rates at the test section. Peripheral resistance was calculated according to the following formula: $Zpr = Pm/Qm$ (McDonald, 1974; Fung, 1984), where $Zpr$ is the input impedance at zero frequency (peripheral resistance), $Pm$ is the mean pressure, and $Qm$ is the mean flow. The average diastolic velocities were computed from the digitized Doppler frequency shift information from a total of 10 cycles. The angle correction was made in computing the diastolic velocities from the frequency shift.

## RESULTS

Examples of different Doppler wave configurations produced by the in vitro circulatory system are shown in Figure 2. The system was capable of producing other configurations including uteroplacental waveforms with or without a dicrotic notch.    The changes in the EDV values secondary to the change in the upstream compliance are presented in Figure 3.   The EDV demonstrated a direct linear relationship with the compliance changes (correlation coefficient of 0.94). It should be noted that these changes occurred when the other circulatory parameters remained constant. The change in the EDV in relationship to the alterations in the peripheral resistance are shown in Figure 4.   As to be expected, there was a high negative correlation between the EDV and the peripheral resistance (correlation coefficient of -0.96).

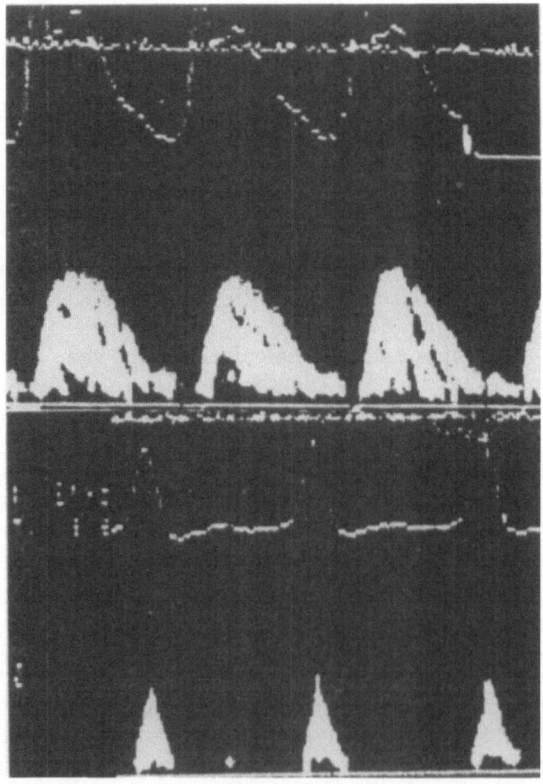

Figure 2.  Samples of the in vivo arterial Doppler frequency shift waveform in the in vitro circulatory model system.   Upper panel demonstrates continuing flow in diastole and the presence of dicrotic notch.   The middle panel presents simulated umbilical arterial flow with low end-diastolic velocity.    The lower panel demonstrates the total absence of end-diastolic velocity.

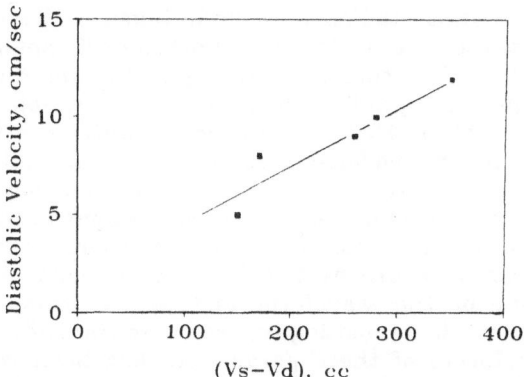

Figure 3. Changes in the downstream end diastolic velocity (cm/sec) secondary to experimentally controlled alterations in the upstream compliance as measured from the systolic and diastolic volume changes (cc). Vs, Volume of the compliance section at peak systolic pressure; Vd, Volume of the compliance section at end-diastolic pressure. Correlation coefficient, 0.94; slope, 0.0296; and intercept, 1.63.

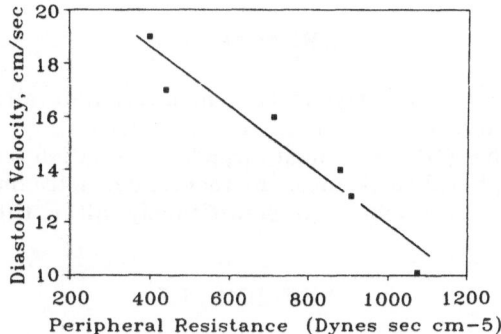

Figure 4. Changes in the upstream end diastolic velocity (cm/sec) following the experimentally induced alterations in the peripheral resistance (dynes·sec· cm⁻⁵). Correlation coefficient, -0.96; slope, -0.0112; and intercept, 23.1.

## DISCUSSION

Although a considerable body of empiric evidence exists for using the Doppler waveform analysis analytic techniques for hemodynamic assessment, there has been a significant dearth of experimental verification of the hemodynamic premises up on which the waveform analytic techniques are based. Fundamental questions, such as the contributions of the up and downstream hemodynamic parameters towards influencing the shape of the waveform and the ability of the indices to unscramble the up and downstream information, remain largely unresolved. In order to address these issues, circulatory simulation for

Doppler and hemodynamic studies were undertaken. The first phase of the investigation was presented at the 9th Rochester Trophoblast Conference (Rochester, NY) in 1983. The changes in the up and downstream PI values were calculated with the pressure gradient changes across a simple resistance unit in the circulation (Maulik et al., 1983). The major limitations of that study were 1. inability to reproduce the in vivo feto-placental or uteroplacental waveforms, and 2. the use of a model too simplistic for expressing complex hemodynamic parameters. The improved circulatory model presented here allowed one to recreate in vivo feto-placental and uteroplacental waveforms. Please note that the EDV can be altered according to experimental requirements (Figure 2); similarly one can also change other characteristics of the waveform and control complex hemodynamic parameters such as compliance and impedance parameters of the system. A more comprehensive description of these parameters has been reported elsewhere (Maulik and Yarlagadda, 1987). These results demonstrate that changes in the EDV can be produced by only compliance changes in the upstream without any changes in the resistive component in the downstream. This finding is important, as there seems to be a tendency to presume that any changes in the EDV must always be related to the downstream circuit. More significantly in this project, it has been shown that the downstream changes, such as reduction in the cross-sectional area of a branching unit, can markedly decrease the EDV. This successful in vitro study also provides the justification for its further use for hemodynamic validation of the Doppler indices.

## SUMMARY

The effect of up and downstream hemodynamic alterations on Doppler derived EDV was investigated in an in vitro circulatory system. The study demonstrated that the EDV has a high negative correlation (correlation coefficient: -0.96) with the peripheral resistance. Moreover, downstream circulation changes in upstream compliance can also significantly alter the EDV (correlation coefficient: 0.94).

## REFERENCES

Blackshear, W., Jr., Phillips, D.J., Chikos, Harley, J.D., Thiele, B.L., and Strandness, D.E., Jr. (1980) Carotid artery velocity patterns in normal and stenotic vessels. *Stroke* 11, 67-71.

Fung, Y.C. (1984) *Biodynamics*, Springer-Verlag, Inc., New York. pp. 127-129.

Gosling, R.G. and King, D.H. (1975) *Ultrasound Angiology, Arteries and Veins*, (eds.), A.W. Marces and L. Adamson, Churchill Livingstone:Edinburgh, pp. 61-98.

Greisen, G., Johansen, K., Ellison, P., Fredrika, P.S., Mali, J., and Fries-Honson, B. (1984) Cerebral blood flow in the newborn infant: comparison of Doppler ultrasound and Xenon clearance. *J. Pediatr.* 104, 411-418.

Maulik, D., Saini, V.D., Nanda, N.C., and Rozensweig, W.S. (1982) Doppler evaluation of fetal hemodynamics. *Ultrasound Med. Biol.* 8, 705-710.

Maulik, D. and Yarlagadda, A.P. (1987) In vitro hemodynamic validation of Doppler waveform indices, In: *Doppler Ulstraound Measurement of Maternal-Fetal Hemodynamics*, (eds.), D. Maulik and D. McNellis, Proceedings from an NICHD Workshop, Perinatatology Press, pp. 257-282.

McDonald, D.A. (1974) *Blood Flow in Arteries*, The Williams and Wilkins Company, Baltimore, pp. 352-353.

Noordergraaf, A. (1978) *Circulatory System Dynamics*, Atlantic Press, New York, pp. 25-26.

Pourcelot, L. (1974) Applications clinicae de l'examen Doppler transcutare, In: Velocimetric Ultrasonore Doppler, (ed.) L. Pourcelot, *INSERM*, Oct., 34, 213-240.

Rochelson, B., Schulman, H., Farmakides, G., Bracero, L., Ducey, J., Fleischer, A., Penny, B., and Winter, D. (1987) The significance of absence of end-diastolic velocity in umbilical artery velocity waveforms. *Am. J. Obstet. Gynecol.*, in press.

Westerhof, N. and Noordergraaf, A. (1970) Arterial viscoelasticity: a generalized model: effect on input impedance and wave travel in the systemic tree. *J. Biomed.* 3, 357-359.

Woodcock, J.B., Gosling, R.G., and Fitzgerald, D.E. (1972) A new non-invasive technique for assessment of superficial femoral artery obstruction. *Br. J. Surg.* 59, 226-231.

# CLINICAL APPLICATIONS

Trophoblast Research 3:293-300, 1988

# DOPPLER ASSESSMENT OF FETOPLACENTAL CIRCULATION

Dev Maulik, Prasad Yarlagadda,
and Lee Willoughby


Department of Obstetrics and Gynecology
University of Missouri
Kansas City School of Medicine
Kansas City, Missouri 64108

## INTRODUCTION

The Doppler principle elucidates the phenomenon of changes in the wave length or the frequency of energy which propogate in waves. This phenomenon is due to the relative motion between the energy source and the receiver. If the source and the receiver are moving toward each other, the frequency will increase. If they are moving apart, the frequency will decrease. Moreover, the magnitude of the frequency change or shift will be proportionate to the velocity of this relative motion. The principle has been utilized to study immensely diverse phenomena, and its biomedical application has led to the development of Doppler ultrasound technology (Satumora, 1957; Franklin et al., 1967; Peronneau et al., 1969; Light and Cross, 1972; Fronek, 1973) which has been used successfully and extensively for assessing blood flow dynamics in humans in a non-invasive manner. More recently, the Doppler ultrasound technique has been extended to investigation of fetal and feto-placental hemodynamics (Fitzgerald and Drumm, 1977; McCallum et al., 1978; Stuart et al., 1980; Gill et al., 1980; Eik-Nes et al., 1980; Maulik et al., 1982; Trudinger et al., 1985).

Doppler ultrasound provides measurement of volumetric flow if the angle of insonation between the ultrasound beam and the vessel axis, and the vessel cross sectional area are known. However, in relation to the feto-placental arterial hemodynamics, small size, spiral course, and relative inaccessibility of the umbilical arteries do not permit measurement of the angle for insonation of the vascular cross sectional area with any degree of accuracy. In order to eliminate these limitations of volumetric flow assessment, alternative techniques have been developed for analyzing Doppler derived arterial flow velocity that do not involve measurement of the beam angle or the vessel cross sectional area (Pourcelot, 1974; Gosling and King, 1975; Stuart et al., 1980; Maulik et al., 1982). Most of these analytic techniques are ratios derived from various combinations of the peak systolic, end diastolic, and mean values of the maximum frequency shift envelope. Several preliminary clinical investigations have demonstrated the potential clinical benefits of these indices (Campbell et al., 1987; Schulman et al., 1987). There is, however, a significant dearth of information on gestation specific distribution characteristics of the Doppler indices measured in a longitudinal manner in a normal population. In order to address this issue, this study was undertaken to characterize the changes in the umbilical arterial Doppler velocity waveform measured longitudinally in a normal pregnant population, and expressed as Doppler indices.

## MATERIALS AND METHODS

### Instrumentation

A continuous wave bidirectional Doppler equipment was used. This includes a 4 mHz transducer, a Fast Fourier Transform (FFT) Spectral Analyzer, and a Video Monitor Display (Angioscan, Ultrasonix, North Yonkers, NY). The instrument performs the FFT processing in real time, stores up to 13 seconds of spectral data continuously, and can average one, two, four, or eight frames of these data. Differential time and frequency measurements are accomplished by moving appropriate cursor lines on frozen frame display of the spectral shift. The results can be printed or can be stored in a microcomputer. The equipment contains a thump filter (300 Hz) which was not used during the current investigation.

### Patient Population

The study population consisted of three hundred and fifty-three pregnant women without any complications of pregnancy and having normal outcome. The Doppler measurements were performed in a longitudinal manner, beginning from 18 weeks to term gestation.

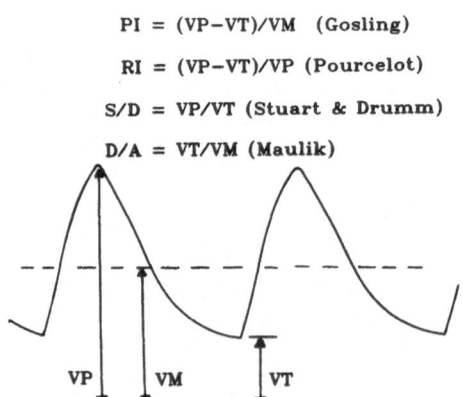

Figure 1. Graphic depiction of the Doppler Indices. PI, Pulsatility Index; RI, Resistance Index; S/D, Systolic to Diastolic Ratio; D/A, Diastolic to Average Ratio; VP, Peak Systolic Velocity; VM, Mean Velocity; VT, End-Diastolic Velocity.

Table 1

Variation in Doppler Indices at Different Stages of Gestation

| Doppler Indices | | Gestation (Weeks) | | | | | | | | | | |
|---|---|---|---|---|---|---|---|---|---|---|---|---|
| | | 18 | 20 | 22 | 24 | 26 | 28 | 30 | 32 | 34 | 36 | 38 |
| RI | Mean | 0.78 | 0.77 | 0.74 | 0.69 | 0.70 | 0.70 | 0.51 | 0.65 | 0.63 | 0.63 | 0.62 |
| | SEM | 0.01 | 0.01 | 0.02 | 0.01 | 0.01 | 0.01 | 0.02 | 0.01 | 0.01 | 0.01 | 0.01 |
| PI | Mean | 1.31 | 1.27 | 1.18 | 1.12 | 1.11 | 1.12 | 1.02 | 0.99 | 0.95 | 0.92 | 0.92 |
| | SEM | 0.03 | 0.03 | 0.03 | 0.05 | 0.03 | 0.03 | 0.04 | 0.03 | 0.04 | 0.02 | 0.03 |
| S/D | Mean | 4.62 | 4.70 | 4.00 | 3.48 | 3.59 | 3.60 | 3.16 | 3.04 | 2.91 | 2.90 | 2.70 |
| | SEM | 0.26 | 0.26 | 0.15 | 0.16 | 0.15 | 0.18 | 0.17 | 0.13 | 0.22 | 0.08 | 0.08 |
| D/A | Mean | 0.38 | 0.37 | 0.41 | 0.44 | 0.46 | 0.46 | 0.51 | 0.52 | 0.53 | 0.56 | 0.55 |
| | SEM | 0.03 | 0.02 | 0.01 | 0.01 | 0.02 | 0.02 | 0.03 | 0.02 | 0.02 | 0.01 | 0.01 |

RI = Resistance Index; PI = Pulsatility Index; S/D = Systolic to Diastolic Ratio;
D/A = Diastolic to Average Ratio; SEM = Standard Error of the Mean

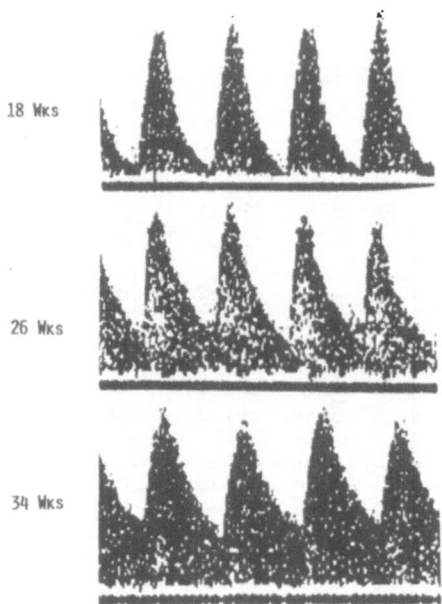

18 Wks

26 Wks

34 Wks

Figure 2.  Changes in the umbilical arterial Doppler frequency shift waveforms with the progression of gestation.

## Procedure

With the patient lying in a modified Fowler's position with left lateral tilt, the Doppler transducer was placed on the maternal abdomen, and was systematically manipulated in order to obtain the umbilical arterial Doppler waveform. The typical configuration of the waveform and the characteristic audio output enabled ready recognition of the umbilical Doppler signal. In order to ensure complete Doppler interrogation of the umbilical cord, care was taken to obtain umbilical venous Doppler shifts (which were in the opposite direction) along with the arterial waveform. If difficulty was encountered in obtaining the signal, real time two-dimensional imaging was used to identify the cord. As Doppler technique can only underestimate and not overestimate the velocity, only maximum frequency shifts with strong spectral power display were chosen for analysis. Doppler data were rejected when fetal movement, fetal breathing, or hiccup interferred with the measurement; this precaution minimized variations in the angle of insonation.

## Doppler Indices

In this study the following indices were chosen for analysis (Figure 1): a) The Pulsatility Index (PI), (Gosling and King, 1975); b) The Resistance Index (RI), (Pourcelot, 1974); c) The Systolic/Diastolic (S/D) ratio, (Stuart et al., 1980 - as A/B ratio); and d) The Diastolic/Average (D/A) ratio (Maulik et al., 1982 - as V1/VM ratio).

## Data Collection and Analysis

The Doppler results and the clinical data were collected in a microcomputer system (IBM PC AT, Boca Raton, FL) and the analysis was performed using SAS statistical analysis softward package (SAS Institute, Inc., Cary, NC). Means and standard error of the means were computed for each gestational week interval. An analysis of variance was conducted using the data for gestational weeks 18, 28, and 38. Duncan's multiple range test was then applied to test significance of the differences among the three groups.

## RESULTS

The umbilical arterial Doppler waveforms in different stages of gestation show progressive increase in the end diastolic frequency shifts (Figure 2). Table 1 presents the gestational age specific distribution of the Doppler indices (mean ± standard error of the mean). The means for gestational weeks 18, 28, and 38 were significantly different (P < .05) as indicated by the Duncan multiple range test. The means for PI, RI, and SD refect a progression from highest at 18 weeks to lowest at 38 weeks. DA, on the other hand, demonstrated a progression from lowest at 18 weeks to highest at 38 weeks.

## DISCUSSION

The significant differences among the means of different Doppler indices at 18, 28, and 38 weeks reflect the remarkable and consistent decline in the flow pulsatility and concomitant progressive increase in the end diastolic flow velocity in the feto-placental circulation. These observations are, in general, consistent with the previous reports on changes in the umbilical Doppler indices during pregnancy (Schulman et al., 1984; Reuwer et al., 1984; Trudinger et al., 1985). There are, however, discrepancies in terms of the detailed characteristics of these changes. The current results contradict the findings of Reuwer et al. (1984) in relation to the values of PI in earlier pregnancy. In the present study, the PI remained below 0.8 throughout the same duration of pregnancy, in contrast to the findings of Reuwer et al. (1984), which demonstrated that the mean value of PI was higher than 1, until 28 weeks of pregnancy. Moreover, the S/D ratio, demonstrated higher mean values at all stages of gestation, than those reported by Trudinger et al. (1985). Obviously, further studies are required to resolve these discrepancies, which may be related to normal biological variations, population differences, or use of different techniques and protocols. The main objective of these approaches in relation to studying the umbilical arterial flow velocity is to obtain an angle-independent measure of the continuing flow in diastole so that one can assess impedence to pulsatile flow in the downstream circulation. This forward diastolic flow is a distinct characteristic of the feto-placental circulation which it shares with other circulations, such as utero-placental, carotid, and pulmonary. Of all the indices, the S/D ratio is the most studied in relation to feto-placental circulation. Its main disadvantage is that its value approaches infinity as the end-diastolic velocity approaches zero. This feature may diminish the utility of S/D ratio precisely in the circumstance where feto-placental perfusion tends to be most compromised. The PI, RI, and D/A ratio remain underinvestigated. Of these, the unique theoretical advantage of the D/A ratio is that it offers a direct, normalized evaluation of the end-diastolic velocity.

The plateau effect observed in the mean Doppler indices (Table 1) during 26 to 28 weeks should be viewed with caution. There are no currently known physiological or morphological changes in the fetal or fetoplacental circulation that can explain these changes. Moreover, the role of random biological variations in the indices in producing this effect cannot be ruled out. Obviously, this finding warrants further investigation.

Other modes of waveform analysis include those of Maulik et al. (1982), Campbell et al. (1983), and Thompson et al. (1985). The common theme of all these techniques is to produce a comprehensive analysis of the Doppler waveform. Maulik et al. (1982) described a method of analysis which involved: a) re-processing of the waveform by coherent averaging in order to reduce spectral variance, and b) a comprehensive measurement of the waveform in both frequency and time domains by using 10 points on the maximum frequency shift envelope. Campbell et al. (1983) described a technique in which the entire waveform is normalized, which thus becomes independent of the angle of insonation, and the length of the cardiac cycle. The normalized waveform is called the Frequency Profile Index (FPI). A waveform is judged abnormal if two or more points are outside the normal range of FPI. Thompson et al. (1985) averaged the waveform, following which an analytic function of the form was fitted to the representative waveform, and a variety of indices were generated. It remains to be shown whether all these approaches are superior to the simpler indices as a clinical tool.

In conclusion, it is apparent that the indices characterizing the umbilical arterial Doppler waveform demonstrate gestation specific changes. This observed trend may, in general, be attributable to progressively decreasing pulsatility and downstream impedance in the feto-placental arterial circulation. Obviously, there are a number of methodological and hemodynamic issues that need further resolution.

## SUMMARY

Doppler velocimetric assessment of the umbilical circulation was performed in 353 fetuses between 18 and 38 weeks of gestation. A continuous wave Doppler instrument with a 4 mHz transducer and an FFT analyzer was used. The indices measured were PI, RI, S/D, and D/A. An analysis of variance employing Duncan's multiple-range test showed statistically significant changes ($P < .05$) in the indices at 18, 28, and 38 weeks. This observation reflects gestation age specific complex hemodynamic alterations in the fetoplacental circulation, and needs further investigation.

## REFERENCES

Campbell, S., Diaz-Recasens, J., Griffin, D., Cohen-Overbeek, T., Pearce, J.M.F., Willson, K., and Teague, M. (1983) New doppler technique for assessing utero-placental blood flow. *Lancet* i, 675-677.

Campbell, S. and Cohen-Overbeek, T.E. (1987) Doppler investigation of the uteroplacental circulation during pregnancy. In: *Doppler Ultrasound Measurement of Maternal-Fetal Hemodynamics*, (eds.), D. Maulik and D.

McNellis, NICHD Research Planning Workshop, Perinatology Press, Ithaca, NY, pp. 147-165.

Eik-Nes, S.H., Marsal, K., Brubakk, A.O., and Ulstein, M. (1980) Ultrasonic measurements of human fetal blood flow in aorta and umbilical vein: influence of fetal breathing movements. In: *Recent Advances in Ultrasound Diagnosis*, (ed.), A. Kurjak, Excerpta Medica, Amsterdam, Vol. 2, pp. 233-240.

Fitzgerald, D.E. and Drumm, J.E. (1977) Non-invasive measurement of the fetal circulation using ultrasound: a new method. *Br. Med. J.* 2, 1450-1451.

Franklin, D.L., Schlegal, W.A., and Rushmer, R.F. (1961) Blood flow measured by Doppler frequency shift of backscattered ultrasound. *Science* 134, 564-565.

Fronek, A., Johansen, K.H., and Dilley, R.B. (1973) Noninvasive physiologic tests in the diagnosis and characterization of peripheral occlusive disease. *Am. J. Surg.* 126, 205-214.

Gill, R.W., Kossoff, B.J., Trudinger, G.J., and Warren, P.S. (1980) Flow velocity in the venous return from the placenta. In: *Recent Advances in Ultrasound Diagnosis*, (ed.), A. Kurjak, Excerpta Medica, Amsterdam, pp. 229-232.

Gosling, P.G. and King, D.H. (1985) *Ultrasound Angiology. Arteries and Veins*, (eds.), A.W. Marcus and L. Adamson, Churchill Livingstone, Edinburgh, pp. 61-98.

Light, L.H. and G. Cross (1972) *Cardiovascular Data by Transcutaneous Aorta Velography. Blood Flow Measurement*, (ed.), R.C. London, Sector Publishing Limited, London.

Maulik, D., Saini, V.D., Nanda, N.C., and Rosenzweig, M.S. (1982) Doppler evaluation of fetal hemodynamics. *Ultrasound Med. Biol.* 8, 705-710.

Maulik, D., Saini, V.D., and Nanda, N.C. (1983) Doppler assessment of fetoplacental circulatory dynamics. *Trophoblast Res.* 1, 149-158.

McCallum, W.D., Williams, C.S., Napel, S., and Daigle, R.E. (1978) Fetal blood velocity waveforms. *Am. J. Obstet. Gynecol.* 132, 425-429.

Peronneau, P., Deloche, A., Bui-Mong-Hung, H. and Hinglais, J. (1969) Debitmetrie ultrasonore: developpements et application experimentales. *Eur. Surg. Res.* 1, 147-156.

Pourcelot, L. (1974) Applications clinique de l'examen Doppler transcutanc, in Pourcelot, Velocimetric Ultrasonore Doppler, *INSERM*, October 34, 213-240.

Reuwer, P.J.H.M., Bruinse, H.W., Stoutenbeek, P., and Haspels, A.A. (1984) Doppler assessment of the fetal placental circulation in normal and growth retarded fetuses. *Eur. J. Obstet. Gynecol. Reprod. Biol.* 18, 199-205.

Satumora, S. (1957) Ultrasonic doppler method for the inspection of cardiac functions. *J. Acount. Soc. Am.* 29, 1181-1185.

Schulman, H., Fleischer, A., Stern, W., Farmakides, G., Jagani, N., and Blattner, P. (1984) Umbilical velocity wave ratios in human pregnancy. *Am. J. Obstet. Gynecol.* 148, 985-990.

Schulman, H., Ducey, J., Rochelson, B., Framakides, G., Bracero, L., and Fleischer, A. (1987) Abnormal umbilical artery waveforms and umbilical vein flow, (eds.), D. Maulik and D. McNellis, In: *Doppler Ultrasound Measurement of Maternal-Fetal Dynamics,* NICHD Research Planning Workshop, Perinatology Press, Ithaca, NY, pp. 141-146.

Stuart, B., Drumm, J., Fitzgerald, D.E., and Duignan, N.M. (1980) Fetal blood velocity waveform in normal pregnancy. *Br. J. Obstet. Gynecol.* 81, 780-785.

Thompson, R.S., Trudinger, B.J., and Cook, C.M. (1985) Doppler ultrasound waveforms in the fetal umbilical artery: quantitative analysis. *Tech. Ultrasound Med. Biol.* 11, 707-718.

Trudinger, B.J., Giles, W.B., Cook, C.M. Bombardier, J., and Collins L. (1985) Fetal umbilical artery flow velocity waveforms and placental resistance: clinical significance. *Br. J. Obstet. Gynaecol.* 92, 23-30

Trophoblast Research 3:301-307, 1988

# DOPPLER MEASUREMENT OF UTERINE BLOOD FLOW IN THE FIRST TRIMESTER OF NORMAL AND COMPLICATED PREGNANCIES

Isabel Stabile[1], Caterina Bilardo, Marco Panella, Stuart Campbell, and J. Gedis Grudzinskas

Academic Units of Obstetrics and Gynaecology
The London Hospital Medical College and King's College
Hospital Medical School
London, United Kingdom

## INTRODUCTION

The technique of doppler ultrasound has revolutionized our understanding of the changes in uteroplacental blood flow impedance that occur in human pregnancy. Several reports in the last few years have examined the use of doppler ultrasound to detect blood velocity changes in maternal (Campbell et al., 1983), umbilical (Trudinger et al., 1986), and fetal vessels (Griffin et al., 1984). Both pulsed (Erskine and Ritchie, 1985) and continuous wave doppler (Trudinger et al., 1985) have been used to study the flow velocity waveforms in normal and abnormal pregnancies. These studies have concentrated on the latter half of pregnancy, in an attempt to assess the potential clinical value of this non invasive test for the screening and subsequent management of high risk pregnancies.

When an ultrasound beam is directed against a moving boundary, the energy backscattered undergoes a change in frequency known as the Doppler shift, which is proportional to the blood velocity and inversely proportional to the cosine of the angle between the doppler beam and the vessel. The doppler shift may be represented by the on-line spectrum analyzer as a visual display, which is representative of all velocities within the sample volume covering the vessel lumen at the time of insonation.

Cohen-Overbeek et al. (1985) studied 10 normal pregnancies longitudinally from 14 to 20 weeks gestation demonstrating an increase in end diastolic velocities with advancing pregnancy. Our aim was to study the changes in doppler assessed uterine blood flow which occur from 6 to 16 weeks in both normal pregnancies and those complicated by threatened miscarriage (TMC).

## MATERIALS AND METHODS

### Equipment

A pulsed wave doppler duplex system with a sector scanner (ATL 600) was used. The equipment comprises a 3 MHz transducer, with a sample volume 2

---

[1]To Whom Correspondence Should be Addressed: 4th Floor, Holland Wing, The London Hospital, Whitechapel, London, United Kingdom.

millimeters in width and variable gate length, permitting full insonation of the uterine vessels. The beam direction and position of the sample gate was displayed on the real time image and could be altered accordingly (Figure 1). A 100 Hz high pass thump filter was in place to remove any interfering vessel wall signals. As the study progressed, signals were obtained using continuous wave (Doptek, UK) doppler with an on-line spectrum analyzer. Although this device cannot discriminate between signals arising from different moving structures along the beam, it is possible to record flow velocity waveforms (FVW's) resembling those previously described as arcuate artery FVW's. This was done with both continuous wave and pulsed wave apparatus in turn, and the waveforms obtained are depicted in Figures 2 and 3.

## Patients

Pregnant women (n = 115) ranging from 6 to 16 weeks gestation were recruited. Women with uncomplicated singleton pregnancies (n = 73) were asked to have a blood flow examination prior to their antenatal clinic visit, and the remaining 42 women were referred from the Casualty Department with threatened abortion. An acceptable waveform was not obtained in 4 patients who were overweight and at 6 to 8 weeks gestation. The study was performed both cross-sectionally and longitudinally. Satisfactory measurements were obtained on 167 occasions in the 111 women. Informed, verbal consent was obtained from all women prior to the examination.

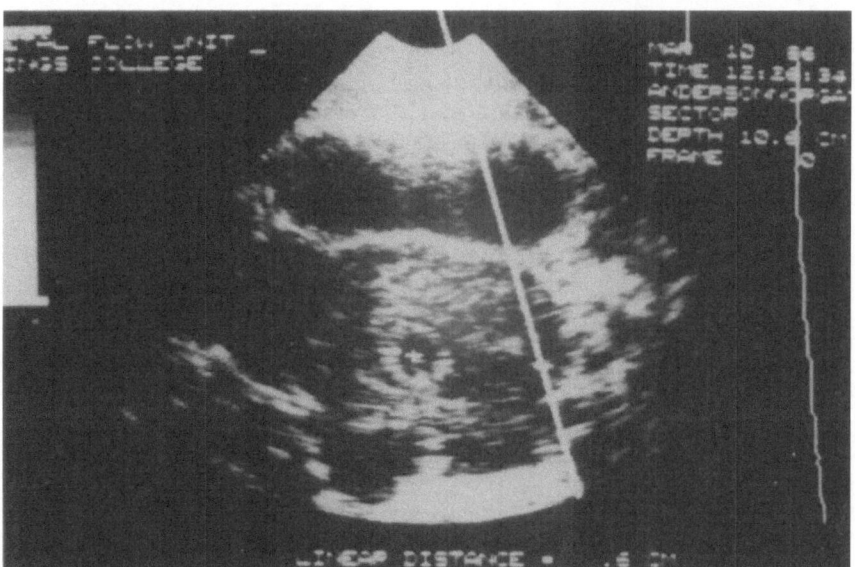

Figure 1. Transverse section of uterus at 6 weeks gestation showing intrauterine fetal pole with a Crown Rump Length (CRL) of 6 mm. The Doppler beam direction and position of sample gate is shown on the right side.

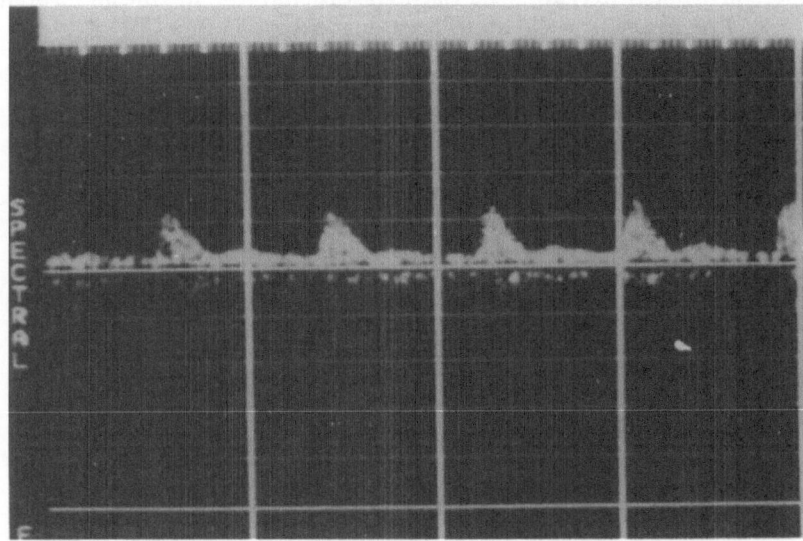

Figure 2. Flow velocity waveforms (FVW's) obtained from the lateral uterine wall at 6 weeks gestation with pulsed wave Doppler.

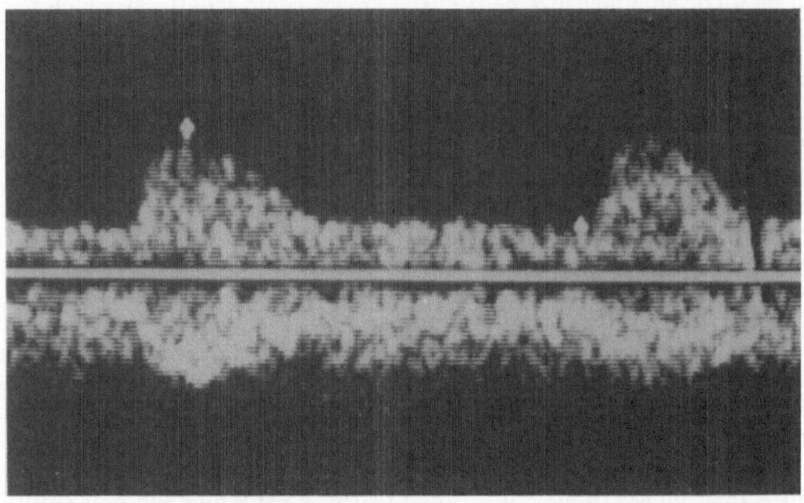

Figure 3. Flow velocity waveforms (FVW's) obtained at the 9th week of an uncomplicated pregnancy with continuous wave Doppler. The FVW's are recognized as being arcuate in origin by their characteristic pattern.

Table 1

Numbers of Women Recruited At Each Gestational Age in Uncomplicated
Pregnancy (n = 73) and Threatened Abortion (n = 38)

| Week of Gestation | Uncomplicated Pregnancy | Threatened Abortion |
|:---:|:---:|:---:|
| 6 | 3 | 2 |
| 7 | 6 | 2 |
| 8 | 11 | 7 |
| 9 | 13 | 2 |
| 10 | 11 | 4 |
| 11 | 10 | 7 |
| 12 | 7 | 1 |
| 13 | 3 | 4 |
| 14 | 5 | 2 |
| 15 | 2 | 4 |
| 16 | 2 | 3 |
| Total | 73 | 38 |

The duration of the pregnancy was determined from menstrual dates and confirmed by ultrasonic measurement of the crown rump length, at which time the fetal heart action was demonstrated. The duration of rest prior to the examination, the time interval since the last meal, and the maternal pulse/blood pressure were recorded on each occassion.

Patients were examined in the supine position with a full bladder in order to visualize the pelvic organs. After locating and measuring the fetus and confirming viability, the transducer was orientated along the transverse axis of the uterus. The doppler beam was then aimed at the lateral wall of the uterus on either side, and the sample gate adjusted accordingly.

The external and internal iliac arteries located, in the pelvic side wall, were easily identified by their typical high pulsatility sonograms. Furthermore, blood flow in these vessels is in the opposite direction to the uterine artery and can therefore be distinguished from the arcuate artery FVW using a bidirectional doppler system.

Off screen photographs were taken of the FVW's and the A/B ratio (Peak systole over peak diastole described by Stuart et al. (1980). Resistance Index (Peak systole minus peak diastole over peak systole described by Poucelot, 1974) were measured using vernier calipers, taking the mean of three cycles. The on-line spectrum analyzer of the Doptek automatically calculated the A/B ratio and Resistance Index (RI). These values for RI and A/B were computerized in order to analyze the data.

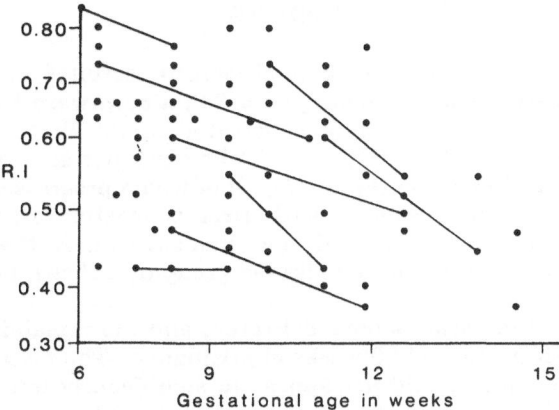

Figure 4. Measurements of resistance index plotted against gestational age in 50 uncomplicated pregnancies. Serial observations in 8 patients are superimposed showing the fall in RI with advancing gestational age.

## REPRODUCIBILITY STUDIES

A difference of 5% between the readings taken with either apparatus in the same patient by the same observer were demonstrated. The within observer coefficient of variation (CV), which was determined by performing the measurements three times in the same individual, was 15%. The between observer CV, which was investigated by asking 4 observers in turn to obtain the waveform without prior knowledge of each others performance, was 12%.

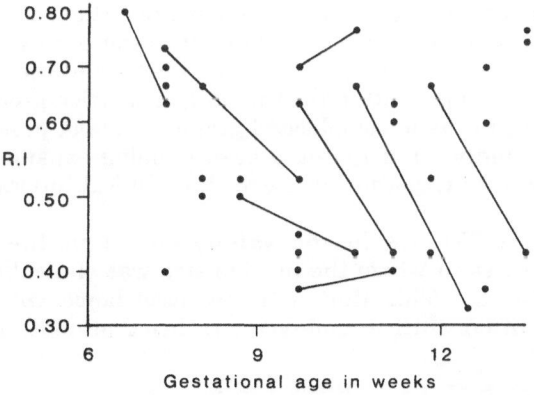

Figure 5. Measurements of resistance index (n = 34) plotted against gestational age in 25 patients with threatened abortion and normal outcome. Serial observations in 6 out of 8 patients demonstrate a more marked rate of change in RI than in the uncomplicated pregnancy group.

## RESULTS

Table 1 summarizes the numbers of women recruited at each gestational age. By studying patients longitudinally (n = 30), a downward trend of resistance from 6 to 16 weeks gestation was demonstrated in the first 50 uncomplicated pregnancies studied successfully (Figure 4). The same pattern was seen in the 38 women with threatened abortion (Figure 5), all of whom progressed uneventfully to 20 weeks gestation. Four women with first trimester losses (anembryonic pregnancy) were also studied. All had measurements that could not be distinguished from those in the uncomplicated group (not shown in Figure 5).

Over 75% of the patients have delivered, and the remaining patients have progressed uneventfully beyond 20 weeks of pregnancy. The maternal condition at the time of the examination did not appear to significantly influence the results obtained.

## DISCUSSION

In the first trimester of pregnancy, there is a complex vascular arrangement within a relatively minute area. The wide range of measurements that were obtained at each gestational age may reflect different degrees of trophoblast invasion in each vessel, as the uteroplacental circulation is not definitively established until the second trimester of pregnancy (Pijenborg and Dixon, 1980). Nevertheless, Doppler signals from this site that visually and audibly resemble those that have been conventionally accepted as arcuate FVW in the second trimester were obtained.

Serial measurements of uteroplacental FVW conducted at 14 day intervals have shown a trend in falling RI values through the first trimester. This pattern represents the early stage of the ongoing process described by Cohen-Overbeek et al. (1985) in the second trimester, which ends when the second wave of trophoblast erosion of the spiral arteries is complete.

There was a great deal of overlap between the values for RI in our uncomplicated and threatened abortion group, since these pregnancies progressed uneventfully to 20 weeks. However, serial measurements in these two groups have shown that the rate of change of RI in the threatened abortion group is more marked (Figures 4 and 5) than in the uncomplicated group. It is not possible to provide an explanation for this finding, but the data base is being expanded to explore this observation which may be of pathophysiological or clinical interest.

No apparent difference in the values for RI in the 4 patients with anembryonic pregnancies in whom the uterine size was clinically compatible with their dates were found. This finding is in accordance with the underlying pathology of the condition which is embryonic rather than maternal in origin.

## SUMMARY

In a prospective study of uterine blood flow of 111 women, it was possible to obtain flow velocity waveforms (FVW's) from as early as 6 weeks of pregnancy. A downward trend in RI with advancing gestational age is seen. Maternal uterine blood flow impedance does not appear to differ in women with threatened abortion who have a normal outcome. The use of this non-invasive technique will help to improve our understanding of the development of the uteroplacental circulation.

## ACKNOWLEDGMENTS

The authors gratefully acknowledge the help of Dr. Titia Cohen-Overbeek in supervising this manuscript. We also thank the staff of the Ultrasound Department at King's College Hospital and the women concerned for permission to carry out this study.

## REFERENCES

Campbell, S., Diaz-Recasens, J., Griffin, D.R., Cohen-Overbeek, T., Pearce, J.M.F., Wilson, K., and Teague, M.J. (1983) New doppler technique for assessing uteroplacental blood flow. *Lancet* i, 675-677.

Cohen-Overbeek, T., Pearce, M., and Campbell, S. (1985) The antenatal assessment of uteroplacental and fetoplacental blood flow using doppler ultrasound. *Ultrasound Med. Biol.* 11, 329-331.

Erskine, R.L.A, and Ritchie, J.W.K. (1985) Umbilical artery blood flow characteristics in normal and growth retarded fetuses. *Br. J. Obstet. Gynaecol.* 92, 605-610.

Griffin, D., Bilardo, C., Masini, L., Diaz-Recasens, J., Pearce, M., Willson, K., and Campbell, S. (1984) Doppler blood flow waveforms in the descending thoracic aorta of the human fetus. *Br. J. Obstet. Gynaecol.* 91, 997-1006.

Pijenborg, R. and Dixon, H.G. (1980) Trophoblastic invasion of human decidua from 8 to 18 weeks of pregnancy. *Placenta* 1, 3-19.

Pourcelot L. (1974) Applications clinique de l'examen doppler trancutanie. In: *Velocimetric Ultrasonor Doppler,* (ed.) Peronneau. P., INSERM, vol. 34, pp. 213-240.

Stuart, B., Drumm, J., Fitzgerald, D.E., and Duigan, N.M. (1980) Fetal blood velocity waveforms in normal pregnancy. *Br. J. Obstet. Gynaecol.* 87, 780-785.

Trudinger, B.J., Giles, W.B., and Cook, C.M. (1985) Uteroplacental blood flow velocity time waveforms in normal and complicated pregnancy. *Br. J. Obstet. Gynaecol.* 92, 39-45.

Trudinger, B.J., Cook, C.M., Jones, L., and Giles, W.B. (1986) A comparison of fetal heart rate monitoring and umbilical artery waveforms in the recognition of fetal compromise. *Br. J. Obstet. Gynaecol.* 93, 171-175.

Trophoblast Research 3:309-323, 1988

# PLACENTAL CORRELATES OF ABNORMAL UMBILICAL DOPPLER INDEX

Catherine Nessmann[1,3], Yolene Huten[1], and Michele Uzan[2]

[1]Laboratoire de Biologie du Developpement et de la Reproduction
CHU Xavier Bichat
16 Rue Henri Huchard
75018 Paris, France

[2]Clinique Baudelocque
123 Boulevard de Port-Royal
75014 Paris, France

## INTRODUCTION

Doppler investigation applied to obstetrics has opened new fields in the knowledge of the fetus and the surveillance of pregnancy. The study of umbilical artery flow velocity profiles has been used to provide an index of blood flow resistance in the fetoplacental circulation.

Various indices have been proposed, based maximum systolic and diastolic velocities. Abnormally high resistance is observed in many maternal pathological conditions associated with arterial hypertension and intrauterine growth retardation (IUGR).

An elevated resistance has also been noted in major fetal anomalies. The placenta was naturally thought to be the site of this high vascular resistance. However, little is known about the morphological basis of placental alterations underlying abnormal Doppler indices. In particular, little attention has yet been paid to the pathology of such placentae, and in addition, morphometric description of the fetal vessels which have been investigated is still missing.

Thus, the present work was more specifically focused on these two aspects of perinatal pathology.

## PATIENTS AND METHODS

Placentae (61) routinely explored by Doppler ultrasound velocimetry were submitted for macro- and microscopic examination. In addition, histomorphometric study was performed on the umbilical vessels.

[3]To Whom Correspondence Should be Addressed

## Patients

Twenty-three originated from normal pregnancies, 38 from complicated pregnancies: 24 hypertension, 14 other pathology, without sustained hypertension (6 IUGR, 3 tobacco smoking, 2 diabetes mellitus, and 3 various).

The condition of the infants at birth can be summarized as follows: 39 were of normal weight, 18 were small-for-dates (less than 10th centile) using the birthweight curve of Leroy and Lefort (1971). There were 4 stillborn.

All the placentae were explored at least once by pulsed Doppler, at the level of umbilical arteries using a DOP 104 apparatus (Compagnie Generale de Radiologie, Meaux, France). The index used in this study was determined by the ratio of D/S, where D represented diastolic velocity (permanent placental blood flow) and S represented the peak systolic velocity. There was a progressive rise of this index during pregnancy which indicates a decrease in peripheral resistance. Curves of normality with means, 10th and 90th centile between 20 and 40 weeks were established by Uzan et al. (1987). The measurements were performed in the days or weeks preceeding delivery (1 day to 8 weeks). All umbilical cords were immediately clamped at delivery.

## Placental Examination

All of the placentae were macroscopically examined after formalin fixation. Placentae were weighed without membranes and cord, and cut into parallel slices at 1 cm intervals.

Placentae of normal weight (300 to 600 g at term) and without any significant lesions were considered normal.

Different aspects of placental pathology have been taken into account: vascular lesions (hypotrophy: less than 300 g at term, infarcts: more than 3, massive or basal perivillous fibrin deposition, retroplacental hematoma); "hypermaturity", estimated by a score which includes 4 stages based upon the sum of 7 parameters (lobation, congestion, septa, subchorial thrombosis, calcifications, subchorial, or marginal perivillous fibrin deposition, and marginal infarct). The last stage characterizes this category; major abnormalities of placental shape (extrachorialis, multipartita), or of the cord (velamentous insertion, single umbilical artery); other anomalies such as hydrops, hypertrophy (more than 600 g at term) were included.

## Histological Examination

Two samples were taken systematically, one from the central part of the placenta (including chorionic and basal plates) in a macroscopically normal area and one from the proximal part of the cord (less than 5 cm from the placental insertion).

After paraffin embedding and hematein-eosin-safran staining, a classic histological study was conducted on villi, fetal vessels of chorionic and stem branches, maternal vessels (infarcts, collapsed intervillous space; uteroplacental arteries were noted), calcifications, and inflammatory lesions (chorioammiotitis, funisitis, villitis).

For the section of the cord, the appearance of the lumen for arteries (narrow or large) and the abundance of Wharton's jelly were described. In the conclusion of the histological examination, three groups were distinguished: normal, subnormal (moderate or focal alterations), and pathological (important or extensive lesion). Lesions related to vascular alterations of maternal or fetal origin were separated. Forty-nine were available for histological study.

Histomorphometric measurements were achieved on umbilical vessels with the help of an Apple II computer programmed to calculate several parameters such as lumen's surface and thickness of the vascular wall. Histological sections were first reproduced via camera lucida (Carl Zeiss). Thirty-one cords underwent such measurements. Statistical assessment involved CHI-Square analysis.

## RESULTS

Clinical aspects are summarized in the first two tables. The Dopper index was normal 52 times, and in particular in 29 complicated pregnancies (Table 1). On the contrary, it was abnormal only in 9 cases, and always in severe pathology (p < 0.05).

Doppler index was normal for all newborns of normal birthweight, but also for 13 of the 18 small-for-dates (Table 2). It was abnormal 9 times. Five cases had a very low index (< 10th centile), two infants were alive and 3 were stillborn. Three cases had a zero diastolic component, two were alive and one was stillborn. In one case, it was the progressive diminution of the index between 25 or 34 weeks, associated with alteration of the fetal cardiac rhythm, which was considered as abnormal, the infant was alive.

In this group, it is interesting to consider that two of these infants were malformed. One was alive with a 21 trisomy, the other had a cerebral malformation diagnosed ultrasonographically, and the pregnancy was medically interrupted. The three other stillborns did not exhibit any malformation, and a maternal diagnosis of severe hypertension was present. No karyotype could be performed on the stillborns.

The conclusions of macroscopic examination of the placenta are regrouped in Table 3. Large and obvious lesions or alterations were observed in 19 out of the 52 cases with a normal Doppler index, whereas they were observed in 8 out of 9 cases with an abnormal Doppler index (p < 0.02). The number of small-for-dates is indicated in brackets for each category of lesions. On the other hand, placental lesions were almost always obvious when the Doppler was abnormal. Nevertheless, one of these placentae was considered normal from the macroscopic point of view.

## Table 1

### Clinical Aspects of Pregnancy

| Pregnancy | Doppler Index | | Total |
|---|---|---|---|
| | Normal | Abnormal | |
| Normal | 23 | - | 23 |
| Hypertension | 18 | 6 | 24 |
| Other Pathologies | 11 | 3 | 14 |
| Total | 52 | 9 | 61 |

## Table 2

### Condition of the Infants at Birth

| Infants | Doppler Index | | Total |
|---|---|---|---|
| | Normal | Abnormal | |
| Normal weight | 39 | - | 39 |
| Small for dates | 13 | 5 | 18 |
| Stillborn | - | 4 | 4 |
| Total | 52 | 9 | 61 |

## Table 3

### Macroscopic Examination of the Placenta

| Placenta | Doppler Index | | Total |
|---|---|---|---|
| | Normal | Abnormal | |
| Normal | 33 (4) | 1 (1) | 34 (5) |
| Vascular lesions | 4 (2) | 6 (6) | 10 (8) |
| Hypermaturity | 7 (4) | 2 (2) | 9 (6) |
| Shape anomalies Cord | 6 (1) | - - | 6 (1) |
| Others | 2 (2) | - - | 2 (2) |
| Total | 52 (13) | 9 (9) | 61 (22) |

Table 4

Histologic Examination of the Placenta

| | Doppler Index | |
| | Normal (n = 41) | Abnormal (n = 8) |
|---|---|---|
| **Villi** | | |
| Hypotrophy | 14 | 6 |
| Capillaries | 19 | 5 |
| Trophoblast | 9 | 5 |
| Other alterations | 10 | 1 |
| **Fetal Vessels** | | |
| Endarteritis | 11 | 6 |
| Arterial Stenosis | 16 | 6 |
| Fibrinous Vasculosis | 10 | 4 |
| Venous Thrombosis | 0 | 1 |
| **Maternal Vessels** | | |
| Infarcts | 5 | 5 |
| Intervillous Space | 4 | 2 |
| **Cord** | | |
| Constricted Arteries | 4 | 4 |
| Large Arteries | 37 | 4* |
| Wharton Jelly | 14 | 6 |
| **Calcifications** | 17 | 0 |
| **Inflammatory Lesions** | | |
| Chorioammiotitis | 5 | 0 |
| Funisitis | 4 | 0 |
| Focal Villitis | 2 | 2 |
| **Conclusions** | | |
| Normal | 13 | |
| Subnormal | 19 (17**) | 1 (1**) |
| Abnormal | 9 (5**) | 7 (7**) |

\* Stillborn
\*\* Hypoxic Lesions

Table 5

Vascular Surfaces of Umbilical Vessels

| Doppler Index | Arteries (mm²) | | Veins (mm²) | |
|---|---|---|---|---|
| | Lumen | Media | Lumen | Media |
| Abnormal n = 4 | 0.030 ± 0.021 | 1.53 ± 0.38 | 0.77 ± 0.75 | 1.35 ± 0.21 |
| Normal n = 5 | 0.13 ± 0.07 | 1.66 ± 0.40 | 1.16 ± 0.58 | 1.87 ± 0.73 |

The results of histological study of the placentae are detailed in Table 4. It was tentatively concluded that the villous or vascular lesions could be related to chronic hypoxia from the other types of pathology (number in brackets). Placentae with normal Doppler indices (17 - 41%) represented mild or moderate alterations of this type. The lesions were extensive in 12% (5) of the placentae. When the Doppler index was abnormal, none of the histology was interpreted as normal. All placentae presented moderate (1 of 8) or extensive (7 of 8) hypoxic lesions ($p < 0.01$). The umbilical arteries appeared constricted in all cases of infants alive who had an abnormal Doppler index (4 of 4), whereas the aspect was only rarely observed in cases with a normal index (4 of 41), $p < 0.01$.

The morphometric study of umbilical vessels is presented in Table 5 and Figure 1. Four stillborn fetuses which were macerated to various degrees were excluded from this part of the study since fetal lethality leads to passive dilatation of the vessels. There was a positive correlation between the surface of the fetal arteries and the Doppler index. The lumen of the umbilical arteries always seemed to be reduced when the index was abnormal. The results were similar regardless of whether the gestational ages were the same (Table 5) or different (Table 6).

## DISCUSSION

The increased vascular resistance measured in the umbilical arteries may have a placental or fetal origin. The fact that it is mainly observed in maternal diseases with hypertension and IUGR prompted the study of the placenta in order to establish the morphological correlate of placental insufficiency.

Table 6

Vascular Surfaces: Lumen of Umbilical Arteries

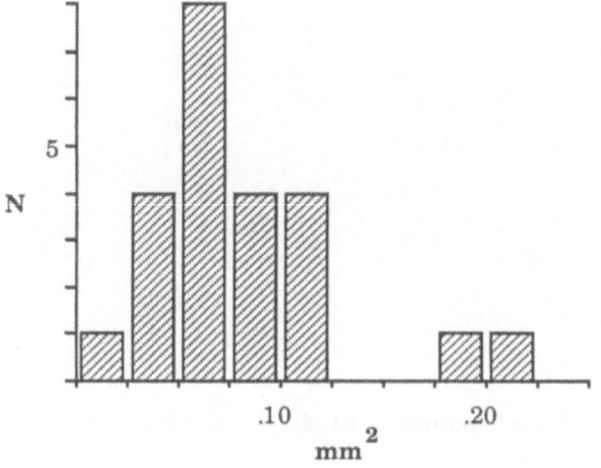

Normal Doppler Index
n = 23
0.082 ± 0.047

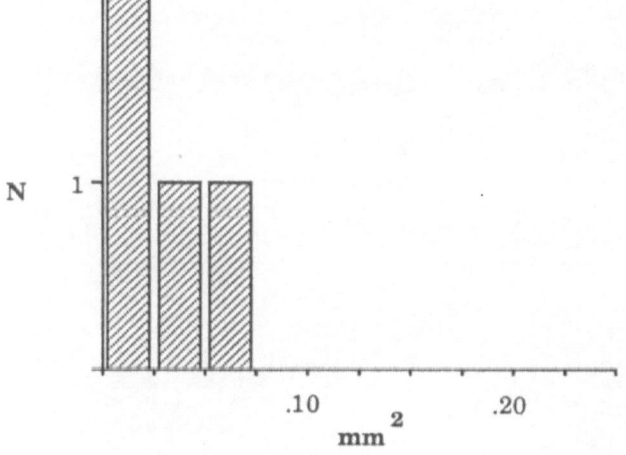

Abnormal Doppler Index
n = 4
0.030 ± 0.021

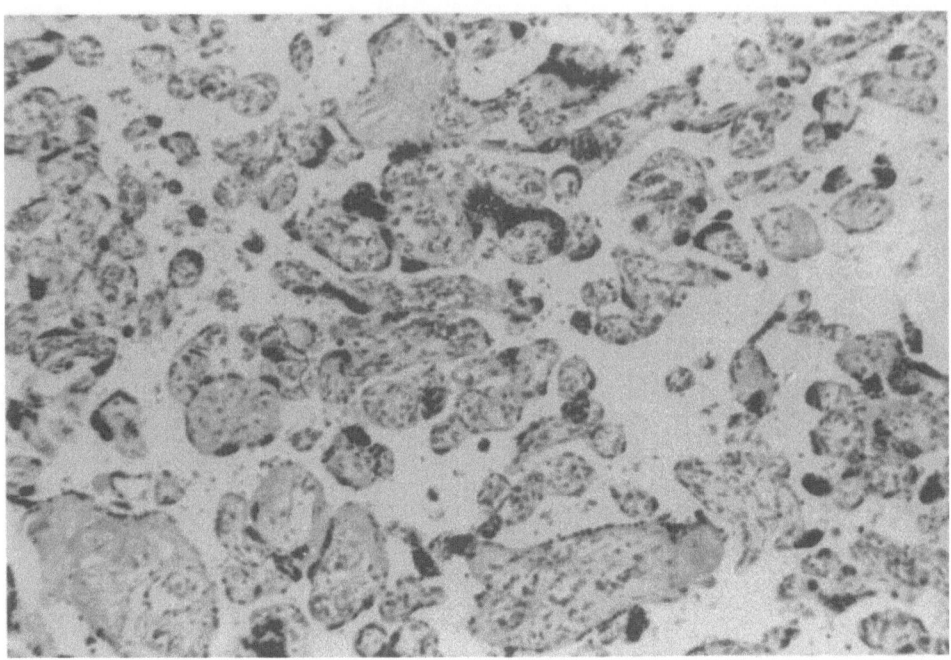

Figure 1.  Villous hypotrophy (X100).

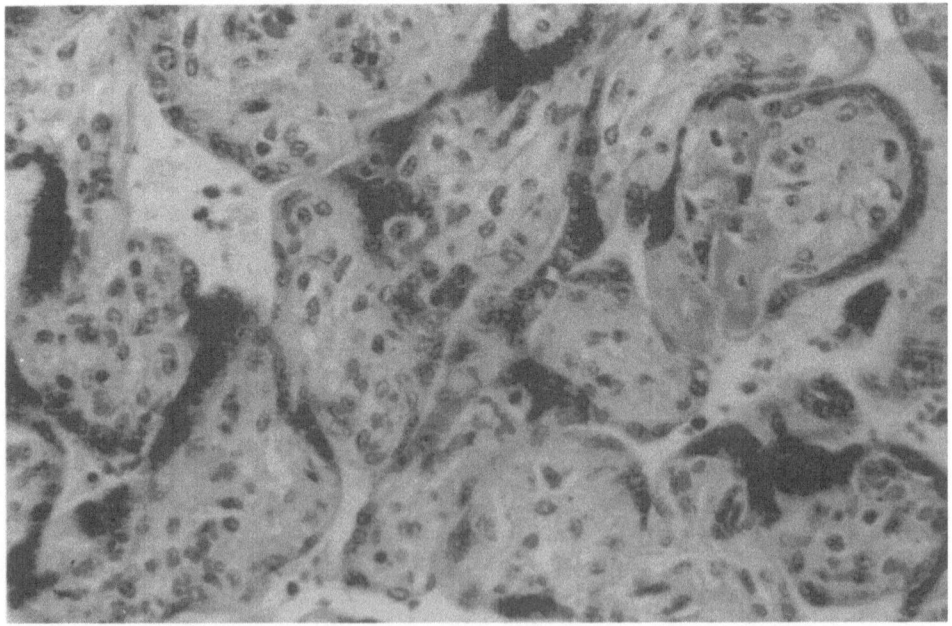

Figure 2.  Excess of villous syncytial sprouts, reduced capillaries, collapsed intervillous spaces (X250).

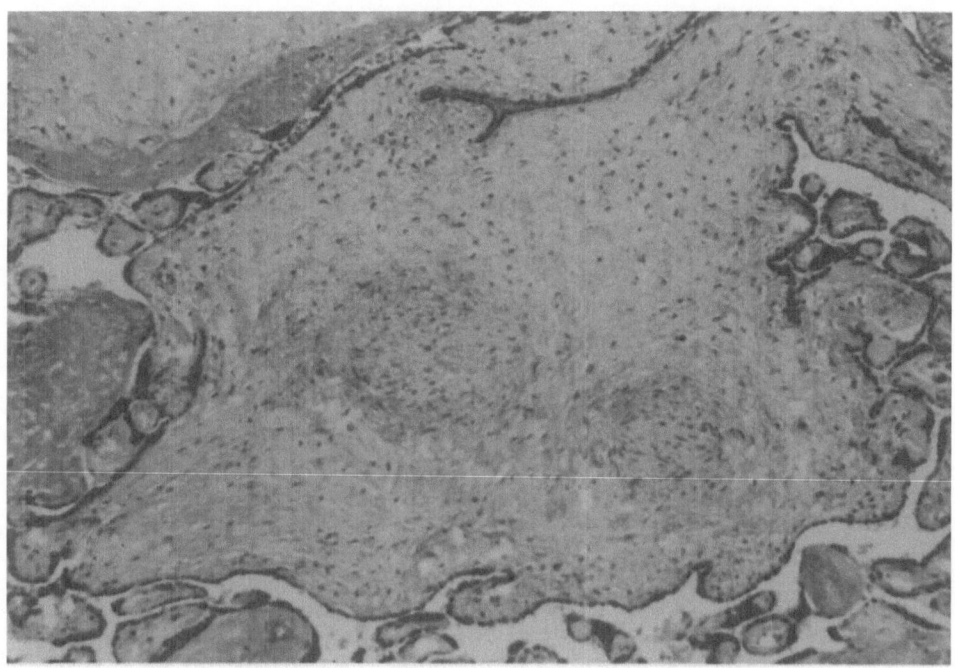

Figure 3. Stem villi: vascular stenosis (X100).

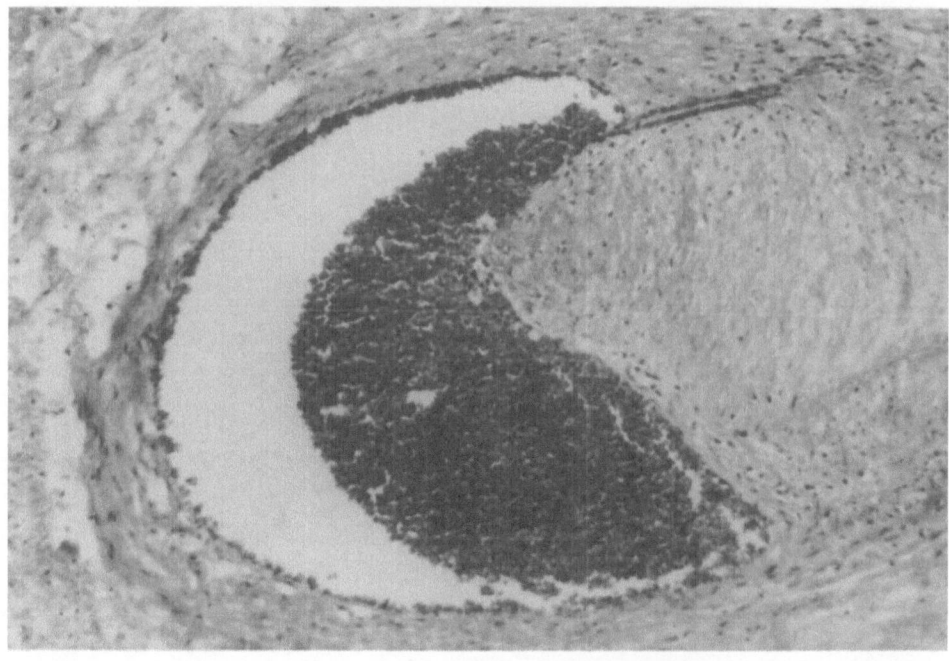

Figure 4. Chorionic vessel: venous cushion (X250).

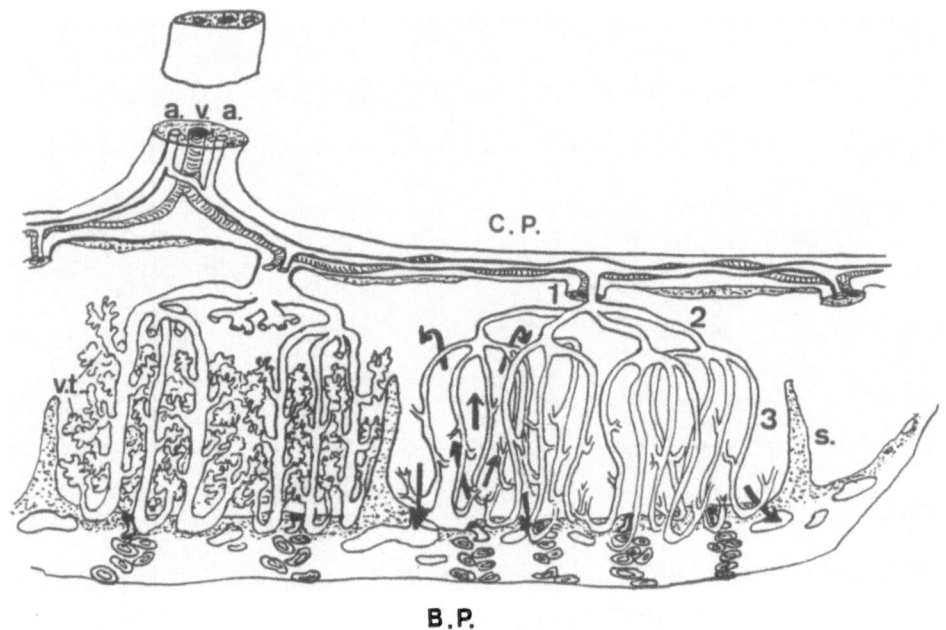

Figure 5. Schematic representation of placental vascularization.  CP = chorionic plate; BP = basal plate; AV = umbilical arteries and vein; 1, 2, 3 = stem villi of 1st, 2nd, and 3rd order.

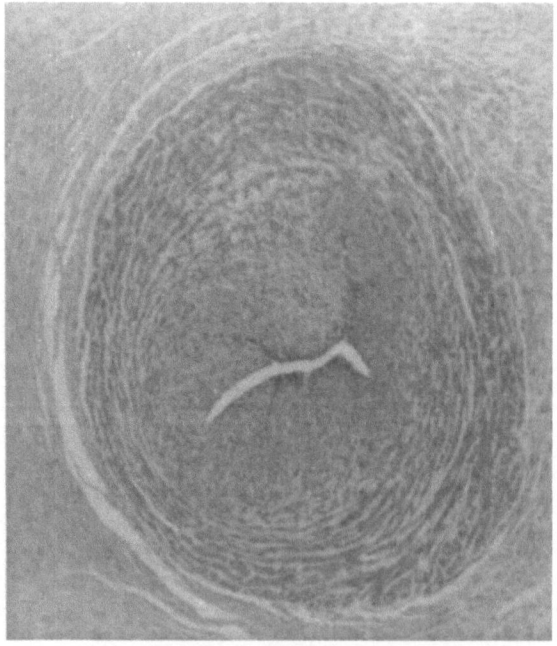

Figure 6. Umbilical artery with constricted lumen (X40).

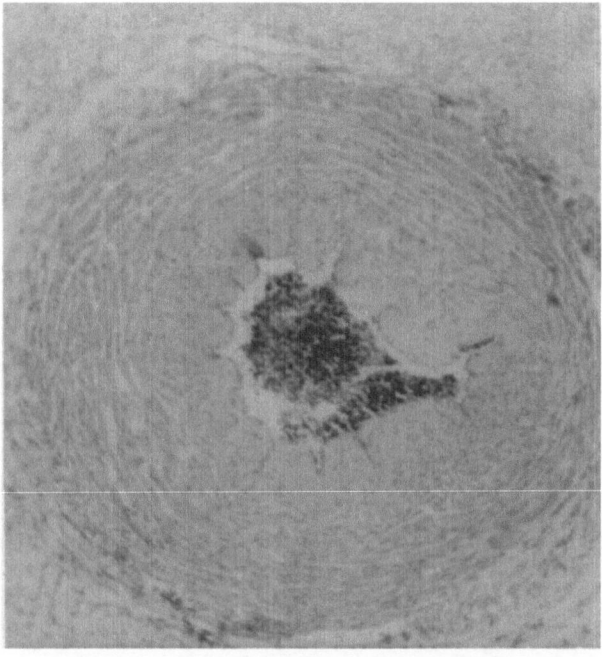

Figure 7. Umbilical artery with large lumen (X40).

Giles et al. (1985) were the first to correlate placental microvascular anatomy with antenatal assessment of umbilical circulation. They reported a reduced number of third order fetal stem arteries, most likely related to a high vascular resistance, and probably secondary to an obliterative process.

This important work can be compared to the study of Las Heras et al. (1985) who observed a diminished diameter in the lumen of these same arteries associated with an excess of syncytial sprouts, in pregnancies complicated by hypertension. These authors suggest that hypoxia can generate both alterations by releasing specific substances into the maternal circulation, which could affect the fetal circulation. Thus, fetal vessels would participate in the process of hypertension in reducing the effective surface of feto-maternal exchanges.

The presence of areas of avascular villi and diminished numbers of villous capillaries due to placental insufficiency as described in earlier work (Gruenwald, 1963; Aladjem, 1970), have probably the same significance.

In the current study, the macroscopic and histologic lesions of placentae antenatally explored by Doppler ultrasound have been conducted. This aspect of perinatal pathology has not been detailed in previous publications. Secondary, a simple, easily reproducible approach to fetal vessels is proposed. This is the reason for which the umbilical vessels were chosen. Little correlation was found between macroscopic lesions or abnormalities of the placenta and the results of Doppler investigation. The latter may be normal despite large and obvious lesions which were present in one third of the cases. The large reserve functional capacity of the placenta can easily explain this initially surprising result.

A variable relationship was found between the histological lesions of the placenta and the results of Doppler investigation. In addition to villous alterations related to hypoxia (Aladjem, 1968, 1970; Fox, 1978) (Figures 1 and 2), special attention was given to the alterations of fetal vessels which are variously name in the literature: obliterative endarteritis, fibromuscular sclerosis, vascular thrombosis (Fox, 1978), fibrinous vasculosis, and venous cushions (Scott, 1983) (Figures 3 and 4). Their significance is still obscure.

This fetal vascular pathology is probably also related to chronic hypoxia, as it has been described with a high incidence in placental insufficiency (Scott, 1983). Such pathology was found very frequently (57%) in the group with normal Doppler index which was partly a high risk group (Table 1), but the lesions were mild to moderate in most of these cases. In contrast, these lesions were always present in the small group with abnormal Doppler index, and they were mild only in one case.

Nevertheless, it is difficult to quantify this aspect of pathology, because of the heterogeneity of placental substance, and of the hazardous character of sampling. This is the reason why this work was focused on umbilical vessels, which reflect the whole placental circulation, and are easy to sample.

The umbilical arteries appeared very constricted upon the histological examination, when the Doppler was abnormal. The morphometric study confirmed this impression. The surface of the lumen of umbilical arteries seems always to be reduced in these cases (Figures 6 and 7). The preliminary results, which were reinforced by a larger series currently under investigation, concur with some recent study. Makila et al. (1983) have shown a direct relationship between fetal blood flow and umbilical prostacyclin production. This production is reduced in pre-eclampsia or complicated pregnancies. Such a reduction has also been reported by Dadak et al. (1982) in the placentae from smoking mothers. As prostacyclin is a vasodilator and anti-aggregatory agent, its diminution may be responsible for vasoconstriction.

Morphological alterations of the intima of umbilical arteries have been described by Asmussen and Kjeldsen (1975) in the case of smoking, and by Dadak et al. (1984) in pre-eclampsia, by electron micrograph studies. These vascular lesions may lead to a disturbed arterial flow, but they also may be indicative of more generalized abnormalities of the whole fetal arterial system. Another hypothesis to explain the reduction in the lumen of umbilical arteries when the Doppler index is abnormal could be a chronic diminution of fetal cardiac blood flow.

Along this line, one can note that a high vascular resistance was not only observed associated with maternal hypertension but also in major fetal abnormalities, as observed in 2 out of the 9 abnormal cases of this series. One fetus presented a cerebral malformation with IUGR. The placenta was macroscopically normal and showed moderate histologic alterations. Histomorphometry could not be performed on the umbilical vessels because of maceration. The other one was a

21 trisomy. The infant was small-for-date, and the placenta was abnormally mature with focal villitis upon histology.

Trudinger and Cook (1985) reported 26 cases of major fetal abnormalities. In 13 cases, fetal blood flow resistance was high, whereas uterine artery waveforms were normal. The placental weights were higher in this group than in the group with a normal fetal blood flow index, but the pathology of these placentae was not detailed. The authors suggested that vascular obliteration could be responsible both for the compensatory overgrowth of the placentae and the high vascular resistance.

Another explanation proposed by Erskine and Ritchie (1985) is the altered blood viscosity frequently observed in growth retarded fetuses. Giles and Trudinger (1986) found an increase in whole blood viscosity at high shear rate, reflecting possibly a change in red cell rigidity as seen in hypoxia, associated with an abnormal pattern in the umbilical artery waveform. They could not yet demonstrate that changes in whole blood viscosity at low shear rates were responsible for the alteration in blood flow resistance.

More studies are necessary to sharpen the predictive value of Doppler index at the level both of the uterine and fetal arteries, and to understand the significance of the high vascular resistances which are observed when the fetus begins to develop a high risk condition.

## SUMMARY

To date, little is known about the morphological relationship to vascular alterations underlying abnormal Doppler indices observed during pregnancy, except for the important work of Giles et al (1985). These authors have reported a reduced number of third order fetal stem arteries, most likely related to a high vascular resistance. However, little attention has yet been paid to the pathology of such placentae, and on the other hand, morphometric description of the fetal vessels which have been investigated, is absent. Thus, the present work was more specifically focused on these two aspects of perinatal pathology. For this purpose, 61 placentae from normal (n = 23) and complicated (n = 38) pregnancies routinely explored by Doppler, were submitted to macro- and microscopic examinations. In addition, histomorphometric studies were achieved on umbilical vessels, with the help of an Apple II computer programmed to calculate several parameters such as the lumen's surface and thickness of the vascular wall.

Tentative conclusions of this combined approach were as follows: 1) surprisingly, there is little correlation between the observed lesions and the results of Doppler investigation, the latter may be normal (n = 52) despite large and obvious lesions (n = 19), or in the case of villous and/or vascular histological alterations, and 2) in contrast, morphometric study revealed a positive correlation between the surface of fetal arteries and the Doppler index. The lumen of umbilical arteries appears to always be reduced when the index was increased. It would be important to determine if this reduction reflected vasoconstriction or diminished blood flow of placental or fetal origin. Along this line, one can note that a high vascular resistance was not only observed associated with hypertension, but also in major fetal abnormalities, as in 2 out of the 9 abnormal cases of this series.

## ACKNOWLEDGEMENTS

We are very grateful to Dr. M.C. Vacher-Lavenue from the Laboratory of Pathologic Anatomy of Hospital Cochin, for the histological documents that she has so generously communicated to us. We thank the staff of Histology of INSERM U. 261 (Institut Pasteur) who familiarized us with the technics of morphometry. We would like to acknowledge Dr. R. Forman for reviewing the english an Dr. G. Breart for statistical advise. This study was partly supported by The Scientific Council of the Medical Faculty of Bichat.

## REFERENCES

Aladjem, S. (1968) An index of syncytial growth in normal and complicated pregnancies. *Am. J. Obstet. Gynecol.* 101, 704-708.

Aladjem, S. (1970) Studies in placental circulation. *Am. J. Obstet. Gynecol.* 107, 88-92.

Asmussen, I. and Kjeldsen, K. (1975) Intimal ultrastructure of human umbilical arteries. Observations of arteries from newborn children of smoking and non-smoking mothers. *Circ. Res.* 36, 579-589.

Campbell, S., Griffin, D.R., Pearce, J.M., Diaz-Recasens, J., Cohen-Overbeek, T.E., Willson, K., and Teague, J.M. (1983) New Doppler technique for assessing uteroplacental blood flow. *Lancet* i, 675-677.

Dadak, C., Kefalides, A., Sinzinger, H., and Weber, G. (1982) Reduced umbilical artery prostacyclin formation and complicated pregnancies. *Am. J. Obstet. Gynecol.* 144, 792-795.

Dadak, C., Ulrich, W., and Sinzinger, H. (1984) Morphological changes in the umbilical arteries of babies born to pre-eclamptic mothers: an ultrastructural study. *Placenta* 5, 419-426.

Erskine, R.L.A. and Ritchies, J.W.K. (1985) Umbilical artery blood flow characteristics in normal and growth-retarded fetuses. *Br. J. Obstet. Gynaecol.* 92, 605-612.

Fox, H. (1978) (ed.) *Pathology of the Placenta*, Saunders, p. 491.

Giles, W.B., Trudinger, B.J., and Baird, P.J. (1985) Fetal umbilical artery flow velocity waveforms and placental resistance: pathological correlation. *Br. J. Obstet. Gynaecol.* 92, 31-38.

Giles, W.B. and Trudinger, B.J. (1986) Umbilical cord whole blood viscosity and the umbilical artery flow velocity time waveforms: a correlation. *Br. J. Obstet. Gynaecol.* 93, 466-470.

Gruenwald, P. (1963) Chronic fetal distress and placental insufficiency. *Biol. Neonat.* 5, 215-265.

Las Heras, J., Baskerville, J.C., Harding, P.G.R., and Daria Haust, M. (1985) Morphometric studies of fetal placental stem arteries in hypertensive disorders ("toxaemia") of pregnancy. *Placenta* 6, 217-228.

Leroy, B. and Lefort, E. (1971) A propos du poids et de la taille des nouveaux nes a la naissance. *Rev. Fr. Gynecol. Obstet.* 66, 391.

Maekilae, U.M., Jouppila, P., Kirkinen, P., Viniikka, L., and Ylikorkala, O. (1983) Relation between umbilical prostacyclin production and blood-flow in the fetus. *Lancet* i, 728-729.

Scott, J.M. (1983) Fibrinous vasculosis in the human placenta. *Placenta* 4, 87-100.

Trudinger, B.J. and Cook, C.M. (1985) Umbilical and uterine artery flow velocity waveforms in pregnancy associated with major fetal abnormality. *Br. J. Obstet. Gynaecol.* 92, 666-670.

Trudinger, B.J., Giles, W.B., Cook, C.M., Bomdardieri, J., and Collins, L. (1985) Uteroplacental blood flow velocity-time waveforms in normal and complicated pregnancy. *Br. J. Obstet. Gynaecol.* 92, 23-30.

Uzan, M., Cynober, E., Uzan, S., Blot, Ph., and Sureau, C. (1987) Doppler en obstetrique: experience de la clinique Baudelocque. *Rev. Fr. Gynecol. Obstet.* 82, 35-43.

Van Der Veen, F. and Fox, H. (1983) The human placenta in idiopathic intrauterine growth retardation: a light and electron microscopic study. *Placenta* 4, 65-78.

Trophoblast Research 3:325-334, 1988

# CORRELATION OF ULTRASONOGRAPHIC MEASUREMENT OF THE UTERO-PLACENTAL AND FETAL BLOOD FLOW WITH THE MORPHOLOGICAL DIAGNOSIS OF PLACENTAL FUNCTION

Etha Jimenez, Martin Vogel, Birgit Arabin,
Gerhard Wagner, and Parwis Mirsalim

Institute of Pathology, Division of
Pediatric Pathology and Placentology
Institute of Perinatal Medicine
Free University Berlin
1000 Berlin, Germany

## INTRODUCTION

Pulsed Doppler sonography of fetal and uteroplacental blood flow velocity is a relatively new method in the diagnosis of fetal distress. It is especially useful in pregnancies with questionable interpretation of the fetal cardiotocogram (Trudinger et al., 1986). Apart from a study of Giles et al. (1985), little is known about the morphological changes in the placenta in cases with disturbed fetoplacental blood flow velocity. The aim of the current examination, therefore, was the correlation of highly pathological blood flow velocity waveforms in the fetal and uteroplacental circulation with a semi-quantitative assessment of placental morphology.

## MATERIALS AND METHODS

Sixty-three placentae of pregnancies were examined in which the velocity of the fetal blood flow (umbilical artery, aorta; and in 14 cases, carotid artery) and maternal blood flow (uteroplacental vessels) had been measured sonographically. A 2 MHz pulsed Doppler ultrasound system (Kranzbuehler 8130 Duplex) with a 150 Hz high-pass filter was used. The time interval between measurement and delivery was less than 4 days.

The cases were subdivided into 3 groups:

1) Unrecordable fetal end diastolic blood flow velocity (n=19).
2) Twin pregnancies with one twin showing unrecordable end-diastolic blood flow velocity (n=3).
3) Normal Doppler flow velocity associated with normal fetal outcome (n=41).

Subgroups 1 and 2 were examined immunohistochemically with the indirect immunoperoxidase method using antibodies against Ulex europeus I lectin (E.Y Labs) and the Avidin Biotin Complex technique (Vector Labs).

The 63 placentae were submitted to a semiquantitative morphological examination.  Prerequisites for a morphological diagnosis of placental function were:

1) The application of quantitative and semiquantitative parameters for macroscopic and histologic examination of the organ.

2) The correlation with normal values for a given gestational age derived from placentae of eutrophic newborns with normal fetal outcome.

These prerequisites were met by the slightly modified criteria of Vogel (1984, 1986) confirmed by an unselected series of 4223 births (Department of Obstetrics, Universitaetsklinikum Charlottenburg, Berlin, see Table 1).

## RESULTS

### Unrecordable End-Diastolic Flow Velocity in the Umbilical Artery and Aorta

The results summarized below are presented in Table 2.  Seventeen of these 19 infants with "zero-flow" suffered from severe intra-uterine growth retardation (birth weight centile less than 3).  Sixteen of them demonstrated the morphological signs of chronic placental insufficiency (n=14) or decreased perfusing capacity (n=2), the other one was a congenital malformation (Pierre Robin Syndrome).

The 2 fetuses with a weight centile less than 25 were stillborn in the 28th week of gestation with a severe amnion infection.  One of them also showed morphological signs of chronic placental insufficiency.  The most common pathological placental findings were decreased weight and decreased basal area in combination with perivillous microfibrinous deposits, villous fibrosis, and chronic circulatory disturbances resulting in changes of the maternal as well as the fetal placenta.  There were 6 cases with normal uteroplacental blood flow velocity which are considered in detail in the discussion following.  Four infants were stillborn, 5 died within the first month of life.  All neonates demonstrated clinical signs of intrauterine asphyxia (pH umbilical artery less than 7.2 and/or one minute's Apgar 7 or less).  The immunohistological examination with UEA I lectin resulted in focal absence of vascular endothelial staining in areas of extensive perivillous microfibrin deposits and villous fibrosis.

### Twin Pregnancies With One Twin Showing Unrecordable End Diastolic Flow Velocity

The results are summarized in Table 3.  Two of three twins with absent end-diastolic velocity were severely growth retarded with a weight centile below 3.  This change agrees with the placental findings which consisted of underweight plus extensive perivillous microfibrinous deposits (case 26 II) or small-for-age placenta combined with medium degree intervillous microfibrinous deposits (case 28 II).  The third twin with absent end-diastolic frequencies of the umbilical artery showed an amnion infection with omphalovasculitis and a weight centile below 10. In Figures 1-4, the findings in fetal blood flow wave-forms and placental histology of one twin pair (case 26) were opposed.

Table 1

Criteria for a Morphological Diagnosis of Placental Function

I. <u>Latent Placental Dysfunction</u>

    1) Reduced Diffusing Capacity
        a) villous immaturity (grade 3)*
        b) villous immaturity (grade 2) + small-for-age placenta

    2) Reduced Perfusing Capacity
        a) small-for-age placenta + reduction of intermediate villi
        b) small-for-age placenta + microfibrinous deposits (grade 2)
        c) microfibrinous deposits (grade 2) + villous immaturity (grade 2)
        d) villous fibrosis (grade 2) + obliterating endangiopathy
          (grade 2) or microfibrinous deposits (grade 2)

II. <u>Manifest Placental Insuffiency</u>

    1) Acute
        a) acute circulatory disturbance (>20 %)
        b) acute circulatory disturbance (> 5 %)
          in a placenta with latent dysfunction
        c) acute circulatory disturbance (> 5 %)
          in chronic placental insufficiency

    2) Chronic
        a) small-for-age placenta + chronic circulatory disturbance
          (> 15 %) + disturbance of villous maturation or villous
          fibrosis (grade 2 or 3)
        b) small-for-age placenta + disturbance of villous maturation
          (grade 3) or microfibrinous deposits (grade 3)
        c) villous fibrosis (grade 3) or obliterating endangiopathy
          (grade 3) + parenchymatous placentitis

*Grade 1,2,3: slight, medium, extensive

Table 2

Correlation of Blood Flow Velocity Waveforms (b.f.v.w.f.) of Fetal and Uteroplacental Vessels With Placental Morphology and Fetal Outcome

| Case No. | Blood Flow Velocity Waveform | | | Placental Morphology | | Fetal Outcome | | | |
|---|---|---|---|---|---|---|---|---|---|
| | Umbilical Artery | Fetal Aorta | Common Carotid Artery | Uteroplacental Vessels | (Numbers of Subgroups See Table 1) | Gest. Wks. at Delivery | Weight Centile | $pH_{ua}$ | Apgar 1 Minute |
| 1 | 0 | 0 | ø | Pathological | CIP (II 2a) | 27/4 | <$P_3$ Stillborn | | |
| 2 | 0 | 0 | ø | Pathological | CIP (II 2b) Omphalovasculitis | 27/6 | <$P_{26}$ Stillborn | | |
| 3 | 0 | 0 | ø | Pathological | CPI (II 2b) | 29 | <$P_3$ Stillborn | | |
| 4 | 0 | 0 | ø | Pathological | I 2 d (reduced perfusing capacity) | 29/2 | <$P_3$ | 7.2 | 3 |
| | | | | | died 7 days post partum | | | | |
| 5 | 0 | 0 | Pathological | Pathological | CPI (II 2b) | 26/5 | <$P_3$ | 7.32 | 6 |
| | | | | | died 28 days post partum | | | | |
| 6 | 0 | 0 | Pathological | Normal | Omphalovasculitis | 27/2 | <$P_{25}$ | Stillborn | |
| 7 | 0 | 0 | ø | ø | CPI (II 2a) | 30/6 | <$p3$ | 7.17 | 8 |
| | | | | | died 7 days post partum | | | | |
| 8 | 0 | Normal | ø | Pathological | CPI (II 2b) | 36/0 | <$P_3$ | 7.2 | 7 |
| 9 | 0 | ø | ø | Pathological | CPI (II 2b) | 32/6 | <$P_3$ | 7.24 | 6 |
| 10 | ø | 0 | Pathological | Normal | Reduced Perfusing/Diffusing Capacity (I 2c and Ib) | 37/2 | <$P_3$ | 7.01 | 2 |
| 11 | 0 | 0 | Pathological | Pathological | Reduced Perfusing Capacity (I 2c) | 36/1 | <$P_3$ | 7.1 | 5 |
| 12 | 0 | 0 | Pathological | Normal | CPI (II 2b) | 35/5 | <$P_3$ | 7.24 | 6 |
| | | | | | died, trisomy 18 | | | | |
| 13 | 0 | 0 | ø | Normal | Acute & Chronic Placental Insufficiency (II 1c) | 37/4 | | 7.22 | |
| 14 | 0 | 0 | ø | Suspicious | CPI (II 2a) | 37/1 | <$P_3$ | 7.33 | 6 |
| 15 | 0 | 0 | ø | Normal | Reduced Diffusing Capacity (I 1b) | 35/3 | <$P_3$ | 7.28 | 5 |
| | | | | | died Pierre-Robin Syndrome | | | | |
| 16 | 0 | 0 | ø | Suspicious | CPI (II 2a) | 37/1 | <$P_3$ | 7.07 | 8 |
| 17 | 0 | 0 | ø | Normal | CPI (II 2b) | 37/5 | <$P_3$ | 7.18 | 9 |
| 18 | 0 | ø | ø | Pathological | CPI (II 2b) | 37/5 | <$P_3$ | 7.28 | 4 |
| 19 | 0 | 0 | Pathological | Pathological | CPI (II 2b) | 36/0 | <$P_3$ | 7.07 | 6 |

$pH_{ua}$ - pH Umbilical Artery; 0 - Unrecordable end diastolic flow velocity (zero flow); ø - Not investigated; Pathological b.f.v.w.f. Common Carotid Artery - Pulsatility Index (PI) < - 2 SD; Pathological b.f.v.w.f. Uteroplacental Vessels - Resistance Index (RI) > + 2 SD; Suspicious b.f.v.w.f. Uteroplacental Vessels - Resistance Index (RI)> + 1 SD; CPI - Chronic Placental Insufficiency; $p_3$ - Below the third weight centile; Gest. Wks. at Deliv. - Gestational weeks at deliver.

Table 3

Correlation of Blood Flow Velocity Waveform (b.f.v.e.f.) of Fetal and Uteroplacental Vessels With Placental Morphology and Fetal Outcome in Twin Pregnancies (Unrecordable End-Diastolic Flow Velocity in One Twin)

| Case No. | | Blood Flow Velocity Waveform | | | | Placental Morphology (Numbers of Subgroups see Table 1) | | Gest. Wks. at Delivery | Weight Centile | Fetal Outcome | |
|---|---|---|---|---|---|---|---|---|---|---|---|
| | | Umbilical Artery | Fetal Aorta | Common Carotid Artery | Uteroplacental Vessels | | | | | $pH_{ua}$ | Apgar 1 minute |
| 26 | I | 0 | Normal | Normal | Normal | Normal | Minimal Changes | 37/3 | $P_{50}$ | 7.34 | |
| | II | 0 | 0 | 0 | Pathological | Normal | CPI (II 2b) | | $<P_3$ | 7.3 | |
| 27 | I | | Normal | Normal | ø | Normal | Minimal Changes | 31/5 | $<P_{25}$ | 7.26 | |
| | II | 0 | 0 | Normal | ø | Normal | Omphalovasculitis | | $<P_{10}$ | 7.21 | |
| 28 | I | | Normal | Normal | Normal | Normal | Minimal Changes | 36 | $<P_{25}$ | 7.25 | |
| | II | 0 | 0 | Suspicious | Pathological | Normal | Decreased Perfusing Capacity (I 2d) | | $<P_3$ | 7.26 | |

$pH_{ua}$ - pH umbilical artery
0 - Unrecordable end diastolic flow velocity (zero flow)
ø - Not investigated
Pathological b.f.v.w.f. Common Carotid Artery - Pulsatility Index (PI) < - 2 SD
Pathological b.f.v.w.f. Uteroplacental Vessels - Resistance Index (RI) > + 2 SD
Suspicious b.f.v.w.f. Uteroplacental Vessels - Resistance Index (RI) > + 1 SD
CPI - Chronic Placental Insufficiency
$P_3$ - Below the third weight centile
Gest. Wks. at Delivery - Gestational weeks at delivery

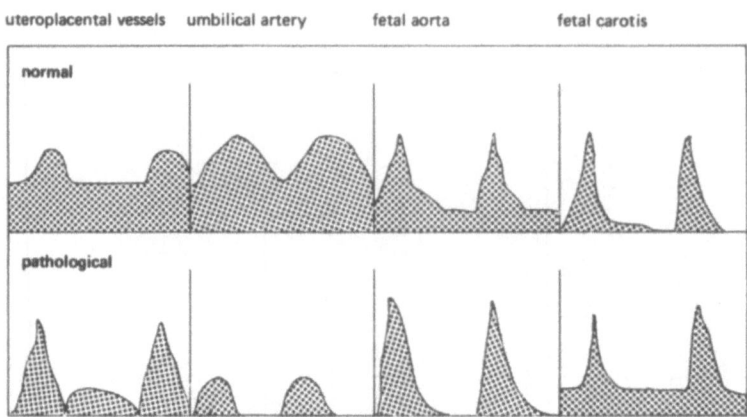

Figure 1. Scheme of normal and pathological blood flow velocity (pulsed Doppler sonography).

## Normal Doppler Blood Flow Velocity Associated With Normal Fetal Outcome

This group consisted of 41 cases (37-40 weeks of gestation). Twenty placentae showed no pathological findings, 21 times "minimal" anatomical changes were found which were quantitatively too small to cause placental dysfunction (combinations of findings of less degree than those listed in Table 1).

## DISCUSSION

In almost all cases (17/19), the loss of end diastolic velocities was associated with severe intrauterine growth retardation and morphological signs of impaired nutritive function of the placenta (Table 2). Unrecordable end diastolic blood flow velocity was diagnosed in 7/19 cases before the 32nd week of gestation. None of them survived, 4 fetuses died antenatally, 3 infants in the neonatal period due to pulmonary hyaline membrane disease or intracranial hemorrhage. All neonates born alive had suffered from intrauterine hypoxia. In twin pregnancies with one twin demonstrating unrecordable end diastolic blood flow velocity, the corresponding placenta showed pathological changes consisting of chronic placental insufficiency, decreased perfusing capacity, and omphalovasculitis, while in three placentae of the healthy twins, only minor morphological variations within normal limits were found. Also the 41 placentae of the cases with normal pulsed Doppler flow patterns and normal neonatal outcome either showed no pathological changes at all (n=20) or minimal changes only (n=21).

These findings are in agreement with the literature. Abnormal flow velocity waveform is known to result in a prevalence of small-for-gestational-age infants and infants with 5 minutes Apgar scores under 7 (Trudinger et al., 1985). Griffin et al. (1983) never found unrecordable end-diastolic flow velocity in normal third trimester pregnancies but rather in 8 of 11 fetuses with intrauterine growth retardation.

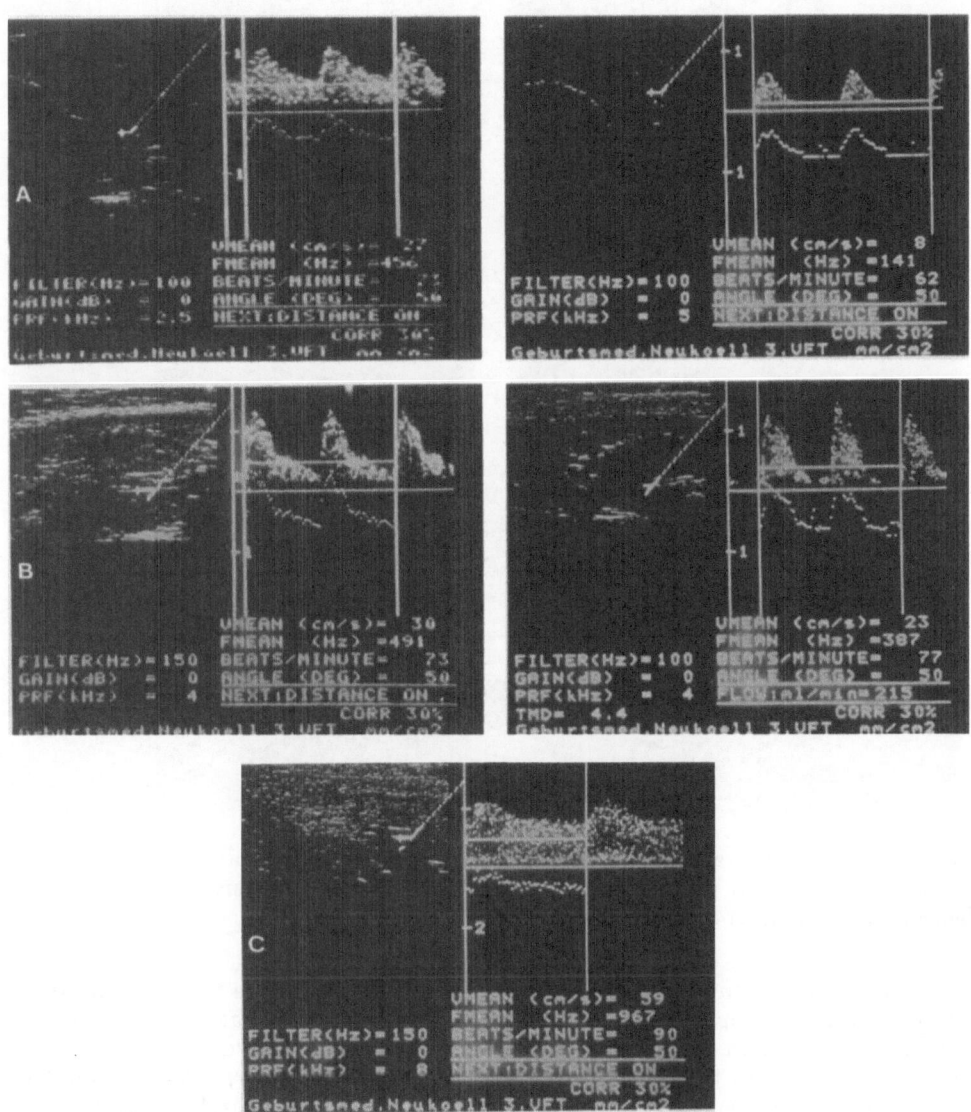

Figure 2. Blood-flow velocity (Doppler sonography) in the umbilical artery (A: first twin, left side; second twin, right side), aorta (B: first twin, left side; second twin, right side), and uteroplacental vessels (C) in twin pregnancy.

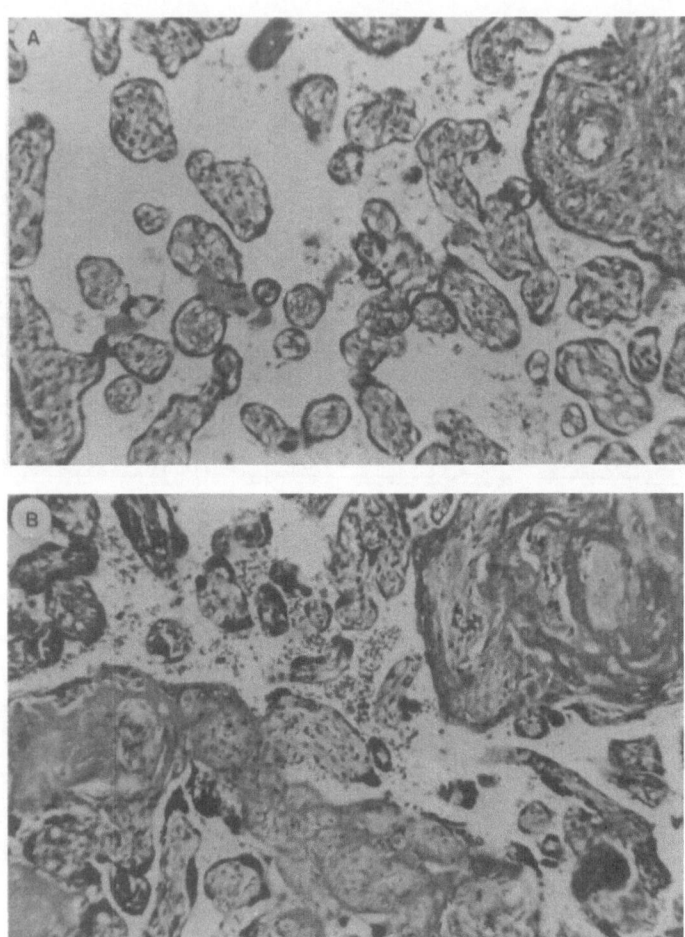

Figure 3.  Representative placental histology in twin pregnancy.  A) Regular villous maturation in placenta of first twin (X150).  B) Extensive microfibrinous deposits in placenta of second twin (X150).

In all of the current cases with the exception of one, the fetal arterial flow velocity and the uteroplacental blood flow were measured.  All cases with abnormal blood flow patterns in the arcuate arteries also showed unrecordable end-diastolic blood flow velocity in the fetal arterial circulation and the morphological signs of chronic placental insufficiency.  The placentae of these severely compromised neonates showed extensive damage of both the fetal and the maternal portions which correlates well with the pathological blood flow waveforms in the fetal and uteroplacental circulation.

While all cases with pathological flow patterns in the arcuate arteries also showed unrecordable end diastolic flow in the fetal circulation, the reverse does not hold true.  There were 6 cases with normal uteroplacental but unrecordable end diastolic fetal blood flow velocity.  Five of these cases (Table 2, Numbers 6, 10, 12,

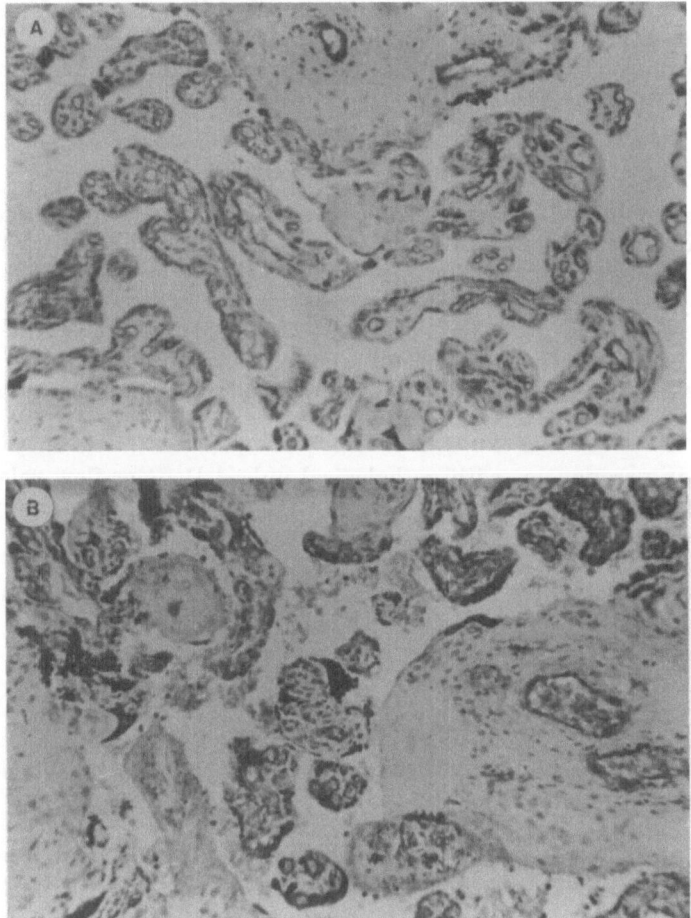

Figure 4. Staining pattern of small stem vessels with UEA I lectin. A) Uniform staining pattern in placenta of first twin (X150). B) Poor UEA I lectin binding in placenta of second twin (X150).

15, and 17) demonstrated no morphological compromise of the maternal placenta but rather the pathological alterations were limited to the fetal placenta. The infants died from an amnion infection syndrome (6), trisomy 18 with placental underweight and extensive villous immaturity (12) and a Pierre-Robin Syndrome with placental underweight and medium degree villous immaturity (15). In the other 2 cases villous stromal fibrosis, obliterating end angiopathy and, to a lesser degree, villous immaturity predominated (10, 17).

Like Giles et al. (1985) an increase of obliterated small arteries in tertiary stem villi was noted in the current study. However, this obliteration was not an isolated pathological change but rather a part of the chronic circulatory disturbances so frequently found in this severely altered placental group.

In future studies, and with further improved Doppler sound technology, it would be essential to correlate placental morphology with abnormal fetal blood flow patterns which are of less severity than the unrecordable end diastolic blood flow velocity used as basis in this study.

## SUMMARY

Unrecordable end diastolic flow velocity measured with pulsed Doppler sonography in the fetal umbilical artery and aorta is associated with the birth of asphyxiated underweight infants and morphological signs of chronic placental insufficiency.

Five of six cases with normal uteroplacental flow velocity waveforms correlated with a morphologically uncompromised maternal placenta and fetal disease.

In twin pregnancies with pathological pulsed Doppler flow velocity in one twin only, morphological signs of placental dysfunction were limited to the compromised twin.

Forty-one cases with normal Doppler flow velocity pattern and normal fetal outcome showed no or minimal pathological changes of the placenta.

## REFERENCES

Giles, W.B., Trudinger, B.J., and Baird, P. (1985) Fetal umbilical artery flow velocity waveforms and placental resistance: pathological correlation. *Br. J. Obstet. Gynaecol.* 92, 31-38.

Griffin, D., Cohen-Overbeek, T., and Campbell, S. (1983) Fetal and utero-placental blood flow. *Clin. Obstet. Gynecol.* 10, 565-602.

Trudinger, B.J., Giles, W.B., Cook, C.M., Bombardieri, J., and Collins, L. (1985) Fetal umbilical artery flow velocity waveforms and placental resistance: clinical significance. *Br. J. Obstet. Gynaecol.* 92, 23-30.

Trudinger, B.J., Cook, C.M., Jones, L., and Giles, W.B. (1986) A comparison of fetal heart rate monitoring and umbilical artery waveforms in the recognition of fetal compromise. *Br. J. Obstet. Gynaecol.* 93, 171-175.

Vogel, M. (1984) Pathologie der Schwangerschaft, der Plazenta und des Neugeborenen. In: *Pathologie (Band 3),* (ed.), W. Remmele, Springer Verlag Berlin, Heidelberg, New York, Tokyo, pp. 509-574.

Vogel, M. (1986) Morphology of Placental Dysfunction. A Contribution to the Recognition of Pathogenetic Factors in Intrauterine Hypoxia and Fetal Growth Retardation. In: *Research in Perinatal Medicine,* (eds.), E.L. Grauel, I. Syllm-Rapaport, and R. Wauer, VEB Thieme, Leipzig, pp. 292-299.

Trophoblast Research 3:335-349, 1988

# ULTRASTRUCTURE OF FETAL STEM ARTERIES OF HUMAN PLACENTA IN HYPERTENSIVE DISORDERS (TOXEMIA) OF PREGNANCY [*]

Jorge Las Heras[1,3] and M. Daria Haust[2]

[1]Instituto de Investigaciones Clinicas
Hospital Paula Jaraquemada
Facultad de Medicina Sur
Universidad de Chile Casilla 226/3
Santiago, Chile

[2]Department of Pathology, Obstetrics/Gynaecology and Paediatrics
The University of Western Ontario
London, Ontario, Canada, N6A 5C1

## INTRODUCTION

During recent years considerable speculation has been forthcoming regarding the status of placental fetal stem arteries in hypertensive disorders (toxemia) of pregnancy. A number of investigators (Isidor and Aubry, 1957; Paine, 1957; Robecchi and Simone, 1965; Fox, 1967; Hoelzl et al., 1974; Las Heras, 1978; Las Heras et al., 1979; Las Heras et al., 1983) have shown that a narrowing of the lumen of those vessels, due to the proliferation and prominence of endothelial cells, the smooth muscle cells, and fibrous tissue of the media was a characteristic feature of placentae from patients with toxemia. The extent of the narrowing was assessed morphometrically by Las Heras et al. (1985) who showed that there was a significant reduction in the ratio of lumen-to-whole-diameter of the fetal stem arteries in toxemia as compared with a normal control group.

Recently, in a study concerned with the morphology of the fetal stem arteries in normal placentaE van der Veen et al. (1982) have suggested that the obliteration of the fetal stem arteries may be due to a combination of vasoconstriction and fixation artefacts.

In an attempt to clarify some of the above problems an ultrastructural study of the fetal stem arteries in placentae from hypertensive disorders of pregnancy was undertaken, and preliminary observations were reported elsewhere (Las Heras and Haust, 1980).

---

[*] Presented in part at the Sixty-Ninth Annual Meeting of the USA/Canadian Division of the International Academy of Pathology, New Orleans, February 25-29, 1980.

[3]To Whom Correspondence Should Be Addressed

## MATERIALS AND METHODS

Fetal stem arteries in placentae of 50 toxemia patients constituted the basis for this study. The criteria for toxemia as employed in the present study was defined elsewhere (Las Heras et al., 1985). The term 'toxemia' of pregnancy, as defined by Page (1972), was applied to a condition of a woman who was over 24 weeks pregnant and who developed hypertension (mean diastolic arterial pressure higher than 105 mm), proteinuria (0.3 gm per 100 ml), and a pathological edema. The term was used in this report interchangeably with 'hypertensive disorder of pregnancy'. Similar arteries in 50 placentae of normal pregnancies served as controls. The placentae were collected at the hospital immediately after delivery, assessed macroscopically, and cut perpendicularly to the basal plate into slices measuring approximately 2.5 cm in width. Upon examination of all slices, tissue blocks were removed from the central area of placentae which appeared normal, and bisected. One portion was processed routinely for light microscopic examination and the other was fixed for 90 minutes at 4°C in 3% buffered glutaraldehyde for electron microscopy. Following fixation in glutaraldehyde and washing in 0.1 M phosphate buffer (pH 7.4), small pieces of tissues (1 to 2 mm) were postfixed for 90 minutes at 4°C in a solution of 1% osmium tetroxide in 0.1 M phosphate buffer (pH 7.4) and for additional 30 minutes at room temperature. Following dehydration the tissues were embedded in Epon-812 according to the method of Luft (1961).

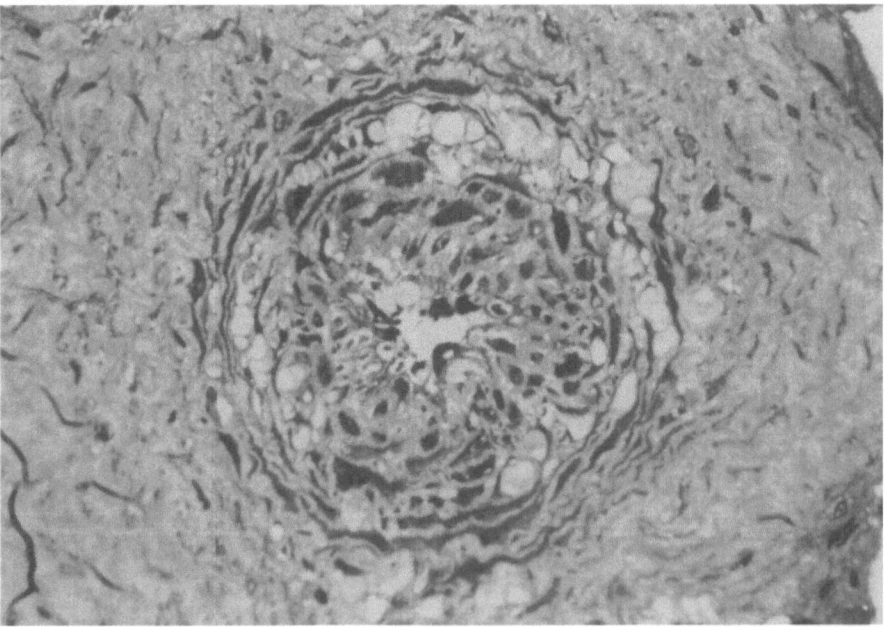

Figure 1. Transverse section of a fetal stem artery from a placenta in toxemia of pregnancy showing the proliferation of smooth muscle cells. Their arrangement appears to be random. There is marked vacuolation in the spaces between the smooth muscle cells. Intimal proliferation with lumen obliteration is also present. Toluidine Blue; Magnification = X256.

One micron thick sections were cut with glass knives on either a Sorvall MI-1/Porter-Blum or a Reichert ultramicrotome. They were stained with alkaline toluidine blue for light microscopy and the selection of fetal stem arteries. Only fetal stem arteries of the third order (Arts, 1961), i.e., measuring 100-300 u in diameter, were the subjects of the present study. Thin sections were cut with a diamond knife, mounted on unsupported copper grids, stained doubly with uranyl acetate and lead citrate, and examined with a Philips EM-300 electron microscope.

## RESULTS

For reference purposes, typical examples of the light microscopic changes present in fetal stem arteries in toxemia of pregnancy are illustrated (Figures 1 and 2). Electron microscopy also demonstrated that the lumen of the fetal stem arteries was either extremely narrowed (Figure 3) or totally obliterated (Figure 4), and the thickness of the wall increased. Several processes accounted for the latter phenomenon. There was an absolute increase in the number of arterial smooth muscle cells (SMC's). Most of these SMC's had a spiral arrangement but some assumed a distinctively circular direction (Figure 3). Moreover, in certain segments of the outer media, there was "crowding" of longitudinally arranged SMC's (Figure 4).

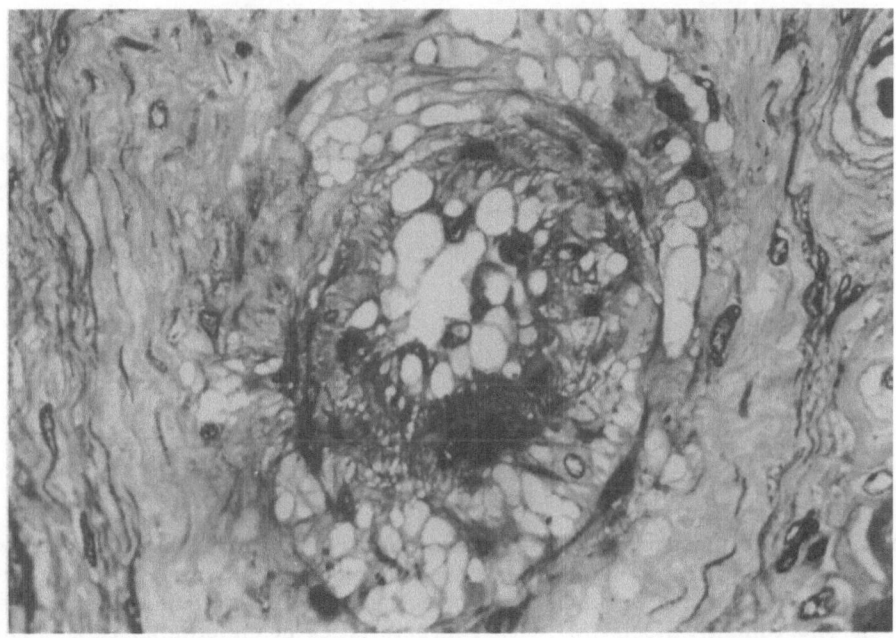

Figure 2. Transverse section of a fetal stem artery from a placenta in toxemia of pregnancy. The advance stage of the medial lesion is characterized by a severe distortion and vacuolization of the smooth muscle cells. The extracellular space contains also many vacuoles. The endothelial cells are prominent and vacuolated, and some of their slender processes form "bridges" across the lumen. Toluidine Blue; Magnification = X256.

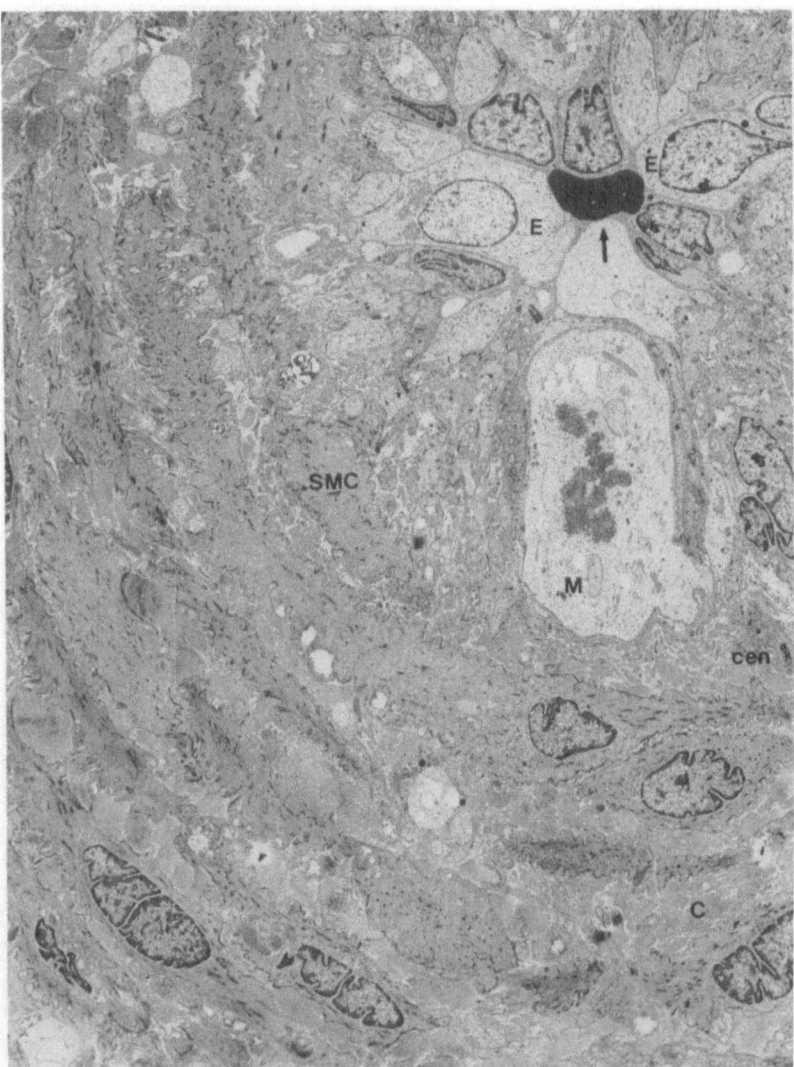

Figure 3. Detail of the intima and inner media of a fetal stem artery of third order from a toxemic patient. The lumen (arrow) of the artery is extremely narrow. The endothelial cells (E) are proliferating towards and impinging upon the lumen. There is one cell in mitosis (M) with characteristics of endothelial cells. The media shows an increase in the number of smooth muscle cells (SMC). The interstitium is occupied by numerous bundles of collagen fibrils (C). Some on the subendothelial smooth muscle cells show the presence of centriolar complex (cen). Magnification = X2800.

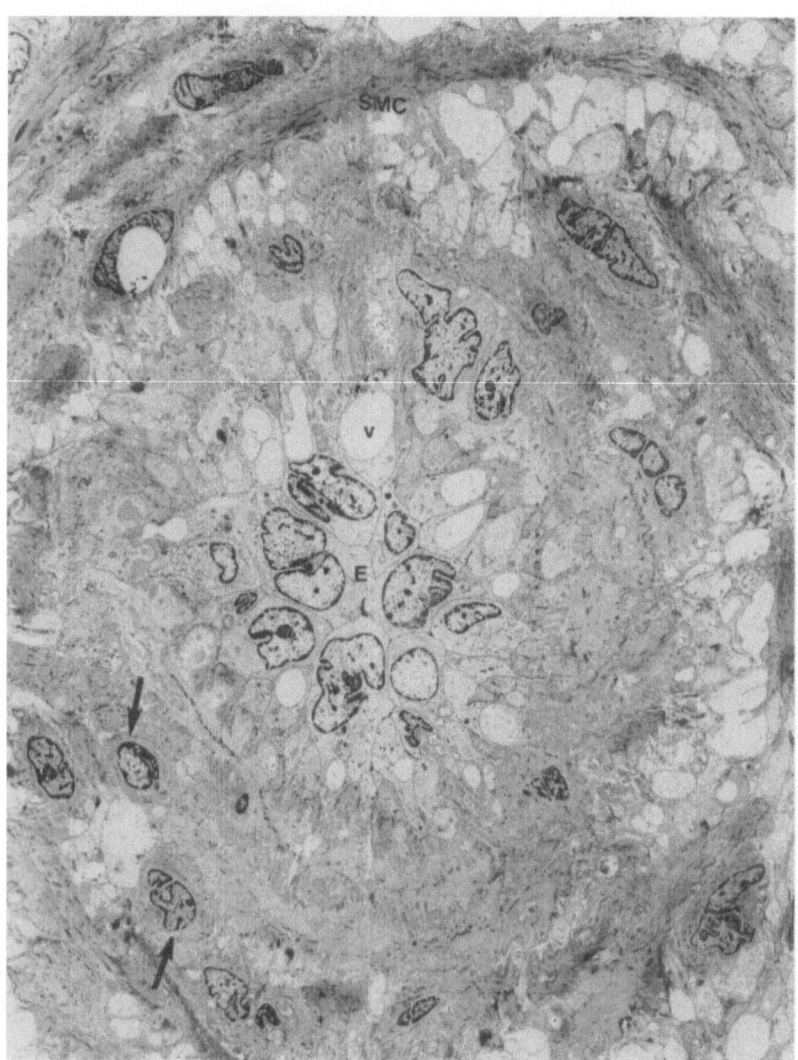

Figure 4. Cross section of a fetal stem artery of third order from a toxemic patient. The lumen is totally obliterated. The proliferating endothelial cells (E) are identified by their cellular features. The smooth muscle cells (SMC) of the medial coat are oriented circularly, tangentially, or longitudinally, contributing by their proliferation to the thickening of the wall. Note numerous vacuoles (v) in the endothelial and medial areas. Magnification = X1700.

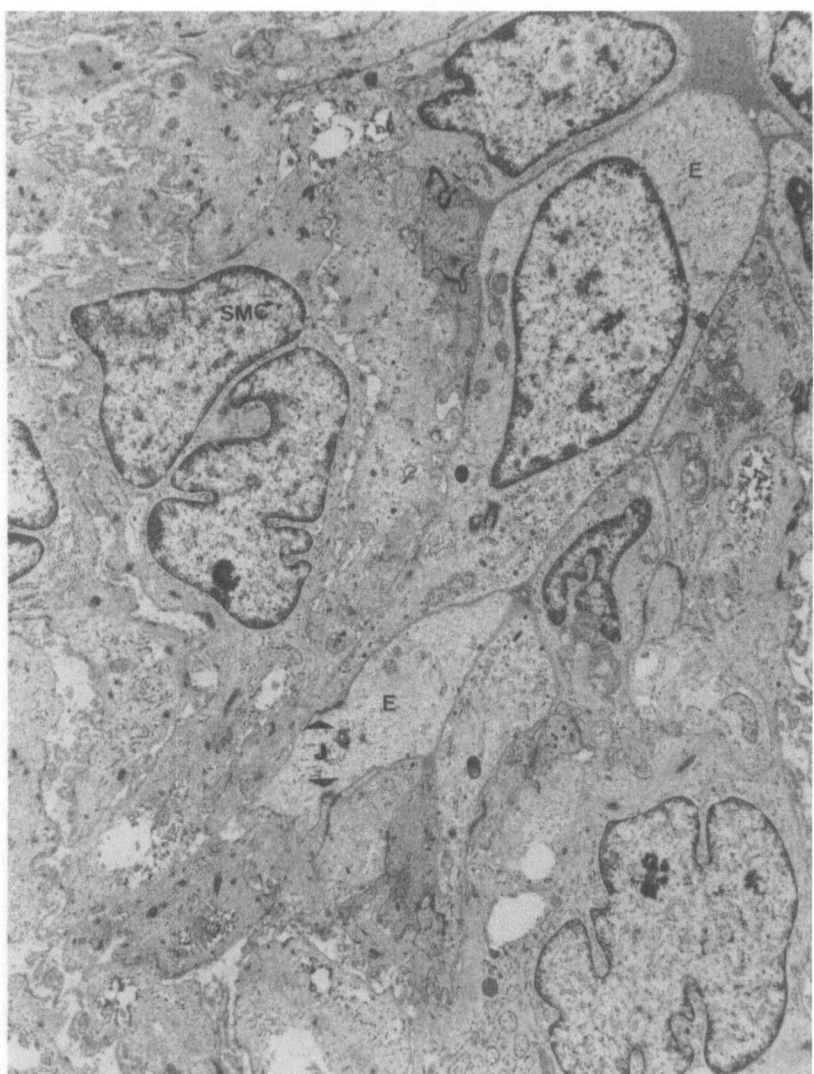

Figure 5. Detail of the intima and innermost media of a fetal stem artery of third order from a toxemic patient. Numerous endothelial cells (E) with distinct and less definitive cellular junctions (J) are seen proliferating towards the lumen; many of these cells are in close contact with smooth muscle cells (SMC). The collagen fibrils commonly found in the interstitial spaces of the media are not present in this area. Magnification = X8000.

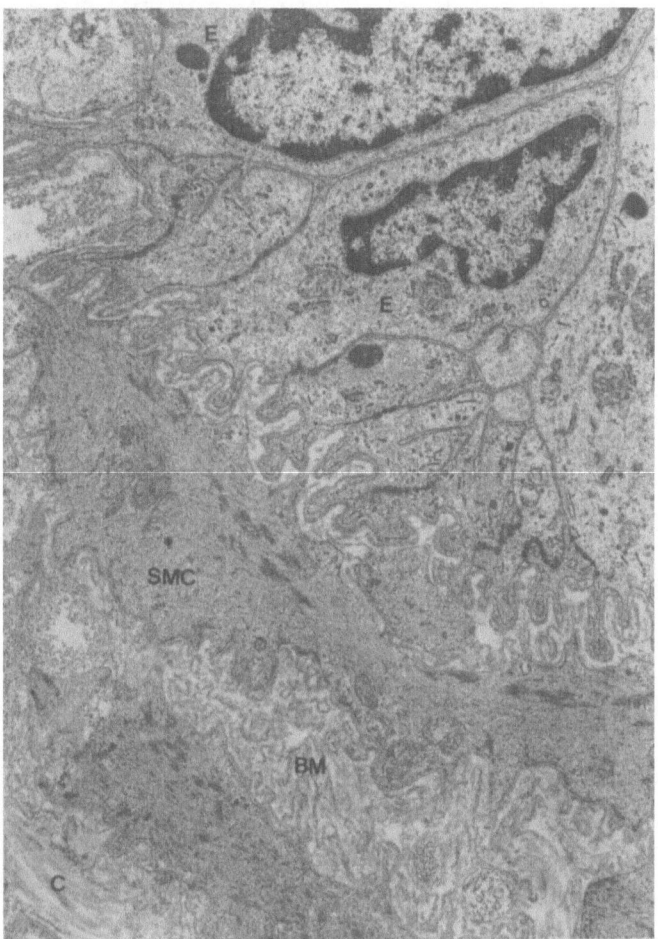

Figure 6. Detail of the intima and media of a fetal stem artery of 3rd order from a toxemic patient. Between the first and second innermost layers of the smooth muscle cells (SMC), there is marked proliferation of basement membrane-like substance (BM). The outer interstitial spaces are also occupied by bundles of collagen fibrils (C). E = endothelial cells. Magnification = X12000.

In addition, there was a definite increase of collagen fibrils in the interstitium with the notable exception of the space between the innermost layer of the SMC's and the endothelium (Figure 5). In addition, there was a considerable proliferation of a basement membrane (BM)-like substance in all spaces. This proliferation was particularly evident between the first and second innermost layers of the SMC's (Figure 6).

In fact, the remarkably intense proliferation of the BM-like substance often created the impression, as if an attempt were made by the second layer of the SMC's to assume the function of the innermost layer of the normal arteries. This hypothesis was especially tempting to postulate in view of the fact that the SMC's of the innermost layer often were oriented tangentially or longitudinally (Figures 4 and 7) rather than circularly as was the case in normal arteries. Finally, proliferation of the innermost cells contributed in large measure to the thickening of the wall (Figure 7). Most of these cells which were proliferating towards and impinging upon the lumen, had unmistakable features of endothelial cells. These proliferating cells were at times "piling up". Their endothelial nature was clearly evident not only by virtue their cellular features, but also by the unequivocal cellular junctions between them (Figures 8 and 9). Whenever present, the Weibel-Palade bodies were helpful in the identification of the endothelial cells, despite the fact that their tubulofibrillar structure often could not be resolved.

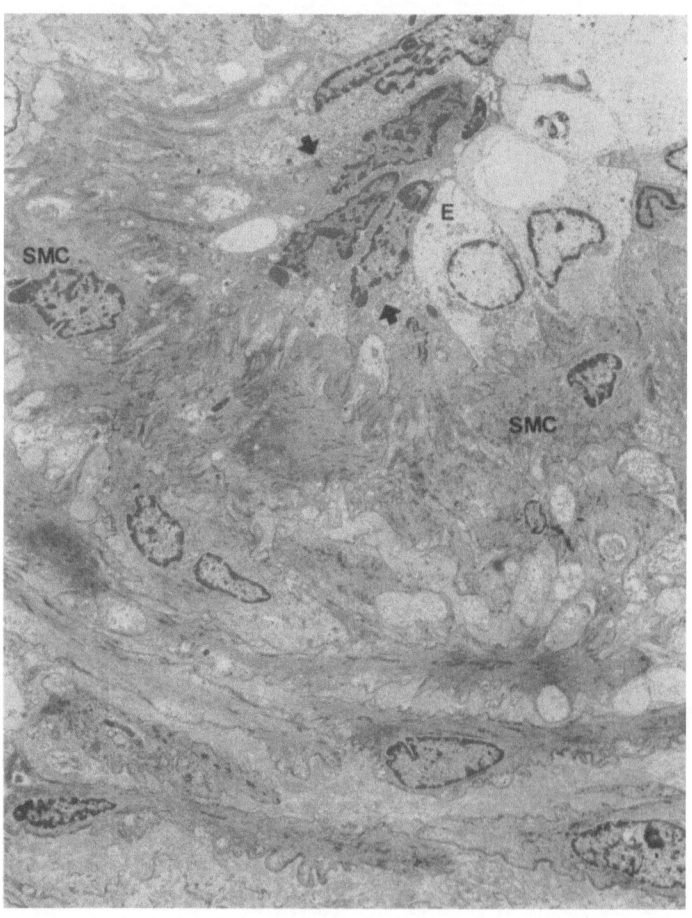

Figure 7. Intima and media of a fetal stem artery of third order from a toxemic patient. There is an increase in the number of medial smooth muscle cells (SMC) which appear to be in close contact with each other. The smooth muscle cells close to the lumen area longitudinally oriented; cells with certain features of SMC's appear with the endothelial cells (E) in the innermost arterial layer (arrows) and thus also impinging upon the lumen. Magnification = X4000.

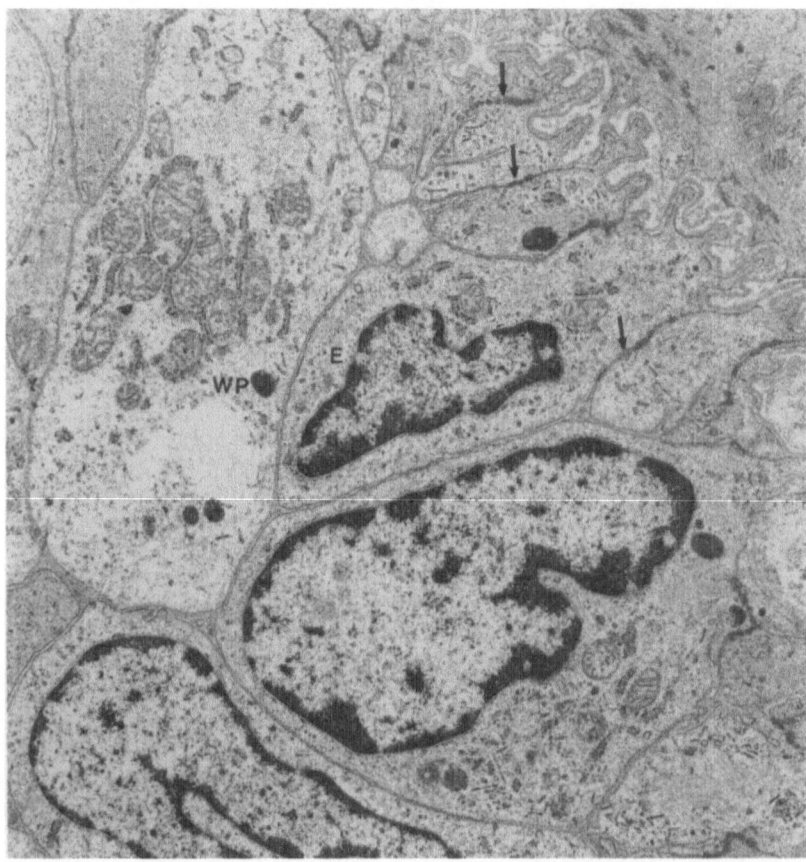

Figure 8. Detail of the intima of a fetal stem artery of third order from a toxemic patient. Some of the proliferating cells have unmistakable features of endothelial cells (E). Note the unequivocal cellular junctions (arrows) between them and the presence of Weibel-Palade (WP) bodies. Magnification = X12000.

At times, some of the proliferating cells had certain features, e.g., the presence of oblong (myofilamentous) densities (Figure 10), that were reminiscent of young SMC's rather than endothelial cells. Often, even cells in mitosis (Figure 3) had characteristics reminiscent of, or even identical with, those of mitotic endothelial cells. These cells could not be identified with certainty as endothelial cells, in the absence of cellular junctional complexes (Figure 3). Many subendothelial SMC's showed the presence of a centriolar complex (Figure 3).

Electron microscopy was of considerable help in the identification of the nature of vacuoles observed by light microscopy within the arterial wall. These vacuoles proved to be intracytoplasmic (Figure 9), involving invariably the peripheral processes of SMC's. The latter feature was observed previously also in normal arterial wall (Las Heras and Haust, 1981). In the luminal area, the edematous SMC's processes (Figure 9) involved those that "participated" in myoendothelial "junctions", whereas in the media the edema affected the slender SMC's extensions (Figure 11). Presumably, when the involvement of either of the two groups of the SMC's processes reached a "saturation" by an edema fluid, the latter could "spill" over into the interstitium. On occasion, a portion of a membrane that was surrounding a vacuole was, indeed, missing. This absence could, however, represent an artefact rather than a true discontinuity of a membrane (Figure 11).

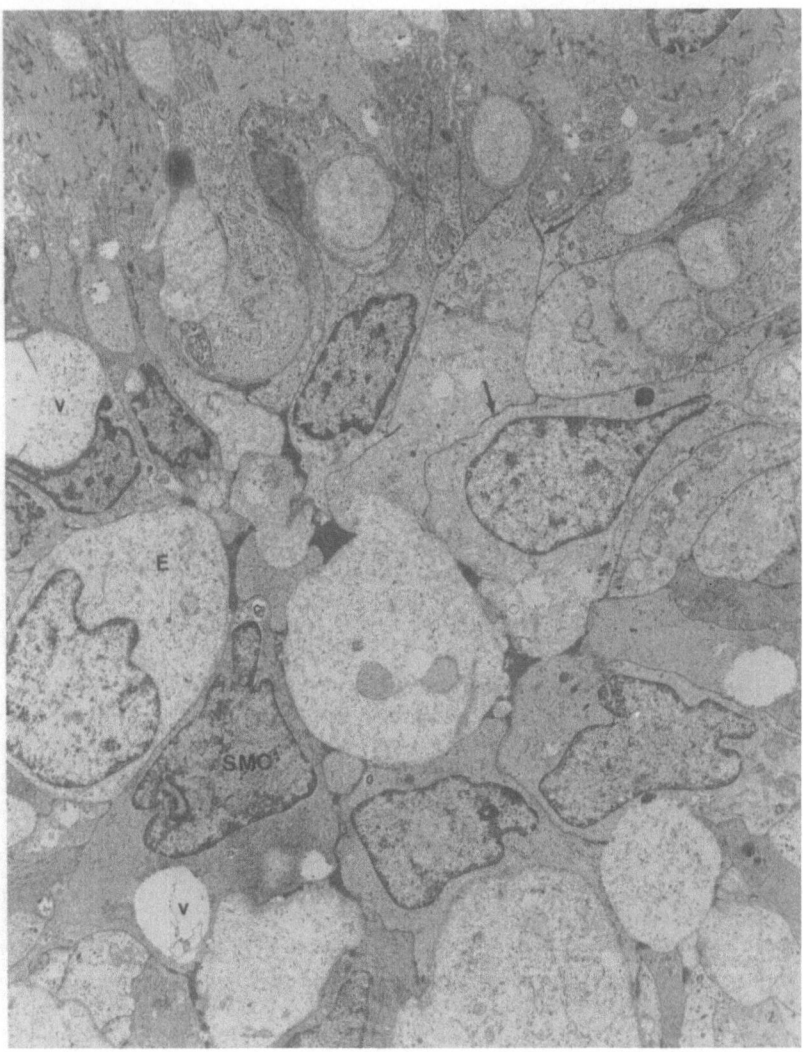

Figure 9. Electron micrograph of the intima of fetal stem artery of third order from a toxemic patient. The lumen is obliterated by the proliferation of endothelial cells (E). There are extensive membrane appositions between the endothelial cells, and at several points they are forming cellular junctions (arrows). Numerous vacuoles (v) are membrane bound and represent swollen processes of smooth muscle cells (SMC). Magnification = X5600.

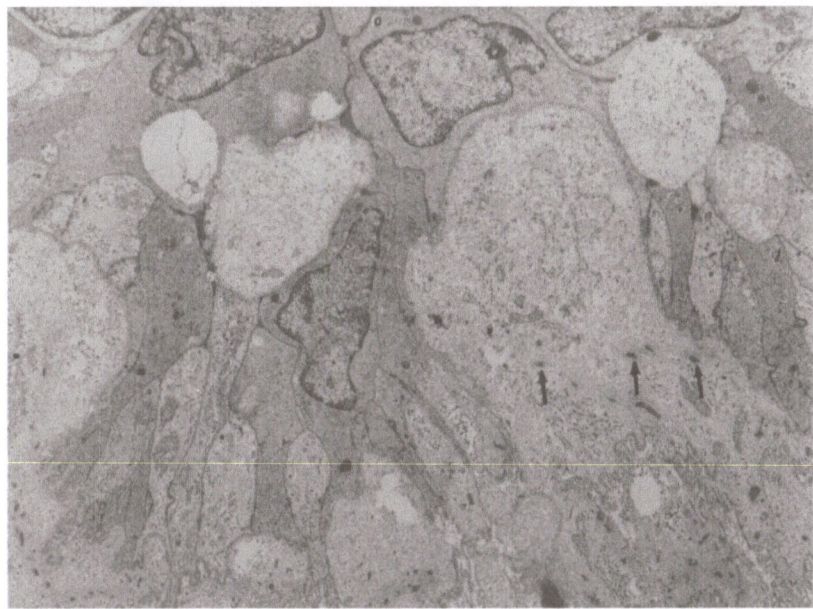

Figure 10. Detail of the intima and innermost media of fetal stem artery of third order from a toxemic patient. The proliferation of the innermost cells results in a complete obliteration of the lumen. Some of the proliferating cells have oblong (myofilamentous) densities (arrows), thus resembling young or dividing smooth muscle cells. Magnification = X5600.

## DISCUSSION

Whereas electron microscopic examination largely confirmed our previous light microscopic observations in fetal stem arteries of the placenta in toxemia of pregnancy (Las Heras et al., 1983), it provided in addition new information concerning the diffuse swelling and haphazard proliferation of the lining endothelial cells, which were features consistently found in the affected vessels of the hypertensive group. On the basal aspect the endothelial cells possessed infoldings and extending, markedly, vacuolated processes. These vacuoles were bound by a double limiting membrane. Such seemingly intraendothelial vacuoles were also identified in fetal vessels of normal pregnancies (Las Heras and Haust, 1981) and were interpreted as representing processes of the SMC's that herniated through the BM and invaginated into the endothelial cells. A similar feature was observed in human and animal arteries by other investigators (Dingemans and Wagenvoort, 1977; Stetz et al., 1979). Much debate ensued as to the significance of these vacuoles, and some authors believe that their apparent intracellular position represents an artefact (van der Veen et al., 1982).

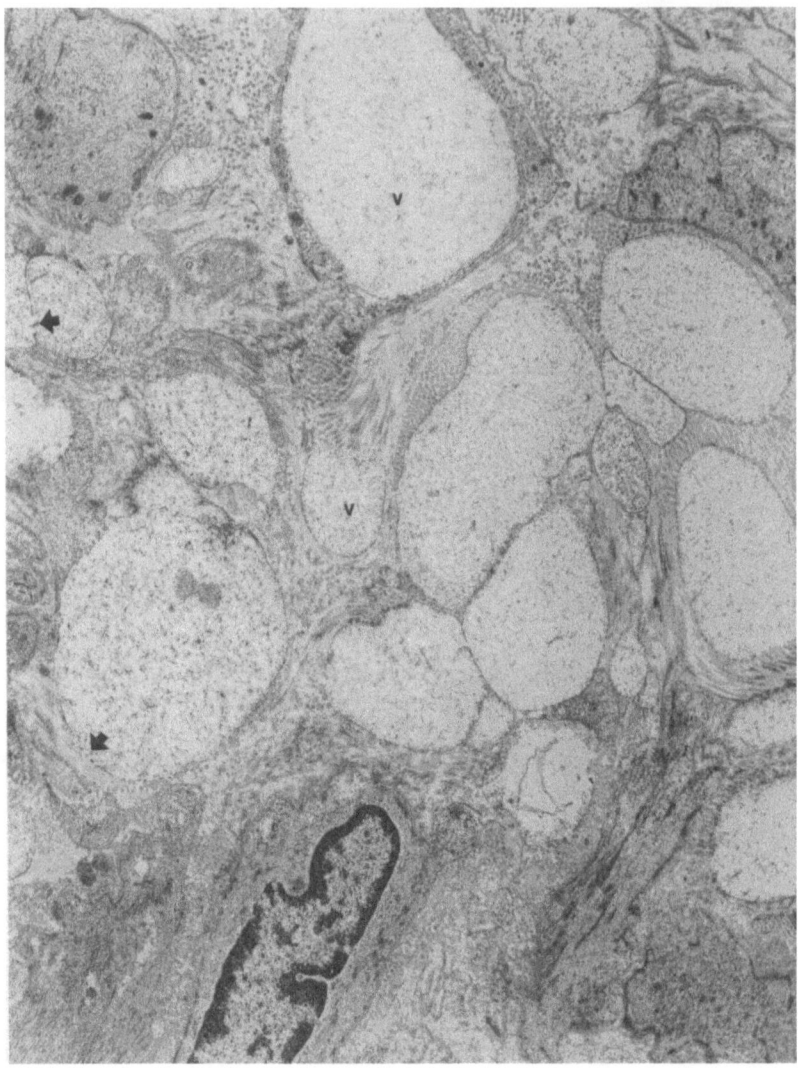

Figure 11. The media of a fetal stem artery of third order from a toxemic patient.
Most of the vacuoles (v) are entirely membrane bound and represent swollen
cellular processes of smooth muscle cells.   Occasionally, a portion of that
membrane is missing (arrows).   The interstitial spaces appear widened and
contain randomly oriented bundles of collagen fibrils (C).   Magnification =
X11000.


    The present study indicated that the media of the compromised arteries in
hypertensive diseases of pregnancy almost always was thickened by proliferating
SMC's and collagen fibrils.  Moreover, there was a marked proliferation of BM-
like substance that was either focally accumulated or duplicated over a

considerable distance. Factors that may induce SMC proliferation and medial hypertrophy are not all known, but one of these was almost certainly a prolonged vasoconstriction or an increase in vascular tone (Wagenvoort and Wagenvoort, 1970). Whether this proliferation was somehow related to the intensity of vasoconstriction, the frequency of vasoconstrictive "bouts" or other factors is unknown. It appeared likely that, as in the systemic circulation, this proliferation may be stimulated by intense vasospasms. Whereas the action of various stimuli may trigger the vasoconstriction, it is possible that in some patients, hypoxia may play the most important role in the mechanism of this vascular alteration. This view was supported by the experimental study of Stock et al. (1980), who have observed a decreased maternal blood flow to the placenta resulting in a marked decrease in fetal-placental blood flow.

The present study demonstrated that the vacuoles, evident by light microscopy in the wall of a stem artery from placenta in toxemia, were edematous cellular processes similar to those SMC-extensions that made contact with the endothelial cells at the myoendothelial junctions. Similar features were observed in studies of isolated SMC's (Fay and Delise, 1973), in the SMC's of the normal arterial tree (Joris and Majno, 1977), and in the SMC's of the fetal stem arteries of placentae in normal pregnancies (Las Heras and Haust, 1981). The presence of the herniating SMC's processes was interpreted by some as a morphological marker of a vascular SMC's contraction (Joris and Majno, 1977). Why these processes tend to swell was not clear. It may be that those portions of the SMC's that were devoid of the basement membrane, either extend to make contact with the endothelial cells or were free in the interstitium as specialized cellular segments. These processes may be capable of absorbing edema fluid that otherwise, if the fluid remained in the interstitium, would damage the extracellular components of the arterial wall.

## SUMMARY

The status of third order fetal arteries of the placenta in hypertensive disorders (toxemia) of pregnancy was evaluated by transmission electron microscopy. In the toxemic placenta there was an absolute increase in the number of arterial smooth muscle cells (SMC's) and a considerable proliferation of a basement membrane (BM)-like substance. The latter was most evident between the first and second innermost layers of SMC's. In addition, there was a definitive increase of collagen fibrils in the interstitial spaces.

Most cells proliferating towards and impinging upon the lumen had unmistakable features of endothelial cells, but some had certain features reminiscent of young SMC's. Numerous, slender, cellular processes were present in the interstitium of arterial media. These processes became distented with edema fluid imparting a vacuolar appearance to the media. Similarly, those SMC extensions which made contact with the endothelial cells also became edematous, giving rise to vacuoles in the endothelial region of the artery. These processes, too, were devoid of the basal lamina of the SMC's. It is postulated that SMC processes that are devoid of BM, and either extend to make contact with the endothelial cells or are in the interstitium, are specialized cellular components.

## ACKNOWLEDGEMENTS

This work was supported by a grant-in-aid of research T.3-11 from the Ontario Heart Foundation (M.D.H.), Toronto, Ontario and a Special Fund from the Department of Obstetrics and Gynaecology, University of Western Ontario. Dr. Las Heras was recipient of a Fellowship from Medical Research Council of Canada while engaged in the initial phases of these investigations. The authors wish to acknowledge gratefully the continuous support provided by Dr. Paul Harding, Professor and Chairman of the Department of Obstetrics and Gynaecology at the University of Western Ontario, who has been collaborating in most phases of the ongoing program on the role of placenta in maternal and perinatal disease processes, and thank Ms. Irena Wojewodzka and Mr. Roger Dewar for their invaluable technical assistance, and Mrs. Betty Gardiner for the efficient typing of the manuscript.

## REFERENCES

Arts, N.F.T. (1961) Investigations on the vascular system of the placenta. Parts 1 and 2. *Am. J. Obstet. Gynecol.* 82, 147-166.

Dingemans, K.P. and Wagenvoort, C.A. (1978) Pulmonary arteries and veins in experimental hypoxia. An ultrastructural study. *Am. J. Pathol.* 93, 353-368.

Fay, F.S. and Delise, C.M. (1973) Contraction of isolated smooth muscle cells; structural changes. *Proc. Natl. Acad. Sci. USA* 70, 641-645.

Fox, H. (1967) Abnormalities of the foetal stem arteries in the human placenta. *J. Obstet. Gynaecol. Brit. Cmwlth.* 74, 734-738.

Hoelzl, M., Luethje, D., and Seck-Ebersbach, K. (1974) Plazenta-Veranderungen bei EPH-Gestose. Morphologischer Befund und Schweregrad der Erkrankung. *Archiv. für Gynaekol.* 217, 315-334.

Isidor, P. and Aubry, B. (1957) A propos d'un type particular d'arteriopathie de la portion foetale du placenta. Essai d'explication pathogenique; ses rapports avec la toxemie grandique et l'anoxie foetale. *Gynecologie et Obstetrique* 56, 152-166.

Joris, I. and Majno, G. (1977) Cell-to-cell herniae in the arterial wall. I. The pathogenesis of vacuoles in the normal media. *Am. J. Pathol.* 87, 375-398.

Las Heras, J. (1978) Morphometry and morphology of fetal stem arteries of human placenta in hypertensive diseases (toxemia) of pregnancy. *Ph.D. Thesis. University of Western Ontario*, London, Canada.

Las Heras, J. and Haust, M.D. (1980) Ultrastructure of third order fetal arteries in normal and toxaemic placentas. *Lab. Invest.* 42, 130-131.

Las Heras, J. and Haust, M.D. (1981) Ultrastructure of fetal stem arteries of human
placenta in normal pregnancy. *Vir. Arch. A. Pathol. Anat. Histol.* 393,
133-144.

Las Heras, J., Harding, P.G., and Haust, M.D. (1979) The morphology of third
order fetal arteries in normal and "toxaemic" placenta. *Lab. Invest.* 40,
260.

Las Heras, J. Haust, M.D., and Harding, P.G. (1983) Morphology of fetal stem
arteries in hypertensive disorders (toxemia) of pregnancy. *Appl. Pathol.* 1,
301-309.

Las Heras, J., Baskerville, J.C., Harding, P.G., and Haust M.D. (1985)
Morphometric studies of fetal placental stem arteries in hypertensive
disorders (toxemia) of pregnancy. *Placenta* 6, 217-228.

Luft, J.H. (1961) Improvements in epoxy resin embedding methods. *Cell Biol.* 9,
409-414.

Page, E.W. (1972) On the pathogenesis of pre-eclampsia and eclampsia. *J. Obstet.
Gynaecol. Br. Cmwlth.* 78, 883-894.

Paine, C.G. (1957) Observations on placental histology in normal and abnormal
pregnancies. *J. Obstet. Gynaecol. Brit. Emp.* 64, 668-672.

Robecchi, E. and Aimone, V. (1965) Osservazioni istologiche sui vasi placentari
nella gestosi-albuminurica-ipertensiva-edemigena. *Minerva
Ginecologica* 17, 994-1003.

Stetz, E.M., Majno, G., and Joris, I. (1979) Cellular pathology of the rat aorta.
Pseudo-vacuoles and myoendothelial herniae. *Vir. Arch. A. Pathol. Anat.
Histol.* 383, 135-148.

Stock, M.K., Anderson, D.F., Pharnetton, T.M., Mclaughlin, M.K., and Rankin,
J.H.G. (1980) Vascular response of the fetal placenta to local occlusion of the
maternal placental vasculature. *J. Develop. Physiol.* 2, 339-346.

van der Veen, F., Walker, S., and Fox, H. (1982) Endarteritis obliterans of the fetal
stem arteries of the human placenta: an eletron microscopic study.
*Placenta* 3, 181-190.

Wagenvoort, C.A. and Wagenvoort, N. (1970) Primary pulmonary hypertension.
A pathologic study of the lung vessels in 156 clinically diagnosed cases.
*Circulation* 42, 1163-1183.

Trophoblast Research 3:351-360, 1988

# EFFECTS OF HIGH ALTITUDE ON THE VASCULARIZATION OF TERMINAL VILLI IN HUMAN PLACENTAE

Moira R. Jackson[1], Terry M. Mayhew[1,3] and Jere D. Haas[2]

[1]Department of Anatomy, Marischal College
University of Aberdeen
Aberdeen AB9 1AS Scotland, United Kingdom

[2]Division of Nutritional Sciences
Martha Van Rensselaer Hall
Cornell University
Ithaca, New York 14853 USA

## INTRODUCTION

The oxygen diffusing capacity of the human hemomonochorial placenta is influenced by the physical dimensions of the tissue components of the materno-fetal interhemal barrier (Laga et al., 1973; Mayhew et al., 1984). Of these tissue components, the villous membrane - comprising trophoblast, villous stroma, and fetal capillary endothelium - makes a major contribution to total placental diffusing capacity (Mayhew et al., 1986a).

It is known that the physical dimensions of the villous membrane are gradually altered during gestation. Thus, the growing fetal mass is served by an expanding villous surface area (Aherne and Dunnill, 1966). Diffusion distances also diminish, partly by a reduction in the relative amount of cytotrophoblast and by attenuation of syncytiotrophoblast but also by dilation and peripheralization of fetal capillaries, especially those within terminal villi. As a consequence of these structural changes, the diffusing capacity of the villous membrane is expected to increase as pregnancy advances (Mayhew et al., 1986a).

Pregnancy at high altitude is associated with fetal growth retardation (Haas, 1980; Haas et al., 1980). For some reason, growth of the villous tree is also retarded in placentae from high-altitude pregnancies (Jackson et al., 1985b, 1986). To compensate for the reduced exchange surface area of villi, there is a decrease in thickness of the villous membrane at high altitude (Mayhew et al., 1986b). As in normal gestation, this is partially attributable to thinning of the trophoblastic epithelium.

The present investigation tests whether or not the villous membrane thinning at high altitude is accompanied by changes in the vascularization of villi. To this end, attention is given not only to the absolute dimensions (volumes, surface areas, lengths, and mean diameters) of fetal capillaries but also to their

[3]To Whom Correspondence Should Be Addressed

proximity to the overlying trophoblast. The stereological analyses are based on term placentae from indigenous and non-indigenous populations of women living at low and at high altitude in Bolivia (Haas, 1980).

## MATERIALS AND METHODS

### Population Sampling

Pregnant women attending ante-natal clinics in Santa Cruz (400 m) and La Paz (3600 m) prior to the seventh month of gestation were screened for possible inclusion in the present investigation. Those finally chosen were considered to be healthy and at no apparent obstetrical risk. In La Paz, all women were born and raised at altitudes beyond 3000 m. This subsample was sufficiently heterogeneous in genetic composition to permit comparisons between two ethnic groups classified on the basis of ancestry of residence at high altitude. Native Amerindians (Quechua and Aymara) had many generations of exposure to high altitudes; non-Indians (Mestizo and European) had more recent exposures and less opportunity to adapt to the primary stressor of hypobaric hypoxia (Haas et al., 1980).

Women of comparable ethnic and socioeconomic status were chosen in Santa Cruz to serve as low-altitude controls. In this subsample, all were born and raised near sea level.

During examinations undertaken in the eighth month, personal records were obtained on maternal age, weight, stature, parity, nutritional status, reproductive history, and smoking habits. Also collected was information on blood biochemistry, hematology and genetic markers. Further details concerning these maternal characteristics and their effects on birth weights can be consulted elsewhere (Haas, 1980; Haas et al., 1980).

Sixty-eight subjects form the basis of this study. The low-altitude subsample comprises 24 mothers of whom 10 were Amerindian and 14 were non-Indian. The high-altitude subsample comprises 16 Amerindian and 28 non-Indian mothers.

### Newborn And Placental Characteristics

All mothers had singleton births; all but four were spontaneous vaginal deliveries. Birth weights were recorded within minutes of each delivery. Weights were significantly smaller at high altitude and native Amerindian mothers tended to deliver heavier babies than non-Indians. Gestational ages were checked using clinical and neurological criteria (Dubowitz et al., 1970) within a few hours of delivery. All newborns were estimated to be between 36 and 41 weeks of gestational age.

Within one minute of delivery (Bouw et al., 1976), clamps were applied to the umbilical cord which was then ligatured and trimmed to within 5 mm of the fetal surface of the placenta. After removing membranes and blood coagula, placentae were weighed. No significant altitudinal or ethnic differences in trimmed placental weights were found.

## Preparation And Sampling Of Placentae

Systematic samples of tissue were excised from two quadrants of each placenta. Tissues were fixed by immersion in isotonic formol saline solution and embedded in paraffin wax. Each of three to five tissue blocks per placenta provided one histological section of random orientation, arbitrary position, and approximately 4 μm in thickness. Sections were stained by the Masson trichrome method.

Fields of view on sections were sampled by a systematic random approach (Weibel, 1979; Mayhew, 1983). Sets of up to 30 fields of view per organ were recorded at two levels of magnification. Black and white micrographs were printed to a final enlargement of X250. Color micrographs were prepared as slide transparencies and projected on to a wall-mounted cardboard screen at X2000. All magnifications were calibrated using stage micrometer scale standards.

## Stereological Methods

The term "villi" used in this study refers to all but stem villi and any terminal or intermediate villi enveloped by fibrin deposits in the maternal vascular space. Sets of micrographs and transparencies were coded and analyzed blind by the same person (MRJ).

1.   Dimensions of fetal capillaries

Volume, surface, and length densities of fetal capillaries were determined for each placenta by point, intersection, and profile counting methods respectively (Weibel, 1979). For this purpose, test lattices were superimposed on each field of view in turn so as to be independently random in both position and orientation.

At the lower magnification, a test lattice of squares of edge length 2 cm was used in order to estimate the volume density of villi within each placenta, $V(v)/V(p)$. At the higher magnification, a similar lattice of spacing 6 cm was employed to calculate the volume density of capillaries within villi, $V(c)/V(v)$. The product of these two volume densities gives the volume density of capillaries in each placenta, $V(c)/V(p)$.

The 6 cm lattice was also adopted to count intersections between test lines and images of the boundaries of fetal capillaries and so provided estimates of the surface density of capillaries within villi, $S(c)/V(v)$. The product of $S(c)/V(v)$ and $V(v)/V(p)$ is an estimate of the surface density of capillaries per placenta, $S(c)/V(p)$. Exactly similar principles were used to calculate the surface density of the inner trophoblast surface per placenta, $S(t)/V(p)$.

Counts of the numbers of capillary profiles per sectional area of placenta provided data on $L(c)/V(p)$, capillary length density per organ. Estimates of the luminal caliber diameter of capillaries, $d(c)$, were derived by dividing $V(c)/V(p)$ by $L(c)/V(p)$ for each organ and treating the resulting area as that of a transverse section through a circular cylinder.

2.    Spatial arrangement of fetal capillaries

The harmonic mean thickness of the villous stroma, T(s), represents the effective diffusion distance from the inner trophoblast surface to the adluminal surface of capillary endothelium.   Values for T(s) were estimated by random intercept length measurements as described in more detail elsewhere (Jackson et al., 1985a).

As an additional expression of the proximity of fetal capillaries to the overlying trophoblast and to assess the proximity of capillaries one to another, a novel test circle pattern analysis method (Cruz Orive, 1976) was employed.  The method relies on a lattice of systematically arranged test circles which is superimposed on to fields of view in an independent random fashion.  For present purposes, test circles of diameter 3 cm were used to analyze color transparencies. Comparing the proportions of circles hitting trophoblast and/or capillaries provides a basis for assessing relative spatial associations.

The following proportions were calculated:

P(t)  - proportion of circles hitting trophoblast alone,

P(c)  - proportion hitting capillaries alone, and

P(t,c) - proportion hitting both together where P(t) + P(c) + P(t,c) = 100%

3.    Absolute quantities

In order to convert volume, surface, and length densities and harmonic mean  thicknesses into absolute quantities ($cm^3$, $m^2$, km and μm, respectively), it was  necessary to take account of tissue shrinkage, placental weight, and placental specific gravity (Laga et al., 1973; Boyd, 1984).  Linear shrinkage factors of 1.27 to 1.42 were used to correct estimates on these preparations. Placental  volumes were calculated from organ weights using a specific gravity of 1.05  $g/cm^3$.

4.    Diffusing capacity of villous stroma

Using a morphometric model described in detail elsewhere (Mayhew et al., 1984, 1986a), estimates of surface areas and harmonic mean thicknesses per placenta were used to calculate a diffusing capacity for oxygen of the villous stroma, D(s):

$$D(s) = (S(c) + S(t)) \cdot (K/2T(s))$$

where S(c) and S(t) are absolute surfaces, T(s) is absolute thickness and K is Krogh's diffusion coefficient for oxygen in placental tissue.  The value taken for K was $2.3 \times 10^{-8}$ $cm^2$/min/torr (Mayhew et al., 1984).

When surfaces are given in $cm^2$ and thickness in cm, the value of D(s) calculated by the equation above has the units ml $O_2$/min/torr.

Table 1

Capillary Volumes, Surface Areas, Lengths, and Mean Diameters
Classified by Altitude and Ethnic Grouping

|  | Low Altitude | | High Altitude | |
| --- | --- | --- | --- | --- |
| Variable | Amerindian | Non-Indian | Amerindian | Non-Indian |
| $V(c)$, cm$^3$ | 41.8 (6.13) | 43.5 (4.70) | 34.7 (3.69) | 31.2 (2.03) |
| $S(c)$, m$^2$ | 5.66 (0.80) | 5.39 (0.56) | 5.52 (0.67) | 4.59 (0.29) |
| $L(c)$, km | 154 (20.8) | 129 (1.11) | 149 (15.9) | 120 (6.53) |
| $d(c)$, μm | 18.6 (0.65) | 20.5 (0.57) | 17.3 (0.37) | 18.2 (0.42) |

Using two-way analyses of variance, the following main effects were significant:
altitudinal - $V(c)$, $P<0.05$; $d(c)$, $P<0.001$; ethnic - $L(c)$ and $d(c)$, $P<0.05$. Values are
group means (standard errors).

Table 2

Variables Characterizing Capillary-Trophoblast Associations
Classified by Altitude and Ethnic Grouping

|  | Low Altitude | | High Altitude | |
| --- | --- | --- | --- | --- |
| Variable | Amerindian | Non-Indian | Amerindian | Non-Indian |
| $T(s)$, μm | 2.29 (0.24) | 2.14 (0.09) | 1.31 (0.06) | 1.35 (0.04) |
| $P(t)$, % | 37.3 (2.20) | 34.7 (1.79) | 33.3 (1.23) | 32.3 (0.80) |
| $P(c)$, % | 24.3 (1.62) | 26.2 (1.34) | 19.7 (1.20) | 20.5 (0.83) |
| $P(t,c)$, % | 38.4 (1.92) | 39.1 (1.25) | 47.0 (1.25) | 47.2 (0.71) |

$T(s)$ denotes harmonic mean thickness of villous stroma; $P(t)$, $P(c)$, and $P(t,c)$
denote proportions of test circles hitting trophoblast, capillaries and trophoblast +
capillaries, respectively. Using two-way analyses of variance, the following main
effects were significant: altitudinal - $P(t)$, $P<0.05$; $T(s)$, $P(c)$ and $P(t,c)$, $P<0.001$.
Group means (standard errors)

## Statistical Evaluations

Values of each variable for individual placentae were used to calculate group means and standard errors, the groups being classified by altitude and ethnic background. Comparisons between groups were performed by two-way analyses of variance (Sokal and Rohlf, 1981) with altitude and ethnic background as the two main effects. The interaction term generated by this test provides an indication as to whether or not altitude influences placentae in both ethnic groups in a similar manner.

## RESULTS

Despite the lack of significant altitudinal and ethnic differences in organ weights, quantitative differences in placental composition and arrangement were demonstrable though not apparent on mere visual inspection of tissue sections. The findings on the physical dimensions of fetal capillaries within villi are summarized in Table 1 for natives and non-natives at low and at high altitude.

No significant interaction terms were found, suggesting that altitude, where it exerts an influence, affects both ethnic groups in the same way. The volume of fetal capillaries was significantly smaller at high altitude, the average organ possessing only 33 $cm^3$ of capillary blood space compared with 43 $cm^3$ at low altitude. No ethnic differences were noted.

The altitude-related decrease in capillary volume appeared to be due to a decrease in mean capillary diameter (17.8 μm versus 19.5 μm) and not to any significant alteration in total length of capillaries. Apparent decreases in capillary surface area at high altitude were not significant.

Table 3

Structural Quantities Influencing Stromal Diffusing Capacity for
Oxygen Classified by Altitude and Ethnic Grouping

| Variable | Low Altitude | | High Altitude | |
|---|---|---|---|---|
| | Amerindian | Non-Indian | Amerindian | Non-Indian |
| S(t), $m^2$ | 6.36 (0.65) | 6.63 (0.55) | 6.42 (0.38) | 5.35 (0.25) |
| S(c), $m^2$ | 5.66 (0.80) | 5.39 (0.56) | 5.52 (0.67) | 4.59 (0.29) |
| T(s), μm | 2.29 (0.24) | 2.14 (0.09) | 1.31 (0.06) | 1.35 (0.04) |
| D(s) | 6.80 (1.14) | 6.54 (0.59) | 10.9 (1.17) | 8.62 (0.46) |

S(t) and S(c) denote inner and outer trophoblast surfaces, respectively; D(s) is the diffusing capacity of the stroma in ml/min/torr. Using two-way analyses of variance, altitudinal differences in D(s) were significant, $P < 0.01$. Group means (standard errors)

Amerindian placentae tended to have smaller caliber diameter capillaries but their total capillary length was greater. Consequently, no ethnic differences in total capillary volume or surface area were demonstrated.

Table 2 provides a summary of the results relating to the spatial association of capillaries and trophoblast. Again, no significant interaction terms were generated. The results demonstrate that the effective diffusion distance across the villous stroma is significantly smaller in highland villi (about 1.3 μm versus 2.2 μm). Evidence that this closer association between capillaries and trophoblast represents a peripheralisation of capillaries can be adduced from the test circle data. The proportion of test circles hitting capillaries and trophoblast together is significantly greater at high altitude (47% versus 39%) while the proportion hitting capillaries alone is significantly smaller (20% versus 25%). No ethnic differences could be detected.

The impact of altitudinal differences in stromal thickness on oxygen diffusing capacity of the stromal component of the villous membrane is illustrated in Table 3. Apparent differences between altitudes in the surface areas of capillaries and inner trophoblast were not significant. However, since stromal harmonic mean thickness is substantially less at high altitude, the oxygen diffusing capacity is significantly greater. At high altitude, the average placenta had a stromal diffusing capacity of roughly 10 ml/min/torr, as compared with only 7 ml/min/torr in lowland controls.

## DISCUSSION

The present study has revealed that high-altitude placentae demonstrate substantial differences in the fetal vascularization of their villi. Decreases in the mean diameter, and hence in the total volume, of capillaries are compensated by changes in the spatial distribution of capillaries which more closely approximate the overlying trophoblastic layer. In consequence, the morphometric diffusing capacity of the stromal component of the diffusion pathway is greater in highland placentae.

The less voluminous fetal capillary space noted at high altitude may be partially compensated by an elevated fetal hematocrit and by an increase in the proportion of total cord hemoglobin made up of fetal hemoglobin (Haas, 1980). These hematological adaptations may be aimed at trying to maintain oxygen tensions in fetal vessels. Studies on sheep at high altitude have shown that lowland oxygen tensions can be conserved on the fetal side despite substantial decreases in oxygen partial pressure gradients (Metcalfe et al., 1962; Barron et al., 1964).

At high altitude, the changes in mean capillary diameter are not associated with significant differences in total capillary length or surface area. Since total length is unaltered, but total villous length is less (Jackson et al., 1985b), it appears that the capillary:villus length ratio must be greater in highland organs. This is consistent with observations made on guinea-pig placentae after maternal hypoxia (Bacon et al., 1984). In this animal model, placentae have smaller but more numerous capillary profiles than in controls. If hypoxia stimulates capillary growth relative to villous growth and so affects villous maturity (Kaufmann et al.,

1985), then the villi in human high-altitude placentae may be regarded as relatively more mature, even though mean villous diameter is not significantly different between altitudes (Jackson et al., 1986).

The smaller diameter of capillaries may represent a shift towards smaller diameter villi at high altitude, the combined lengths of the smallest villi being maintained at the expense of larger villi (Jackson et al., 1986). An alternative interpretation is that a reduction in capillary diameter is a generalized phenomenon designed to increase resistance to blood flow and so allow more time for materno-fetal exchanges. Decreasing the size of small vessels is known to counter the tendency for blood viscosity to increase as blood flow rates diminish. This is of some physiological interest given the greater hematocrit at high altitude (Haas, 1980) and the relationship between hematocrit and blood viscosity.

An increased capillary:villus length ratio at high altitude would be consistent with the finding that capillaries tend to lie closer to the trophoblast. The increased association at high altitude between capillaries and trophoblast points to a greater degree of capillary peripheralization and suggests that thinning of the villous membrane (Mayhew et al., 1986b) arises from both attenuation of trophoblast and margination (but not dilation) of fetal vessels within villi. The mechanism by which peripheralization occurs is not yet clear, but it is more likely to reflect differences in the relative growths of capillaries and villi than physical migration of vessels through the villous stroma.

The combined effect of changes in the dimensions and spatial arrangement of capillaries is to increase the oxygen diffusing capacity of the stroma. Coupled with changes in maternal and fetal hematocrits (Haas, 1980), in the volume of the maternal vascular space (Jackson et al., 1985b) and in the harmonic mean thickness of the trophoblast (Mayhew et al., 1986b), the noted increase in stromal diffusing capacity may be seen as part of a set of adaptations to maintain total placental diffusing capacities at values found in low-altitude organs.

## SUMMARY

Stereological studies have been performed on term placentae delivered by Amerindian and non-Indian mothers residing at 400 m and at 3600 m in Bolivia. Attention is focused on the physical dimensions (volume, surface, length, diameter) of fetal capillaries and on their spatial relationships with each other and to the overlying trophoblast.

Ethnic differences were few and confined to the diameter and length of capillaries. High-altitude placentae had a smaller volume of capillaries due to a reduction in capillary diameter rather than capillary length. Capillaries were also more peripherally disposed in highland organs, harmonic mean stromal thicknesses being considerably less than in lowland placentae. These structural differences indicate a higher stromal diffusing capacity for oxygen at high altitude and form part of a set of adaptations to maintain placental diffusive performance at lowland levels.

## ACKNOWLEDGEMENTS

We are pleased to acknowledge the help afforded by the many individuals who made this study possible. The work has been funded by The Leverhulme Trust, The Anatomical Society of Great Britain and Ireland and The National Science Foundation (BNS 76-12312). This is a research report from the U.S. Agricultural Experiment Station, Cornell University.

## REFERENCES

Aherne, W. and Dunnill, M.S. (1966) Quantitative aspects of placental structure. *J. Path. Bact.* 91, 123-139.

Bacon, B.J., Gilbert, R.D., Kaufmann, P., Smith, A.D., Trevino, F.T., and Longo, L.D. (1984) Placental anatomy and diffusing capacity in guinea pigs following long-term maternal hypoxia. *Placenta* 5, 475-488.

Barron, D.H., Metcalfe, J., Meschia, G., Huckabee, W., Hellegers, A. and Prystowsky, H. (1964) Adaptations of pregnant ewes and their fetuses to high altitude. In: *The Physiological Effects of High Altitude,* (ed.), W. Weihe, Oxford: Pergamon Press, pp. 115-125.

Bouw, G.M., Stolte, L.A.M., Baak, J.P.A., and Oort, J. (1976) Quantitative morphology of the placenta. I. Standardization of sampling. *Eur. J. Obstet. Gynaecol. Reprod. Biol.* 6, 325-331.

Boyd, P.A. (1984) Quantitative structure of the normal human placenta from 10 weeks of gestation to term. *Early Human Develop.* 9, 297-307.

Cruz Orive, L.M. (1976) Quantifying "pattern": a stereological approach. *J. Microscop.* 107, 1-18.

Dubowitz, L.M.S., Dubowitz, V., and Goldberg, C. (1970) Clinical assessment of gestation age in the newborn infant. *J. Pediatr.* 77, 1-20.

Haas, J.D. (1980) Maternal adaptation and fetal growth at high altitude in Bolivia. In: *Social and Biological Predictors of Nutritional Status, Physical Growth and Neurological Development,* (eds.), L.S. Greene and F.S. Johnston, New York: Academic Press, pp. 257-290.

Haas, J.D., Frongillo, E.A., Stepick, C.D., Beard, J.L., and Hurtado, L. (1980) Altitude, ethnic and sex differences in birth weight and length in Bolivia. *Human Biology* 52, 459-477.

Jackson, M.R., Joy, C.F., Mayhew, T.M., and Haas, J.D. (1985a) Stereological studies on the true thickness of the villous membrane in human term placentae: a study of placentae from high-altitude pregnancies. *Placenta* 6, 249-258.

Jackson, M.R., Mayhew, T.M., and Haas, J.D. (1985b) Altitude, ethnic and sex effects on the microscopical morphometry of human term placentae.

Abstracts of XII Intern. Anat. Congr. London, A324.   Cambridge: Cambridge University Press.

Jackson, M.R., Mayhew, T.M., and Haas, J.D. (1986) The human placenta at high altitude in Bolivia. I. Reduced growth of villi. J. Anat. 146, 238-239.

Kaufmann, P., Bruns, U., Leiser, R., Luckhardt, M., and Winterhager, E. (1985) The fetal vascularisation of term human placental villi. II. Intermediate and terminal villi. Anat. Embryol. 173, 203-214.

Laga, E.M., Driscoll, S.G., and Munro, H.N. (1973) Quantitative studies of human placenta. I. Morphometry. Biol. Neonate 23, 231-259.

Mayhew, T.M. (1983) Stereology: progress in quantitative microscopical anatomy. In: Progress in Anatomy 3, (eds.), V. Navaratnam and R.J. Harrison, Cambridge: Cambridge University Press, pp. 81-112.

Mayhew, T.M., Jackson, M.R., and Haas, J.D. (1986a) Microscopical morphology of the human placenta and its effect on oxygen diffusion: a morphometric model. Placenta 7, 121-131.

Mayhew, T.M., Jackson, M.R., and Haas, J.D. (1986b) The human placenta at high altitude in Bolivia. II. Compensatory changes in thickness of the villous membrane. J. Anat. 146, 239.

Mayhew, T.M., Joy, C.F. and Haas, J.D. (1984) Structure-function correlation in the human placenta: the morphometric diffusing capacity for oxygen at full term. J. Anat. 139, 691-708.

Metcalfe, J., Meschia, G., Hellegers, A., Prystowsky, H., Huckabee, W. and Barron, D.H. (1962)  Observations on the placental exchange of the respiratory gases in pregnant ewes at high altitude. Quart. J. Exp. Physiol. 47, 74-92.

Sokal, R.R. and Rohlf, F.J. (1981) Biometry. The Principles and Practice of Statistics in Biological Research.  San Francisco: W.H. Freeman and Co.

Weibel, E.R. (1979) Stereological Methods, Volume 1, Practical Methods for Biological Morphometry. London: Academic Press.

# LIST OF CONTRIBUTORS

Debra F. Anderson
Department of Physiology, L334
Oregon Health Sciences University
3181 SW Sam Jackson Park Road
Portland, Oregon 97201

Augustin Aoki
Centro de Microscopia Electronica
Universidad Nacional de Cordoba
Casilla Postal 362
5000 Cordoba, Argentina

Birgit Arabin
Institute of Pathology, Division of
    Pediatric Pathology and
    Placentology
Institute of Perinatal Medicine
Free University Berlin
1000 Berlin, Germany

Karol F. Bauman
Department of Anatomy
St. George's Hospital Medical School
University of London
Cranmber Terrace
London, SW 17 OPE, United Kingdom

Henning M. Beier
Department of Anatomy
    and Reproductive Biology
RWTH University Aachen
Melatener Strasse 211
D5100 Aachen, FR Germany

Caterina Bilardo
Academic Units of Obstetrics
    and Gynaecology
The London Hospital Medical College
    and King's College
Hospital Medical School
London, United Kingdom

John Bonnar
Trinity College
Department of Obstetrics and
    Gynecology
Sir Patrick Dun Research Centre
St. Jame's Hospital
Dublin 8, Ireland

Jakob Briner
Department of Pathology
University of Zürich
Frauenklinikstrasse 10
CH8091 Zürich, Switzerland

Ivo A. Brosens
Department of Obstetrics and
    Gynecology
University of Hospital Gasthuisberg
Leuven, Belgium

Stuart Campbell
Academic Units of Obstetrics
    and Gynaecology
The London Hospital Medical College
    and King's College
Hospital Medical School
London, United Kingdom

Anthony M. Carter
Department of Physiology
University of Odense
Campsuvej 55
DK5230 Odense M, Denmark

Poul Christensen
Department of Physiology
University of Odense
Campsuvej 55
DK5230 Odense M, Denmark

Carolyn Coulam
Magee-Women's Hospital and
Pittsburgh Nuclear Magnetic
    Resonance Institute
Pittsburgh, Pennsylvania

Vibeke Dantzer
Department of Anatomy
Royal Veterinary and Agricultural
    University.
Bülowsvej 13
DK1870 Copenhagen V. Denmark

Martin W. Donner
Department of Radiology and
    Radiological Science
Johns Hopkins Medical Institutions
Baltimore, Maryland

J. Job Faber
Department of Physiology, L334
Oregon Health Sciences University
3181 SW Sam Jackson Park Road
Portland, Oregon 97201

J. Anthony Firth
Department of Anatomy and Cell
    Biology
St. Mary's Hospital Medical School
University of London
Norfolk Place
London W2 1PG, United Kingdom

Jørgen Grønlund
Department of Physiology
University of Odense
Campsuvej 55
DK5230 Odense M, Denmark

J. Gedis Grudzinskas
Academic Units of Obstetrics
    and Gynaecology
The London Hospital Medical College
    and King's College
Hospital Medical School
London, United Kingdom

Jere D. Haas
Division of Nutritional Sciences
Martha Van Rensselaer Hall
Cornell University
Ithaca, New York 14853

M. Daria Haust
Department of Pathology, Obstetrics
    and Gynaecology and Paediatrics
The University of Western Ontario
London, Ontario, Canada N6A 5C1

Herbert Hees
Institut für Physiologie
Institut für Anatomie
Universität Regensburg
8400 Regensburg, FR Germany

Dirk Heinrich
Universitäts-Frauenklinik
    Heidelberg
Vosstr. 9
D6900 Heidelberg, FR Germany

Randy B. Howard
Department of Pharmacology,
    Toxicology and Therapeutics, and
Ralph Smith Research Center
University of Kansas Medical Center
39th and Rainbow Blvd.
Kansas City, Kansas 66103

T. Hosokawa
Department of Pharmacology,
    Toxicology and Therapeutics, and
Ralph Smith Research Center
University of Kansas Medical Center
39th and Rainbow Blvd.
Kansas City, Kansas 66103

Bae-Li Hsi
INSERM U210
Faculté de Médecine
Avenue de Vallombrose
06034 Nice-Cedex, France

Jean Hustin
Institute of Histopathology
Allée des Templiers 41
B6288 Loveral, Belgium

Yolene Huten
Laboratorie de Biologie du
    Developpement.et de la
    Reproduction
CHU Xavier Bichat
16 Rue Henri Huchard
75018 Paris, France

Moria R. Jackson
Department of Anatomy
Marischal College
University of Aberdeen
Aberdeen AB9 1AS, Scotland

Etha Jimenez
Institute of Pathology, Division of
    Pediatric Pathology and
    Placentology
Institute of Perinatal Medicine
Free University Berlin
1000 Berlin, Germany

Peter Kaufmann
Abt. Anatomie
Melatener Strasse 211
D5100 Aachen, FR Germany

René Lambotte
Department of Obstetrics and
    Gynecology
University of Liege
Bd de la Constitution, 81
B4020 Liege, Belgium

Jorge Las Heras
Instituto de Investigaciones Clinicas
Hospital Paula Jaraquemade
Facultad de Medicina Sur
Universidad de Chile Casilla 226/3
Santiago, Chile

Rudolf Leiser
Department of Animal Anatomy
University of Bern
Postfach 2735
CH3001 Bern, Switzerland

Andreas Lenz
Institut für Physiologie
Institut für Anatomie
Universität Regensburg
8400 Regensburg, FR Germany

Frank Leone
Magee-Women's Hospital and
Pittsburgh Nuclear Magnetic
    Resonance Institute
Pittsburgh, Pennsylvania

Michael Luckhardt
Universitäts-Frauenklinik Hamburg
Martinistrasse 52
D2000 Hamburg 20, West Germany

M. Helen Maguire
Department of Pharmacology,
    Toxicology and Therapeutics, and
Ralph Smith Research Center
University of Kansas Medical Center
39th and Rainbow Blvd.
Kansas City, Kansas 66103

M. Maier
Section of Gynecology Morphology
Department of Obstetrics and
    Gynecology
University of Ulm
Ulm, FR Germany

Dev Maulik
Department of Obstetrics and
    Gynecology
University of Missouri
Kansas City School of Medicine
Kansas City, Missouri 64108

Terry M. Mayhew
Department of Anatomy
Marischal College
University of Aberdeen
Aberdeen AB9 1AS, Scotland

Jürgen Metz
Anatomisches Institut der
    Universität Heidelberg
Im Neuenheimer Feld 307
D6900 Heidelberg, FR Germany

Parwis Mirsalim
Institute of Pathology, Division of
    Pediatric Pathology and
    Placentology
Institute of Perinatal Medicine
Free University Berlin
1000 Berlin, Germany

Waldemar Moll
Institut für Physiologie
Institut für Anatomie
Universität Regensburg
8400 Regensburg, FR Germany

Catherine Nessman
Laboratorie de Biologie du
    Developpement et de la
    Reproduction
CHU Xavier Bichat
16 Rue Henri Huchard
75018 Paris, France

Andrzej Nienartowicz
Institut für Physiologie
Institut für Anatomie
Universität Regensburg
8400 Regensburg, FR Germany

Marco Panella
Academic Units of Obstetrics
    and Gynaecology
The London Hospital Medical College
    and King's College
Hospital Medical School
London, United Kingdom

Maurice Panigel
Reproductive Biology
University P. and M. Curie
Paris, France

Celia Podesta
Magee-Women's Hospital and
Pittsburgh Nuclear Magnetic
    Resonance Institute
Pittsburgh, Pennsylvania

Alan M. Poisner
Department of Pharmacology,
    Toxicology and Therapeutics, and
Ralph Smith Research Center
University of Kansas Medical Center
39th and Rainbow Blvd.
Kansas City, Kansas 66103

Elizabeth M. Ramsey
3420 Que Street NW
Washington, DC 20007

Claudio Redaelli
Department of Pathology
University of Zürich
Frauenklinikstrasse 10
CH8091 Zürich, Switzerland

Jean P. Schaaps
Department of Obstetrics and
    Gynecology
University of Liege
Bd de la Constitution, 81
B4020 Liege, Belgium

Henning Schneider
Department of Obstetrics and
    Gynecology
University of Berne
Schanzeneckstrasse 1
CH3012 Berne, Switzerland

Holger Schmid-Schönbein
Department of Physiology
Klinikum der RWTH Aachen
D5100 Aachen, FR Germany

R. Schuhmann
Section of Gynecology Morphology
Department of Obstetrics and
    Gynecology
University of Ulm
Ulm, FR Germany

Brian L. Sheppard
Trinity College
Department of Obstetrics and
    Gynecology
Sir Patrick Dun Research Centre
St. Jame's Hospital
Dublin 8, Ireland

Colin P. Sibley
Departments of Child Health
    and Physiology
University of Manchester
St. Mary's Hospital
Hathersage Road
Manchester, M13 OJH,
    United Kingdom

Isabel Stabile
4th Floor
Holland Wing
The London Hospital
Whitechapel
London, United Kingdom

F. Stoz
Section of Gynecology Morphology
Department of Obstetrics and
    Gynecology
University of Ulm
Ulm, FR Germany

Jan Stulc
Department of Pharmacology
Faculty of Pediatrics
Charles University
Albertov 4
12800 Prague 2, Czechoslovakia

Michele Uzan
Clinique Baudelocque
123 Boulevard de Port-Royal
75014 Paris, France

Martin Vogel
Institute of Pathology, Division of
    Pediatric Pathology and
    Placentology
Institute of Perinatal Medicine
Free University Berlin
1000 Berlin, Germany

Gerhard Wagner
Institute of Pathology, Division of
    Pediatric Pathology and
    Placentology
Institute of Perinatal Medicine
Free University Berlin
1000 Berlin, Germany

Lee Willoughby
Department of Obstetrics and
    Gynecology
University of Missouri
Kansas City School of Medicine
Kansas City, Missouri 64108

Gerald Wolf
Magee-Women's Hospital and
Pittsburgh Nuclear Magnetic
    Resonance Institute
Pittsburgh, Pennsylvania

Karl-Heinz Wrobel
Institut für Physiologie
Institut für Anatomie
Universität Regensburg
8400 Regensburg, FR Germany

Prasad Yarlagadda
Department of Obstetrics and
    Gynecology
University of Missouri
Kansas City School of Medicine
Kansas City, Missouri 64108

Chang-Jing G. Yeh
INSERM U210
Faculté de Médecine
Avenue de Vallombrose
06034 Nice-Cedex, France

Anthony Zeleznik
Magee-Women's Hospital and
Pittsburgh Nuclear Magnetic
    Resonance Institute
Pittsburgh, Pennsylvania

# INDEX

All page numbers listed below represent the first page of each chapter,
where the subject is located